MOLECULAR ASPECTS OF HUMAN DISEASE
Volume 2

MOLECULAR ASPECTS OF HUMAN DISEASE

Volume 2

Editors:
JOHN W. GORROD
Head of the Chelsea Department of Pharmacy
King's College London

OTTAVIO ALBANO and SERGIO PAPA
University of Bari, Italy

ELLIS HORWOOD LIMITED
Publishers · Chichester

Halsted Press: a division of
JOHN WILEY & SONS
New York · Chichester · Brisbane · Toronto

First published in 1989 by
ELLIS HORWOOD LIMITED
Market Cross House, Cooper Street,
Chichester, West Sussex, PO19 1EB, England
The publisher's colophon is reproduced from James Gillison's drawing of the ancient Market Cross, Chichester.

Distributors:
Australia and New Zealand:
JACARANDA WILEY LIMITED
GPO Box 859, Brisbane, Queensland 4001, Australia
Canada:
JOHN WILEY & SONS CANADA LIMITED
22 Worcester Road, Rexdale, Ontario, Canada
Europe and Africa:
JOHN WILEY & SONS LIMITED
Baffins Lane, Chichester, West Sussex, England
North and South America and the rest of the world:
Halsted Press: a division of
JOHN WILEY & SONS
605 Third Avenue, New York, NY 10158, USA
South-East Asia
JOHN WILEY & SONS (SEA) PTE LIMITED
37 Jalan Pemimpin # 05–04
Block B, Union Industrial Building, Singapore 2057
Indian Subcontinent
WILEY EASTERN LIMITED
4835/24 Ansari Road
Daryaganj, New Delhi 110002, India

British Library Cataloguing in Publication Data
Molecular aspects of human disease. Vol. 2
1. Man. Diseases. Molecular biology
I. Gorrod, J.W. (John W.) *1931–*
II. Albano, Ottavio III. Papa, S. (Sergio) *1935–*
616.07

Library of Congress data available

ISBN 0–7458–0587–6 (Ellis Horwood Limited)
ISBN 0–470–21303–5 (Halsted Press)

Printed in Great Britain by Hartnolls, Bodmin

Contents of Volume 2

Part 10: Diagnostic probes

Contents of Volume 1

Preface

The International Conference on Molecular Approaches to Human Diseases, the proceedings of which are collected in this two volume work, represents the first congress and scientific activity of the International Biomedical Institute, an association founded in Bari, Italy in 1986 for the promotion and development of scientific research in biological sciences and medicine. The conference was structured to cover fundamental aspects of major human diseases. The topics covered, were on purpose, quite diverse.

The unifying theme of these books is provided by the fact that they deal predominantly with the *molecular* basis of the aetiology, pathogenesis, and treatment of the different diseases. This approach provides a unifying language by which the outstanding specialists from various fields convened for the conference, could easily communicate and identify the essential progresses achieved in different areas and to foresee important perspectives for the immediate future.

Thus the conference expanded easily from metabolism dysfunctions, genetic, neoplastic, immune, viral, and cardiovascular diseases, antiviral and antiblastisc chemiotherapy, molecular mechanism of drug toxicity, defence and repair mechanism, and diagnostic probes.

The conference was essentially intended to gather a critical number of experts so as to collect the most advanced information, inputs, and strategic priorities and establish the future scientific activity of the International Biomedical Institute.

Judging from the contributions presented and the interest raised, the present volumes represent an up-to-date and comprehensive coverage of important progress and perspectives in many advanced areas, which may be of significant help to investigators interested in attacking human diseases from their essential nature rather than merely from their symptoms. They provide one more example of how essential it is to proceed in biological science with the rigorous and interdisciplinary application of basic sciences. The volumes contain substantial reviews on the major areas of interest, supplemented with short reports which derived from oral or poster contributions. Thus the volumes contain a contemporary view of molecular approaches to human disease.

The Editors

J. W. Gorrod
O. Albano
S. Papa

Part 6
Antiviral and antiblastic chemotherapy

6.1 The antiviral and immunomodulatory actions of Methisoprinol (inosine pranobex) in relation to its effects on HIV infection

Claudio De Simone†

The discovery and characterization of HIV (human immunodeficiency virus) have prompted the search for effective and non-toxic antiviral agents. Methisoprinol demonstrated an *in vitro* activity against HIV and immunorestorating properties *in vitro* and *in vivo*. The combination of antiviral and immunomodulatory activities seemed an appropriate rationale for employing Methisoprinol in clinical trials on HIV+ subjects.

6.1.1 INTRODUCTION

Methisoprinol (isoprinosine, inosiplex, inosine pranobex) is a synthetic compound formed from the *p*-acetamidobenzoic salt of *N*,*N*-dimethylamino-2-propanol and inosine in a 3:1 molar ratio (Fig. 1).

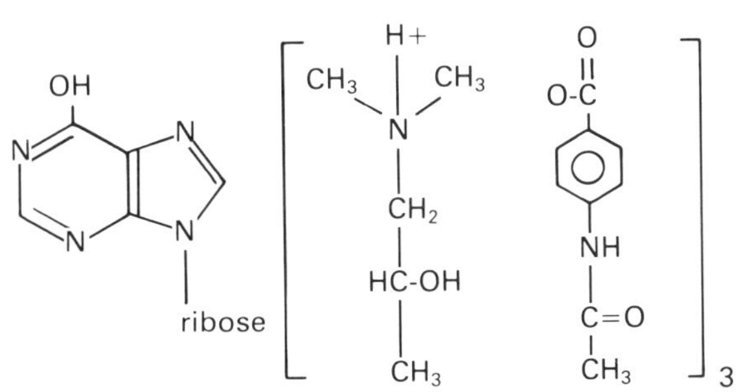

Fig. 1.—Structural formula of Methisoprinol

Methisoprinol has been reported to inhibit viral growth and to enhance host's immunocompetence (for a review, see De Simone 1985, Campoli-Richards 1986, De Simone & Hadden 1987). The efficacy of the drug complex depends on the presence of inosine, and *in vitro* it is potentiated by the simultaneous addition of adenine,

† Insegnamento di Malattie Infettive. Facoltà di Medicina e Chirurgia. Università degli Studi dell'Aquila degli Abruzzi. 67100 L'Aquila, Italy.

adenosine, and interferons (Chany & Cerutti 1977, Fomina *et al.* 1980, Munoz *et al.* 1986). Studies aiming at a comparison between the biological properties of the intact complex and those of the separate components, inosine and DIP-PAcBA, have shown that inosine possesses less antiviral and immunomodulating activity than the complex. The intact complex is essential for the *in vivo* activity perhaps because, otherwise, inosine would be rapidly metabolized. The 1:3 ratio of inosine:DIP-PAcBA is the only one, among those examined (from 3:1 to 1:30), which seems to be significantly effective when assayed by different *in vitro* systems (Ginsberg & Hadden 1984). The elimination half-life of the inosine moiety is about 50 minutes following an oral dose, and the major excretion product is uric acid, so that gout or renal dysfunction are contraindications to the drug administration. The recommended adult oral dosage of Methisoprinol is 1 g four times daily, and in children 50 mg/kg per day. However, dosages up to 10 g daily have been occasionally reported, without major patient's complaints (De Simone 1985, De Simone & Hadden 1987).

6.1.2 ANTIVIRAL ACTIVITY

The *in vitro* antiviral activity of Methisoprinol is somewhat limited in comparison with typical antiviral drugs. However, its *in vivo* action against viral infections in animals and man has been reported to be encouraging. Methisoprinol increased the survival of mice infected experimentally with influenza A or B viruses, including animals having artificially-induced immunodepression. In addition, the drug caused a significant enhancement in the responses of splenocytes from normal mice experimentally infected with *Herpex simplex* virus type I or influenza-infected mice, using the infecting virus as antigen (for a review, see Ginsberg & Hadden 1984). Combined therapy with Methisoprinol plus interferon (IFN) improved the IFN-mediated protection of mice against encephalomyocarditis virus and Forest Spring encephalitis (Munoz *et al.* 1986). In humans, a treatment with Methisoprinol was associated with a reduced virus shedding in nasal washes from volunteers (influenza A/Victoria) or in semen from homosexuals (*cytomegalovirus*) (Longley *et al.* 1973, Conant *et al.* 1986). Recently, Methisoprinol in association with acyclovir proved to be of clinical benefit in those patients infected with *Varicella zoster* and with some degree of immunodepression (Tanphaichitra & Srimmang 1987).

It has been proposed that the mechanism of action of Methisoprinol involves one component of the drug or the drug complex linking to the ribosomes of the host's infected cells (Onhishi *et al.* 1982). The consequence is a sterical modification or rearrangement which renders an advantage to cellular RNA over viral RNA in the competition for the linkage with ribosome combining sites without altering the cellular protein synthesis from a qualitative point of view. The result would be a non-reading or incorrect reading of viral DNA, with incorrect transcription of the viral genetic code. The replication of *Herpex simplex*, *cytomegalovirus*, *adenovirus*, *vaccinia*, *poliovirus*, influenza types A and B, ECHO, *rabies*, *rhinovirus*, *encephalomyocarditis* virus resulted in inhibition by Methisoprinol in tissues cultures (for a review, see Campoli-Richards *et al.* 1986).

6.1.3 IMMUNOMODULATING ACTIVITY

In general, Methisoprinol augments immunological events initiated by other triggering agents such as antigens, lymphokines, and mitogenic substances (Ballet *et al.* 1982). Many, but not all, activities of the drug can be termed 'thymomimetic' (De Simone & Hadden 1987). In addition to inducing T cell differentiation and to modulating mature T cell function, Methisoprinol induces B lymphocyte differentiation, increases natural killer (NK) cell activity, potentiates γ-IFN, interleukin (IL)-1 and IL-2 production, and augments phagocytic cell function (Balestrino *et al.* 1983, Hersey *et al.* 1984). These actions can be explained by assuming that the drug acts through one or more receptors not restricted to T lymphocytes, but common to B cells, NK cells, granulocytes, macrophages, and that it induces modifications of the still poorly known cellular enzymatic pathways. It has been hypothesized that Methisoprinol is agonistic for an inosine-like P receptor or, alternatively, like methylxanthines, it may turn out to be antagonistic for R type receptors (De Simone & Hadden 1987) (Fig. 2).

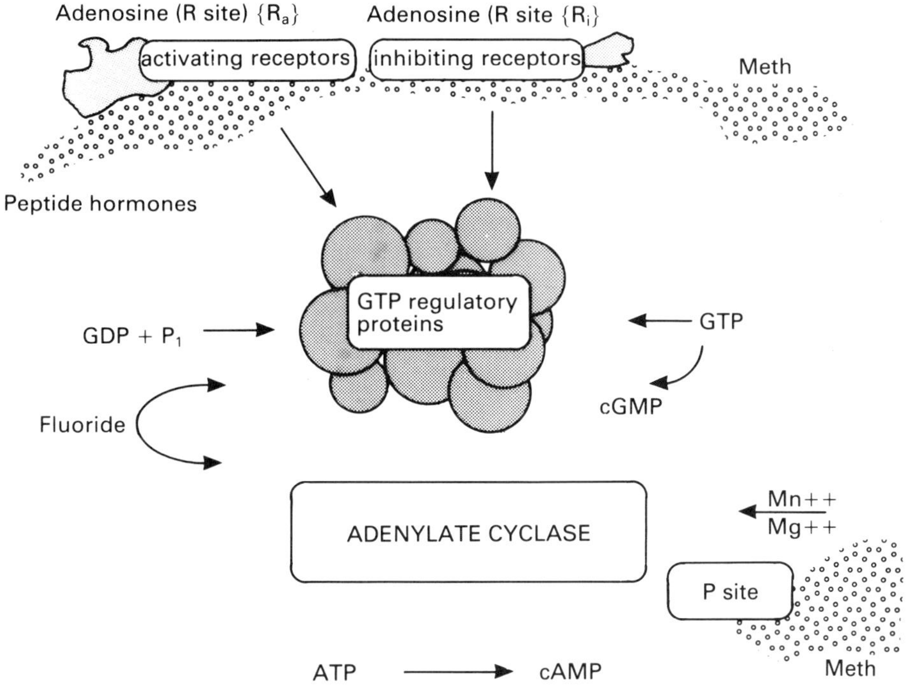

Fig. 2.—Proposed mechanism(s) of action of Methisoprinol (Meth.) on immunocompetent cells

Methisoprinol could be an allosteric modifier of inosine or hypoxanthine-utilizing enzymes giving rise to active analogues of xanthine and uric acid which regulate in turn the activity of adenosine deaminase (ADA), purine-nucleoside phosphorilase (PNP), 5′-nucleotidase inosine dehydrogenase, or hypoxantine-guanine phosphoribosyltransferase (HGPRT). Recently, studies conducted with the quantitative freeze–fracture technique have shown that the drug induces modifications of the density of the intramembranous particles (IMPs) on the external fracture face (EF) of the lymphocyte plasma membrane (De Simone *et al.* in preparation).

Clinically, Methisoprinol reduces the number of recurrences of *Herpes simplex* type I infection, the length and the outcome of acute measles infections, and it has beneficial effects on the course of subacute sclerosing panencephalitis (SSPE), which is thought to be caused by a paramyxovirus, and of viral hepatitis, type B (Bradshaw & Summer 1977, Jones *et al.* 1982, De Simone 1985). In general, the drug's activity is even more evident when the host's immune responses are depressed following viral infection (Binderup 1985).

6.1.4 THE HIV INFECTION AND ITS PHARMACOLOGICAL CONTROL

The aetiological agent of AIDS is an exogenous C-type retrovirus termed HIV (human immunodeficiency virus). The disease can be considered as a human viral infection associated with a selective depletion of CD4+ T helper/inducer lymphocytes and concomitant complications of immunodeficiency such as opportunistic infections and Kaposi's sarcoma (Dalglish *et al.* 1984, McDougal *et al.* 1985, Coffin *et al.* 1986). It is unclear what determines who will and who will not develop severe opportunistic infections after HIV infections, but there is a general agreement that the depression of CD4+ T cells correlates well with the progression of HIV infection. Since CD4+ T cells recognize and proliferate in response to antigens, release lymphokines, modulate the activities of NK cells, macrophages and B cells, efficient CD4+ T lymphocyte function appears central to most of the functional defects observed in HIV-infected subjects (Fig. 3). Moreover, relatively constant features of AIDS are the host's decreased capability to secrete γ-IFN and IL-2 upon T cell stimulation,

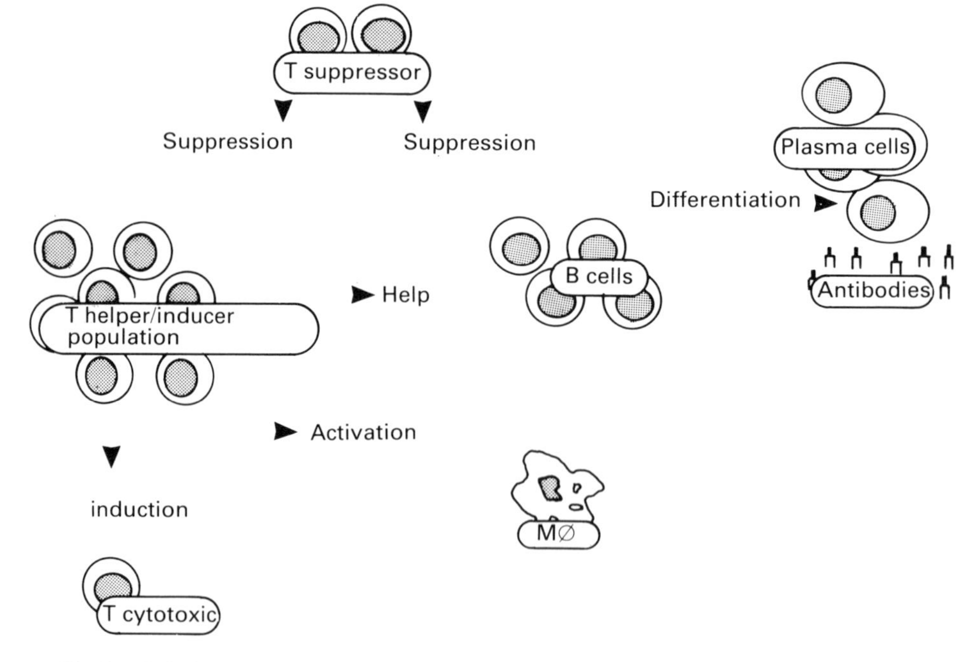

Fig. 3.—Relations and interactions of the T helper/inducer (CD4+) lymphocytes with the other cell subsets

and a reduced Tac (T-activated antigen; IL-2) receptor cxprcssion on activated T cells (Donnelly *et al.* 1986).

Actually, to control the disease from its early stages (HIV seropositivity, without clinical symptoms) to the full-blown manifestations (AIDS), two major approaches are under extensive experimentation:

(a) specific inhibition of HIV replication;
(b) immunological restoration of the infected host.

Many compounds of widely different types are being screened for anti-HIV activitiy *in vitro*. For example, a number of nucleoside derivatives analogous to 3′-azido-3′-deoxythimidine are under investigation for antiretroviral activity. These agents are expected to be able to eliminate the retrovirus from the host or suppress virus replication and maintain a state of latency, allowing the immune system to regenerate and eliminate the retrovirus infected-cells. However, since a prolonged therapy is likely to be necessary to control HIV infection, synergistic drug combinations, as in cancer chemotherapy, may be required to reduce the dose of the individual agents below toxic levels and to prevent the emergence of drug-resistant mutants.

A number of immunomodulatory agents are also under study in HIV-infected subjects (e.g. thymic humoral factors, cyclosporin A, IL-2). These drugs are expected to enhance or reconstitute the host's immune system, allowing immunomediated elimination of virus infected-cells with the ultimate result of spontaneous complete regeneration of the immune system.

Methisoprinol presents an advantage in respect to the above cited agents, in the sense that it has both antiviral and immunomodulatory properties. Moreover, it is burdened by a low toxicity for the host's cells, is orally or i.v. administrable, and penetrates the central nervous system.

6.1.5 METHISOPRINOL AND HIV

As reported in the preceding paragraphs, Methisoprinol protects the host's cells through two different mechanisms: (1) by inhibiting viral growth by suppressing the viral RNA synthesis, and (2), by potentiating the synthesis of lymphocyte RNA that is depressed following viral infection. In other words, Methisoprinol has a combination of direct and indirect antiviral activity which could be used advantageously in the therapy of HIV infection.

As far as the first point is concerned—inhibition of the viral growth—*in vitro* experiments have shown that co-incubation of PBL (peripheral blood lymphocytes) from ARC (AIDS-related complex) patients with Methisoprinol (100 and 200 μg/ml) resulted in an inhibition of reverse transcriptase and of p15 and p24 expression on the lymphoid cell surface (Pompidou *et al.* 1985a). Similar experiments have been carried out in our laboratory but differing in the fact that, instead of lymphocytes from HIV-infected subjects, *in vitro* acutely HIV-infected lymphocytes from healthy donors were employed. A dose-dependent inhibition of the p24 and gp120 antigen expression on the lymphocyte surface as assessed by flow cytometry and of the reverse transcriptase was observed on day 12 of cell culture. No anti-HIV activity was detected when chronically infected H9 cells were so-incubated with Methisoprinol, even at high dosages (400 μg/ml) (De Simone *et al.* in preparation). These data suggest that

Methisoprinol has a direct activity against HIV which is inferior to that observed for other anti-HIV drugs (e.g. 3′-azido-3′-deoxythimidine), similar to that of sodium diethylditiocarbamate (imuthiol), and superior to that of many biological augmenting agents.

In vitro experiments and preliminary clinical trials suggest that Methisoprinol may be useful in the treatment of HIV infection because it improves normal function of HIV-infected patients. In Con A (concanavalin A)-stimulated cultures of PBL from AIDS patients, increased IL-2 production and number of IL-2 (Tac) receptor-bearing lymphocytes in the presence of Methisoprinol has been reported (Tsang *et al.* 1984a). Studies performed in our laboratory have shown that, when the drug is encapsulated in liposomes, it is a 2–3 fold more effective with respect to the free form in promoting an increase in the percentage of Tac+ lymphocytes (De Simone, unpublished results) (Fig. 4). Moreover, when PBL from 72 prodromal

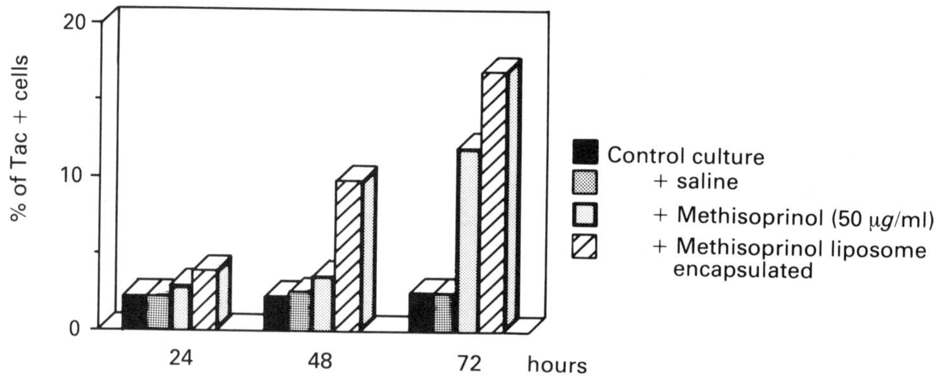

Fig. 4.—Influence of Methisoprinol and Methisoprinol liposome encapsulated on the peripheral blood lymphocytes of ARC patients

homosexuals and 23 AIDS patients were analysed following PWM (pokeweed mitogen) blastogenesis by dual colour flow cytometry, a reduction in the number and percentage of Leu 3+ (CD4+) and an increase of Leu 2+ (CD8+) lymphocytes in comparison with healthy heterosexual subjects was observed. Among prodromal homosexuals with mild symptoms, *in vitro* treatment with Methisoprinol was able to augment the number of helper T cells (CD4+), reducing at the same time the number of effector suppressor lymphocytes and activated suppressor lymphocytes. It is interesting to note that among AIDS patients with severe symptoms, the co-incubation of their lymphocytes with the drug reduced the number of the elevated subset of Leu 2+ Leu 8 lymphocytes but was ineffective in modulating the differentiation and the activities of the other cell subsets (Tsang *et al.* 1987). These data are further substantiated by the observation that Methisoprinol induced an early chromatin activation in PBL from ARC patients (Pompidou 1985b).

Preliminary clinical trials performed on male homosexuals or i.v. drug users at risk of developing AIDS, which were classified as LAS (lymphadenopathy syndrome) and immunodepressed (CD4+/CD8+ ratio <1.5; T lymphocytes $<700\ mm^3$) and treated with Methisoprinol at a dosage of 3 g/day for 28 days have shown an improvement in 52% of the recipients. These improvements, which on day 180 were still present, were characterized by an increased sense of well being, by a reduction of night sweats and lymph node pain, lesser weight loss and skin rashes. From the immunological point of view, there was increase of total T cells, T helper cells (CD4+) and NK cells (Grieco *et al.* 1984, Wallace & Bekesi 1986, Tsang *et al.* 1987).

Early observations from other double-blind placebo-controlled clinical trials appear to confirm the above results. A 24 month randomized study utilizing a dosage of 4 gr/day of Methisoprinol and encompassing over 1500 Italian HIV+ individuals has been initiated to determine the drug's clinical efficacy. Similar multicentre studies are in progress in the USA, Australia, and Denmark.

6.1.6 CONCLUDING REMARKS

Many attempts are in progress to combine antiviral drugs with immunomodulating compounds in order to promote both virus eradication and immune reconstitution. Preliminary evidence seems to suggest that Methisoprinol, inhibiting reverse transcriptase and stimulating T lymphocytes, could be a candidate for HIV infection therapy, even in association with other compounds. One of the major controversial points is that the concentration of Methisoprinol requested for an effective anti-HIV effect, at least *in vitro*, is rather high. However, it is important to emphasize that, if the concentration required for the above effect is achievable *in vivo*, and if Methisoprinol is nontoxic for normal host cells at that concentration, then the absolute concentration is unimportant. On this basis, more studies on the pharmacological characteristics of the compound (e.g. absorption, distribution, metabolism, mode of delivery and synergy with other anti-retroviral drugs) on HIV patients are needed.

REFERENCES

Balestrino, C., Montesoro, E., Nocera, A., Ferrarini, M., & Hoffman, T. (1983) Augmentation of human peripheral blood natural killer activity by methisoprinol. *Journal of Biological Response Modifiers* **2,** 577–585

Ballett, J. J., Morin, A. M., & Agrapart, M. (1982) Effect of isoprinosine on *in vivo* proliferative responses of human lymphocytes stimulated by antigen. *International Journal of Immunopharmacology* **4,** 151–157

Binderup, L. (1985) Effect of isoprinosine in animals models of depressed T-cell function. *International Journal of Immunopharmacology* **7,** 93–101

Bradshaw, L. J. & Summer, H. L. (1977) *In vitro* studies on cell-mediated immunity in patients treated with inosiplex for herpes virus infection. *Annals of the New York Academy of Sciences* **284,** 196–196

Campoli-Richards, D. M., Sorkin, E. M., & Heel, C. R. (1986) Inosine pranobex. A preliminary review of its pharmacodynamic and pharmacokinetic properties and therapeutic efficacy. *Drugs* **32,** 383–424

Cerutti, I., Chany, C., & Schlumberger, J. F. (1979) Isoprinosine increases the antitumour action of interferon. *International Journal of Immunopharmacology* **1,** 59–63

Chany, C. & Cerutti, I. (1977) Enhancement of antiviral protection against encephalomyocarditis virus by a combination of isoprinosine and interferon. *Archives of Virology* **55,** 225–231

Coffin, J., Haase, A., Levy, J. A., Montagnier, L., & Orozzlan, S. (1986) Human immunodeficiency viruses. *Science* **232,** 697

Conant, M., Illeman, M., Glasky, A. J., & Drew, L. (1986) A double blind placebo controlled trial of isoprinosine in volunteers shedding cytomegalovirus in semen. Abstract *2° World Congress of Sexually Transmitted Diseases, Paris,* June 25–28

Dalgleish, A. G., Beverly, P. C. L., & Claphan, P. R. (1984) The CD4 (T4) antigen is an essential component of the receptor for the AIDS retrovirus. *Nature* **312,** 763–767

De Simone, C. (1985) Immunopharmacological profile and clinical trials with methisoprinol. *EOS Journal of Immunology and Immunopharmacology* **5,** 83–87

De Simone, C. & Hadden, J. W. (1987) Prohost modulation of immunity by isoprinosine and NPT 15392. In: *Antibiosis and host immunity* (eds Szentivanyi, A., Friedman, H., & Gilissen, G.) Plenum Press, New York, NY, 289–290

Donnelly, R. P., Tsang, K. Y., Galbraith, G. M. P., & Wallace, J. I. (1986) Inhibition of the IL-2 induced T cell proliferation by sera from patients with AIDS. *Journal of Clinical Immunology* **6,** 92–101

Fomina, A. N., Grigorian, S. S., Nikolaeva, O. V., & Erhov, F. I. (1980) Combined use of isoprinosine and an interferon inducer in experimental viral infection. *Antibiotiki* **25,** 854–856

Ginsberg, T. & Hadden, J. W. (1984) Immunopharmacology of methisoprinol. In: *Immunomodulation: new frontiers and advances* (eds by Fudenberg, H. H., Whitten, H. D., & Ambrogi, F.) Plenum Press, New York, NY, 331–348

Grieco, H. H., Reddy, M. M., Monvar, D., Ahuja, K. K., & Moriarty, M. L. (1984) *In vivo* immunomodulation by isoprinosine in patients with AIDS and ARC. *Annals of International Medicine* **101,** 206–207

Hersey, P., Bindon, C., Bradley, M., & Hasic, E. (1984) Effect of isoprinosine on interleukin 1 and 2 production and on suppressor cell activity in PWM stimulated cultures of B and T cells. *International Journal of Immunopharmacology* **6,** 315–320

Jones C. E., Dyken, P. R., Huttenlocher, P. R., Jabbour, J. T. & Maxwell, K. W. (1982) Inosiplex therapy in subacute sclerosing panencephalitis. *Lancet* **1,** 1034–1036

Longley, S., Dumming, R. C., & Waldmann, R. H. (1973) Effect of isoprinosine against challenge with A(H3N2)/Hong Kong influenza virus in volunteers. *Antimicrobial Agents and Chemotherapy* **3,** 506–509

MCDougal, J. S., Kennedy, M. S., Sligh, J. M., Cort, S. P., Maude, A., & Nicholson, J. K. A. (1985) Binding of HTLVIII/LAV to T4+ T cells by a complex of the 110K viral protein and the T4 molecule. *Science* **231,** 382

Munoz, A., Garcia, R. A., & Perez-Aranda, A. (1986) Potentiation by levamisole, methisoprinol and adenine or adenosine of the inhibitory activity of human interferon against encephalomyocarditis virus. *Antimicrobial Agents Chemotherapy* **30,**182–195

Onhishi, H., Kosozuma, H., Inaba, H., Okura, M., & Morita, Y. (1982) Mechanism of host defense suppression induced by viral infection: mode of action of inosiplex as an antiviral agent. *Infection and Immunity* **38,** 243–250

Pompidou, A., Zagury, D., Gallo, R. C., Sun, D., & Thronton, A. (1985a) *In vitro* inhibition of LAV-HTLVIII infected lymphocytes by dithiocarb and inosine pranobex. *Lancet* **2,** 1423

Pompidu, A., Delsaux, M. C., Telvi, L., Mace, B., & Coutance, F. (1985b)

Isoprinosine and imuthiol. Two potentially active compounds in patients with AIDS-related complex symptoms. *Cancer Research* **45,** 4671–4673

Tauphaichitra, D. & Srimuang, S. (1987) Efficacy of acyclovir combined with immunopotentiating agents in the treatment of varicella zoster. *Journal of Antimicrobial Chemotherapy* **19,** 255–262

Tsang, K. Y., Fudenberg, H. H., & Galbraith, M. P. (1982a) *In vitro* augmentation of IL-2 production and lymphocytes with the Tac antigen marker in patients with AIDS. *New England Journal of Medicine* **310,**987

Tsang, P. H., Tanguavarad, K., Solomon, S., & Bekesi, J. G. (1984b) Modulation of T and B lymphocyte functions by isoprinosine in homosexual subjects with prodromata and in patients with AIDS. *Journal of Clinical Immunology* **4,** 469–478

Tsang, P. H., Robson, J. P., & Bekes, J. G. (1987) Isoprinosine induced modulation of immune responses in HIV infected patients: *in vivo* and *in vitro* studies. EOS *Journal of Immunology and Immunopharmacology* **4,** 134–138

Wallace, J. & Bekes, J. G. (1986) A double blind clinical trial of the effects of inosine pranobex in immunodepressed patients with prolonged lymphadenopathy. *Clinical Immunoloy and Immunopathology* **39,**179–186

6.2 Bleomycin: studies of the mechanism of action of an antitumour antibiotic

Sidney M. Hecht†

A study of the mechanism of DNA cleavage by bleomycin resulted in several findings, including: bleomycin-mediated DNA degradation involves the formation of two sets of products; one set of products involves DNA strand scission, with the formation of a base propenal, a 3′-fragment terminating with a 5′-phosphate and a 5′-fragment terminating with a 3′-phosphoroglycolate moiety;
a second set of products consists of a free base and alkali labile lesion, the latter of which is a C-4′ hydroxyapurinic acid;
both lesions are formed preferentially at pyridimine nucleosides that are part of the sequence $^{5'}$-G · pyr-$^{3'}$;
platination of a DNA oligonucleotide with an analog of *cis*-platinum resulted in dramatic alteration of DNA sequence cleavage specificity by bleomycin, due to a conformational alteration of DNA structure.

6.2.1 INTRODUCTION

The bleomycins (BLMs) are structurally related antitumour antibiotics used clinically for the treatment of squamous cell carcinomas and malignant lymphomas (Crooke 1978, Carter 1978, Umezawa 1979). The bleomycins have been used in the clinic as a mixture of congeners, blenoxane, purified from *Streptomyces verticillus* (Umezawa 1978, Hecht 1979). Blenoxane consists primarily of bleomycin A_2 (~60–65%; Fig. 1) and bleomycin B_2 (~30%), although several other congeners are also present in lesser abundance.

Biochemical studies have identified a number of cellular loci at which bleomycin may act to exert its therapeutic effects; however, the accumulated evidence suggests that the primary locus is DNA. Bleomycin mediates DNA damage in a reaction that is oxygen and metal ion dependent (Ishida & Takahashi 1975, Sausville *et al.* 1978a,b, Oppenheimer *et al.* 1979). While the initial work carried out with bleomycin involved an Fe(II)·BLM complex, it has now been shown that the Cu(I) (Ehrenfeld *et al.* 1985, 1987), Mn(II) (Ehrenfeld *et al.* 1984, Burger *et al.* 1984), and VO(IV) (Kuwahara *et al.* 1985) complexes also mediate DNA damage. In addition, Co(III)·BLM has also been reported to degrade DNA in a light-dependent reaction that does not seem to require oxygen (Chang & Meares 1984). It is generally assumed that the Fe(II)

† Departments of Chemistry and Biology, University of Virginia, Charlottesville, Virginia 22901, USA

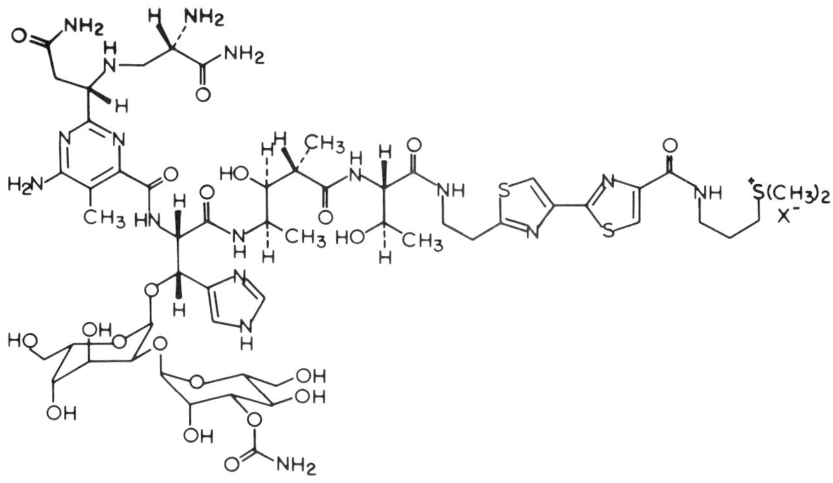

Fig. 1.—Structure of bleomycin A_2

complex of BLM is responsible for the therapeutic effects of the drug; however, the finding that other metal complexes of bleomycin can mediate DNA strand scission raises the possibility that one of these could function therapeutically.

When Form I DNA (i.e., supercoiled covalently closed circular (ccc)DNA) is used as a substrate for cleavage by bleomycin, it is observed that the DNA is converted both to nicked circular (Form II) DNA and to linear duplex (Form III) DNA (Figs 2, 3). The conversion to linear duplex DNA has been shown to be significantly in excess of what would be predicted on the basis of the random accumulation of single-strand breaks, and is believed to occur by a specific mechanism (Haidle *et al.* 1979). The ability of cells to repair such breaks is of interest both from a mechanistic and therapeutic perspective.

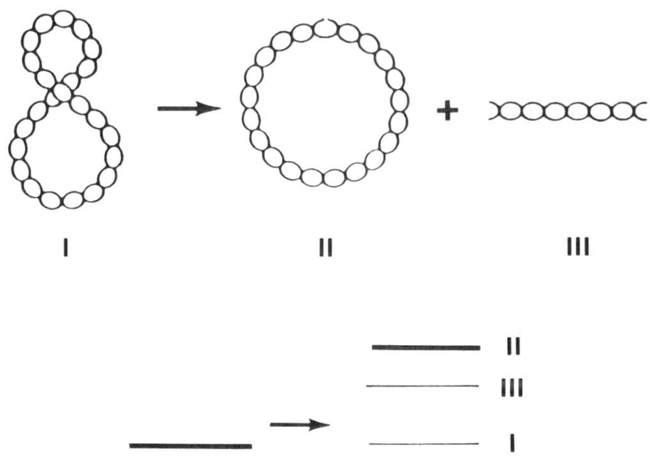

Fig. 2.—Conversion of supercoiled (Form I) cccDNA to nicked circular (Form II) DNA and linear duplex (Form III) DNA

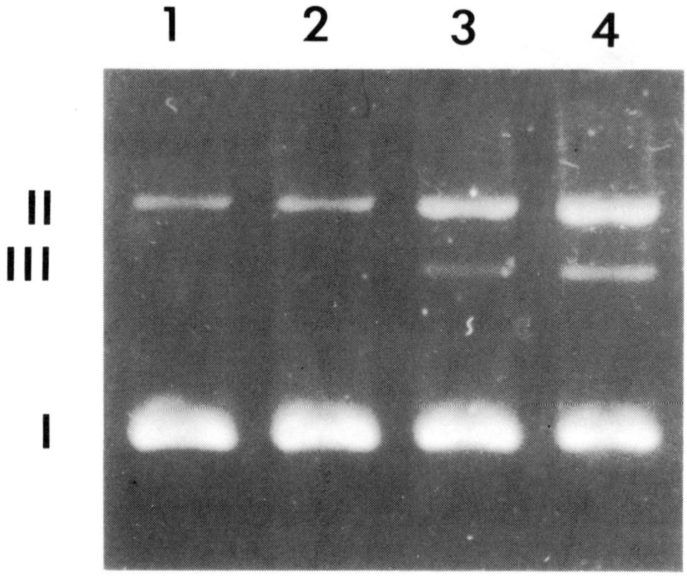

Fig. 3.—Conversion of SV40 Form I DNA to Form II and Form III DNA by treatment with 0 (lane 1), 0.2 μM, (lane 2), 0.5 μM (lane 3) or 1.0 μM Fe(II)·BLM A_2

Bleomycin-mediated DNA strand scission proceeds with considerable sequence selectivity for $^{5'}GC^{3'}$ and $^{5'}GT^{3'}$ sequences (D'Andrea & Haseltine 1978, Takeshita *et al.* 1978, Mirabelli *et al.* 1983) and is generally unaltered for congeners of bleomycin that differ structurally only within the C-terminal substituent. Although some alterations of sequence specificity have been documented using bleomycin congeners that differed more substantially in structure (Kross *et al.* 1982, Mirabelli *et al.* 1982, Shipley & Hecht 1988), or by the use of DNA substrates having altered conformations (Hertzberg *et al.* 1985, Mascharak *et al.* 1983), the molecular basis of sequence specificity is not well understood at present.

6.2.1.1 DNA degradation products formed by bleomycin

The identification of products resulting from DNA degradation by metallobleomycins is central to the development of an understanding of the mechanism of DNA degradation by this drug. Products identified in early studies included free bases especially thymine and cytosine, and the four possible base propenals (e.g., 3-(thymin-1′-yl)propenal (**1**)) (Burger *et al.* 1980, Giloni *et al.* 1981), the latter of

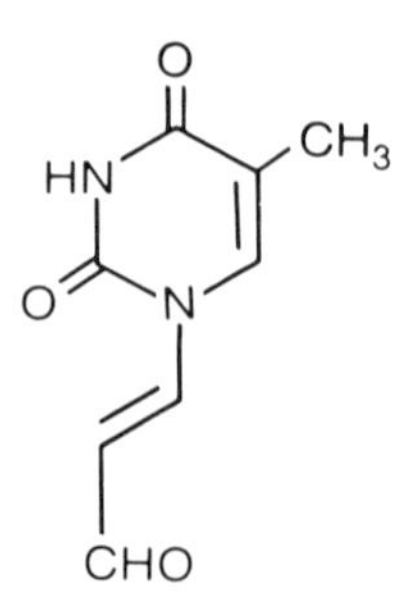

1

which are formed specifically as the *trans*-isomers (Murugesan *et al.* 1985). Also indicated was the formation of DNA fragments ending at their 3′-termini with some group other than a 3′-OH group or phosphate (D'Andrea & Haseltine 1978, Takeshita *et al.* 1978, Kross *et al.* 1982). Studies in a number of laboratories subsequently demonstrated that the 3′-termini contained groups resulting from alteration of the deoxyribose moiety concomitant with production of the observed free bases or base propenals.

To facilitate the identification of bleomycin cleavage products still covalently attached to the substrate nucleic acid, we designed a DNA target that we believed would afford products readily amenable to structure analysis. Specifically, we employed the self-complementary dodecanucleotide d($^{5'}$CGCTTTAAAGCG$^{3'}$) as a target for Fe·BLM, in the hope that cytidine$_3$ would be modified readily and afford products of the form $^{5'}$CpGpx$^{3'}$. Based on the appearance of the base propenals upon treatment of DNA with bleomycin, and the knowledge that this species was derived from the base and C-1′–C-3′ of deoxyribose (Giloni *et al.* 1981), it seemed logical to anticipate that the deoxyribose C-4′ and C-5′ carbon atoms might remain attached to the 3′-terminus of the remaining oligonucleotide at the site of the strand scission event. In fact, glycolic acid had been observed upon successive treatments of DNA with Fe·BLM and strong acid (Giloni *et al.* 1981), suggesting that **2** might be formed from d(CGCTTTAAAGCG) upon treatment with Fe(II)·BLM + O_2 (Scheme I).

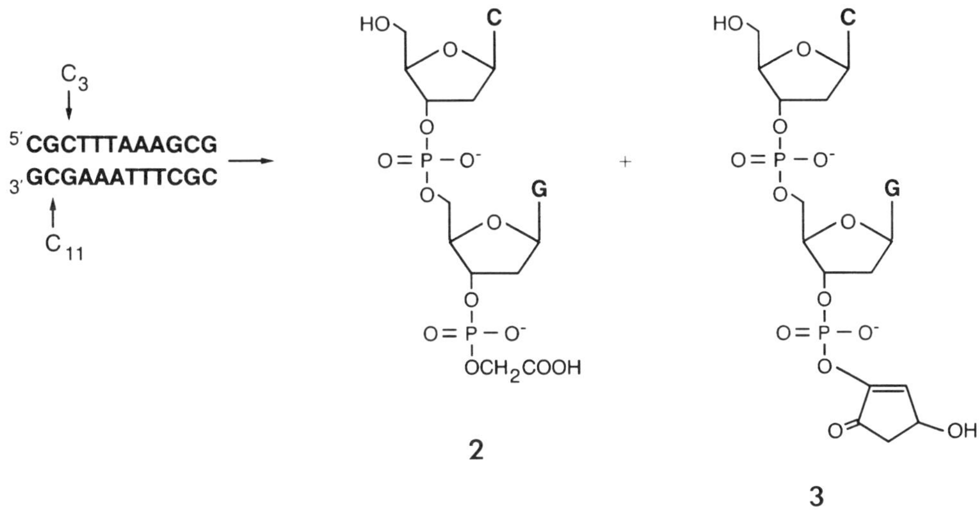

Scheme I.—Fe·BLM—mediated formation of CpGpx's 2 and 3 from d(CGCTTTAAAGCG)

Identification of **2** among the reaction products formed from the dodecanucleotide was accomplished readily by synthesis of an authentic sample, as outlined in Scheme II (Murugesan *et al.* 1985, Sugiyama *et al.* 1985a). The authentic and dodecanucleotide-derived samples of **2** were shown to have identical properties under a number of conditions when analysed by anion exchange and reverse phase hplc.

In addition to the formation of base propenals with concomitant DNA strand scission, it is known that a second type of DNA damage also occurs. This DNA modification involves the formation of a free base and an alkali-labile lesion (Hecht

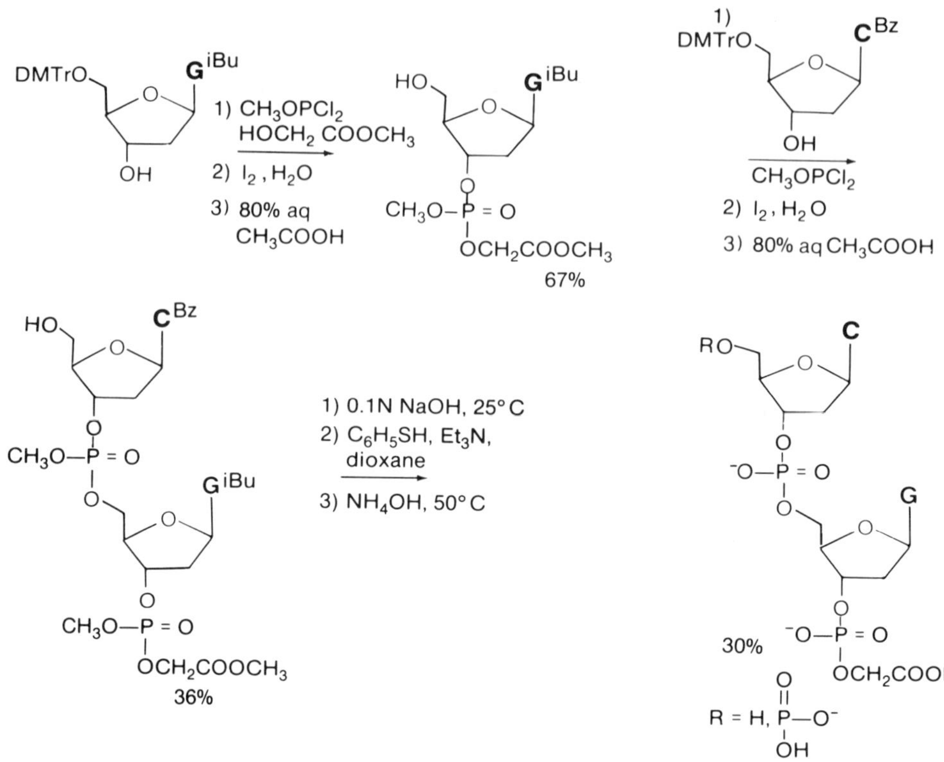

Scheme II.—Chemical synthesis of CpGpx 2

1979, Burger *et al.* 1982). Although the formation of this lesion does not produce DNA strand scission *per se*, subsequent treatment with base has been found to produce DNA cleavage. By the use of d(CGCTTTAAAGCG) as a target for Fe(II)·BLM, followed by treatment with alkali, a new product of the form CpGpx was obtained. The identification of this dinucleotide as diastereomeric **3** was accomplished by comparison with an authentic synthetic sample (Sugiyama *et al.* 1985b); their properties on anion exchange and reverse phase hplc were shown to be identical.

The production of **3** from d(CGCTTTAAAGCG) upon successive treatments with Fe(II)·BLM + O_2 and then with alkali suggested the possible intermediacy of a C-4′ OH derivative of deoxyribose formed at $cytidine_3$ (Sugiyama *et al.* 1985b). An intermediate of this type would be expected to produce a C-4′ hydroxyapurinic acid with the loss of free base. Alkali treatment of the C-4′-hydroxyapurinic acid should afford **3** in analogy with known chemical transformations (Scheme III) (Büchi *et al.* 1971, Stork *et al.* 1975, Floyd 1978).

6.2.1.2 Alteration of the sequence specificity of DNA strand scission

There have been two reports of alteration of the pattern of DNA strand scission as a result of prior DNA modification. One of these involved the observed diminution of strand scission in proximity to some cytidine moieties that had been methylated

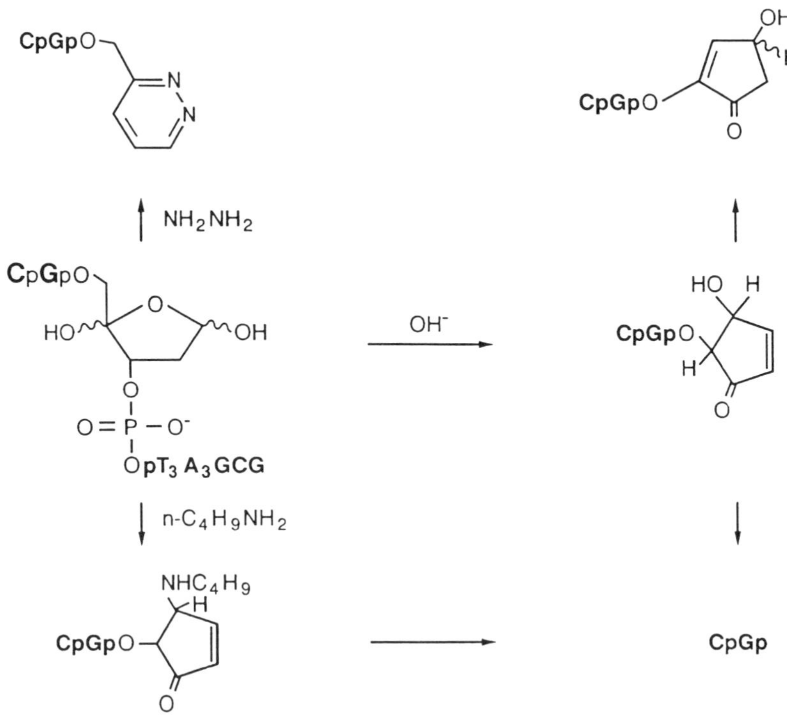

Scheme III.—Chemistry of the alkali-labile lesion

with restriction methylases (Hertzberg *et al.* 1985). No new sites of DNA strand scission were noted in this study.

The second report involved the sequence specificity of Fe · BLM-mediated strand scission of pBR322 DNA-derived restriction fragments that had intially been platinated with *cis*-diamminedichloroplatinum (*cis*-DDP) (Mascharak *et al.* 1983); alterations included the appearance of new sites of DNA cleavage, as well as the suppression of sites normally preferred in the absence of platination. The actual sites of platination were not reported, however. Because bleomycin and *cis*-DDP are often used in combination chemotherapy for the treatment of the cancers, the interaction of these two agents at their common therapeutic locus seemed of considerable interest and we decided to study platinum-induced alteration of BLM cleavage sites in a well defined system. This was accomplished by the use of the complementary oligonucleotides d($^{5'}$CGCTTTAAAGG$^{3'}$) and d($^{5'}$CCTTTAAAGCG$^{3'}$), the former of which could be specifically platinated with *cis*-dichloro(ethylenediamine)platinum(II) (*cis*-DEP) at its 3′-terminal GG sequence. As shown in Scheme IV, the unplatinated duplex derived from these two oligonucleotides underwent BLM-mediated modification primarily at C_{21}. Remarkably, platination at $G_{10}G_{11}$ redirected BLM cleavage primarily to T_6 and constitutes the first example of preferred cleavage at a TT site in a well controlled system (Gold *et al.* in preparation). That the position of BLM-mediated oligonucleotide cleavage was altered as a result of conformational changes resulting from platination of the DNA can be appreciated from the distances between the metal centre and the C-4′ H's of the deoxyribose moieties of cytidine$_{21}$, and thymidine$_6$ (Scheme IV). Clearly, the distances involved preclude the direct,

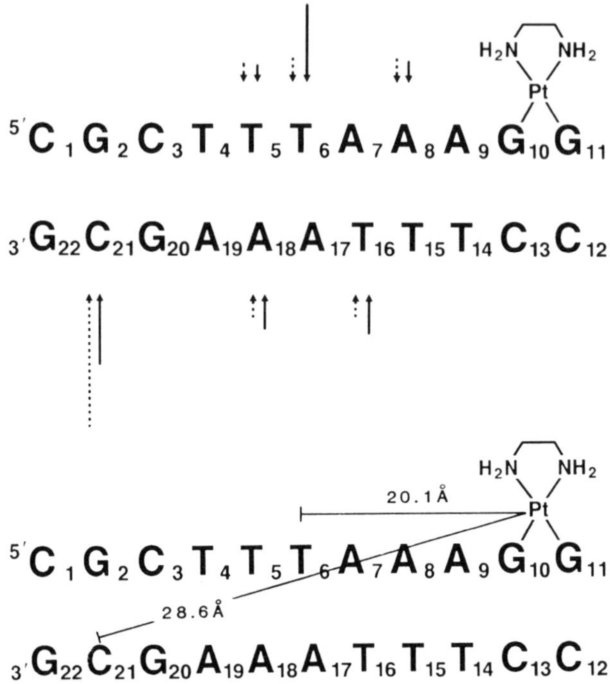

Scheme IV.—Cleavage of a platinated (↑) and unplatinated (⇡) DNA duplex by Fe(II)·BLM A_2 (upper duplex); distances from the metal centre to C-4′ H of thymidine$_6$ and cytidine$_{21}$ (lower duplex)

simultaneous steric involvement of BLM with the platinum centre and either of the affected cleavage sites.

ACKNOWLEDGEMENT

The study was supported by Public Health Service Grant CA38544, awarded by the National Cancer Institute, DHHS.

REFERENCES

Büchi, G., Minster, D., & Young, J. C. F. (1971) A new synthesis of rethrolones. *J. Am. Chem. Soc.* **93,** 4319–4320.

Burger, R. M., Berkowitz, A. R., Peisach, J., & Horwitz, S. B. (1980) Origin of malondialdehyde from DNA degraded by Fe(II)·bleomycin. *J. Biol. Chem.* **255,** 11832–11838.

Burger, R. M., Peisach, J., & Horwitz, S. B. (1982) Effects of O_2 on the reactions of activated bleomycin. *J. Biol. Chem.* **257,** 3372–3375.

Burger, R. M., Freedman, J. H., Horwitz, S. B., & Peisach, J. (1984) DNA degradation by manganese (II)-bleomycin plus peroxide. *Inorg. Chem.* **23,** 2215–2217.

Carter, S. K. (1978) In: *Bleomycin: current status and new developments* (eds. Carter, S. K., Crooke, S. T., & Umezawa, H.) pp. 9–14, Academic Press, New York.

Chang, C.-H. & Meares, C. F. (1984) Cobalt-bleomycins and deoxyribonucleic acid: sequence-dependent interactions, action spectrum for nicking, and indifference to oxygen. *Biochemistry* **23,** 2268–2274.

Crooke, S. T. (1978) In: *Bleomycin: current status and new developments* (eds. Carter, S. K., Crooke, S. T., & Umezawa, H.) pp. 1–8, Academic Press, New York.

D'Andrea, A. S. & Haseltine, W. A. (1978) Sequence specific cleavage of DNA by the antitumor antibiotics neocarzinostatin and bleomycin. *Proc. Natl. Acad. Sci. USA* **75,** 3608–3612.

Ehrenfeld, G. M., Murugesan, N., & Hecht, S. M. (1984) Activation of oxygen and mediation of DNA degradation by manganese-bleomycin. *Inorg. Chem.* **23,** 1496–1498.

Ehrenfeld, G. M., Rodriguez, L. O., Hecht, S. M., Chang, C., Basus, V. J., & Oppenheimer, N. J. (1985) Copper(I)-bleomycin: structurally unique complex that mediates oxidative DNA strand scission. *Biochemistry* **24,** 81–92.

Ehrenfeld, G. M., Shipley, J. B., Heimbrook, D. C., Sugiyama, H., Long, E. C., van Boom, J. H., van der Marel, G. A., Oppenheimer, N. J., & Hecht, S. M. (1987) Copper-dependent cleavage of DNA by bleomycin. *Biochemistry* **26,** 931–942.

Floyd, M. B. (1978) Prostaglandins and congeners. 18. Synthesis of cyclopentenolone precursors to prostaglandins from 2,5-dihydro-2,5-dimethoxyfurans. *J. Org. Chem.* **43,** 1641–1643, and references therein.

Giloni, L., Takeshita, M., Johnson, F., Iden, C., & Grollman, A. P. (1981) Bleomycin-induced strand scission of DNA. *J. Biol. Chem.* **256,** 8608–8615.

Gold, B., Dange, V., Moore, M., Eastman, A., van der Marel, G. A., van Boom, J. H., & Hecht, S. M. (in preparation).

Haidle, C. W., Lloyd, R. S., & Robberson, D. L. (1979) In: *Bleomycin: chemical, biochemical and biological aspects* (ed. Hecht, S. M.) pp. 222–243, Springer-Verlag, New York.

Hecht, S. M. (1979) In: *Bleomycin: chemical, biochemical and biological aspects* (ed. Hecht, S. M.) p. 1–23, Springer-Verlag, New York.

Hertzberg, R. P., Caranfa, M. J., & Hecht, S. M. (1985) DNA methylation diminishes bleomycin-mediated strand scission. *Biochemistry* **24,** 5285–5289.

Ishida, R. & Takahashi, T. (1975) Increased DNA chain breakage by combined action of bleomycin and superoxide radical. *Biochem. Biophys. Res. Commun.* **66,** 1432–1438.

Kross, J., Henner, W. D., Hecht, S. M., & Haseltine, W. A. (1982) Specificity of deoxyribonucleic acid cleavage by bleomycin, phleomycin and tallysomycin. *Biochemistry* **21,** 4310–4318.

Kuwahara, J., Suzuki, T., & Sugiura, Y. (1985) Effective DNA cleavage by bleomycin-vanadium(IV) complex plus hydrogen peroxide. *Biochem. Biophys. Res. Commun.* **129,** 368–374.

Mascharak, P. K., Sugiura, Y., Kuwahara, J., Suzuki, T., & Lippard, S. J. (1983) Alteration and activation of sequence-specific cleavage of DNA by BLM in the presence of the antitumor drug *cis*-diamminedichloroplatinum(II). *Proc. Natl. Acad. Sci. USA* **80,** 6795–6798.

Mirabelli, C. K., Ting, A., Huang, C.-H., Mong, S., & Crooke, S. T. (1982) Bleomycin and talisomycin sequence-specific strand scission of DNA: a mechanism of double-strand cleavage. *Cancer Res.* **42,** 2779–2785.

Mirabelli, C. K., Huang, C.-H., & Crooke, S. T. (1983) Role of deoxyribonucleic acid topology in altering the site/sequence specificity of cleavage of deoxyribonucleic acid by bleomycin and talisomycin. *Biochemistry* **22,** 300–306.

Murugesan, N., Xu, C., Ehrenfeld, G. M., Sugiyama, H., Kilkuskie, R. E., Rodriguez, L. O., Chang, L.-H., & Hecht, S. M. (1985) Analysis of products formed during bleomycin-mediated DNA degradation. *Biochemistry* **24,** 5735–5744.

Oppenheimer, N. J., Rodriguez, L. O., & Hecht, S. M. (1979) Structural studies of 'active complex' of bleomycin: assignment of ligands to the ferrous ion in a ferrous–bleomycin—carbon monoxide complex. *Proc. Natl. Acad. Sci. USA* **76,** 5616–5620.

Sausville, E. A., Peisach, J. & Horwitz, S. B. (1978a) Effect of chelating agents and metal ions on the degradation of DNA by bleomycin. *Biochemistry* **17,** 2740–2746.

Sausville, E. A., Stein, R. W., Peisach, J., & Hortwitz, S. B. (1978b) Properties and products of the degradation of DNA by bleomycin and iron(II). *Biochemistry* **17,** 2746–2754.

Shipley, J. B. & Hecht, S. M. (1988) Bleomycin congeners exhibiting altered DNA cleavage specificity. *Chem. Res. Toxicol.* **1,** 25–27.

Stork, G., Kowalski, C., & Garcia, G. (1975) A route to prostaglandins via a general synthesis of 4-hydroxylyclopentenones. *J. Am. Chem. Soc.* **97,** 3258–3260.

Sugiyama, H., Kilkuskie, R. E., & Hecht, S. M. (1985a) An efficient, site-specific DNA target for bleomycin. *J. Am. Chem. Soc.* **107,** 7765–7767.

Sugiyama, H., Xu, C., Murugesan, N., & Hecht, S. M. (1985b) Structure of the alkali-labile product formed during iron(II)-bleomycin-mediated DNA strand scission. *J. Am. Chem. Soc.* **107,** 4104–4105.

Takeshita, M., Grollman, A. P., Ohtsubo, E., & Ohtsubo, H. (1978) Interaction of bleomycin with DNA. *Proc. Natl. Acad. Sci. USA* **75,** 5983–5987.

Umezawa, H. (1978) In: *Bleomycin: current status and new developments* (eds. Carter, S. K., Crooke, S. T., & Umezawa, H.) pp. 15–19, Academic Press, New York.

Umezawa, H. (1979) In: *Bleomycin: chemical, biochemical and biological aspects* (ed. Hecht, S. M.) pp. 24–36, Springer-Verlag, New York.

6.3 Recent developments in antiviral drug targeting

K. L. Powell, G. K. Darby, D. J. M. Purifoy, M. Tisdale, D. K. Stammers, & B. Larder†

(1) The various approaches to the discovery of drugs to combat virus infections are introduced to demonstrate the role that molecular biology has in this process.
(2) The derivation of drugs through a detailed knowledge of the biochemistry of virus replication is illustrated with reference to the antiherpes drug acyclovir, and the anti-AIDS drug azidothymidine.
(3) The progress of our work on the AIDS virus (HIV) reverse transcriptase is described. Purification of the enzyme in milligram quantities is possible through the expression of the enzyme in prokaryotic systems.
(4) Finally, the aim of our work—the derivation of the three-dimensional structure of the HIV reverse transcriptase—is discussed in relation to its use in the design of new antiviral agents.

The aim of this paper is to discuss the current position regarding the use of some selective antiviral drugs and to examine how the search for such compounds can be simplified by the progress that has been made in the molecular biology of virus infections.

6.3.1 THE BEGINNINGS

Antiviral drugs, or the search for them, has gone through various levels of popularity, depending on the perception of the difficulty in obtaining *specific* compounds. Thus the early demonstration in the 1950s of antiviral activity of simple 5-substituted uracils gave hope of obtaining antiviral drugs which were dashed by the realization that the compounds were either toxic or non-potent. Thus the clinical use of these early compounds against viruses was limited to the topical treatment of herpetic keratitis, first with 5-iododeoxyuridine (Kaufman *et al.* 1962), then with 5-trifluorothymidine (Galasso 1981). Useful though these were to the patients, the markets were too small to be of great interest to the drug companies, and there was a general waning of interest during the late 60s and early 70s.

6.3.2 EARLY SUCCESSES

Those who pursued the idea of specific antiviral drugs during more recent times have concentrated to a large part on either the 5-substituted pyrimidines or on acyclic

† The Wellcome Research Laboratories, Langley Court, Beckenham, Kent BR3 3BS, UK

nucleosides as anti herpes-virus drugs. Particular interest was evoked (Elion 1986) by the 5-halovinyl deoxyuridines and the 2′-fluoro-2′-arabino-furanosyl derivatives of 5-iodocytosine (FIAC) and thymine (FMAU). These compounds exhibit very good selectivity *in vitro* with specificity being conferred by the viral thymidine kinase which could phosphorylate compounds which were not substrates for the cell enzymes. No therapeutically useful drug has yet emerged from studies of these compounds, owing to unexpected problems with toxicity or mutagenecity.

Meanwhile, in the purines the description of the antiviral activity of adenine arabinoside led Gertrude Elion and her colleagues at Wellcome's USA subsidiary to synthesise, and D. J. Bauer and P. Collins in the UK to test, the antiviral activities of purines. During this exercise Howard Schaeffer in the same laboratories was examining the changes that could be made in the ribose moiety of adenosine whilst retaining the ability to interact with adenosine deaminase. The acyclic derivatives of adenine, 2,6-DAP, and guanine were thus included in the antiviral testing programme, the latter being 100× more active than the 2,6-DAP and 400× more than the adenosine (Elion 1986). Thus acyclovir was discovered, and has led to intensive programmes in many companies to derive active drugs with similar properties.

6.3.2.1 Mechanism of action of acyclovir

The mechanism of acyclovir is perhaps one of the most surprising attributes of this drug; though it resembles deoxyguanosine, missing only the 2′carbon and 3′carbon and hydroxyl groups, it is phosphorylated predominantly by the herpes virus induced thymidine kinase and not by cellular enzymes (Fyfe *et al.* 1978). This property of the drug gives it a dramatic therapeutic ratio, there being approximately a 3000-fold difference in the ID_{50} for Vero cells and that for HSV-1 (0.1 μM). Once the drug has been phosphorylated to the monophosphate it is further phosphorylated by cellular enzymes to the di- and tri-phosphate forms (Miller & Miller 1980, 1982). In uninfected cells very small levels of ACV triphosphate are produced following limited production of the monophosphate by a 5′-nucleotidase at high drug concentrations (Keller *et al.* 1985). Further selectivity then occurs, owing to differential affinities of the cell and viral DNA polymerases for the ACV triphosphate. For example, the Ki of ACV-triphosphate for HSV-1 DNA polymerase is 0.08 μM, and for Vero cell α DNA polymerase is 2.2 μM. Once HSV DNA polymerase has reacted with ACV triphosphate it is inactivated (Furman *et al.* 1984) and, further, any incorporation of ACV into growing DNA chains results in chain termination due to the lack of the 3′-hydroxyl (Furman *et al.* 1979).

An important feature of the elucidation of this mode of action was the isolation in cell culture in a wide variety of laboratories of virus mutant which were resistant to the drug (Larder & Darby 1984). These *in vitro* resistant viruses were shown to be of three types having (i) no thymidine kinase, (ii) an altered thymidine kinase with restricted substrate specificity, or (iii) an altered DNA polymerase. These mutants have been paralleled in the clinical situation not from 'normal' patients but from patients with compromised immune systems. These patients most commonly have virus with altered tk genes, but recently Peter Collins in our department has discovered an isolate from an immunocompromised patient which has an altered DNA polymerase activity.

6.3.2.2 Current status of acyclovir

Acyclovir has been, and continues to be, a very successful drug both commercially and in the clinic. Studies are continuing on new therapeutic uses for the drug which has proved uniquely safe and effective as an antiviral agent. There can be little doubt that the success of acyclovir has brought about much more interest in the possibility of producing antiviral drugs and in their use.

6.3.3 AZIDOTHYMIDINE

The emergence of the AIDS epidemic has brought new challenges to those interested in the control of virus infections. The fact that the causitive agent of the disease, the human immunedeficiency virus (HIV), was identified early (Barré-Sinoussi *et al.* 1983) has concentrated much effort on the various gene products of this virus which might act as targets for antiviral drugs. The virus belongs to the retrovirus group and has an RNA genome. A feature of the replication of these viruses is the conversion of their genomes to double stranded DNA by a virus-encoded reverse transcriptase present within the virus particles. This enzyme has been studied extensively in animal RNA tumour viruses. Several inhibitors of the enzyme that were discovered were known before the advent of AIDS. The most interesting of these is Azidothymidine which is now being widely used as an anti-AIDS drug (Mitsuya *et al.* 1985). Azidothymidine is closely related to thymidine, and is currently made by using this natural substance as starting material.

6.3.3.1 Mode of action of Azidothymidine (Furman *et al.* 1986)

Azidothymidine is phosphorylated in infected or uninfected cells by the same enzymes that are responsible for the phosphorylation of thymidine. The drug is a good substrate for cellular thymidine kinase, but on phosphorylation to the monophosphate it is bound strongly by the cell thymidylate kinase but is converted slowly by this enzyme to the diphosphate. Thus the monophosphate may be considered as a substrate based inhibitor of the cell TMP-kinase. Intracellular levels of AZT-MP have been recorded as high as 800 μM in cells treated with 50 μM AZT. This level of the monophosphate greatly exceeds the level of the triphosphate which is the level at which specificity occurs. Inhibition of the AIDS virus reverse transcriptase occurs at very low levels of AZT-triphosphate. Using cloned HIV RT we have measured the IC_{50} of the drug on the enzyme as <0.1 μM (Lardner *et al.* 1987b). Although the drug does have inhibitory effects on cell enzmes, these occur at a level hundreds of times higher than that required to inhibit the viral enzyme.

6.3.3.2 Clinical experience with AZT

The results of preliminary phase 1 and phase 2 trials with AZT are well known, and I will just touch on them here (Yarchoan *et al.* 1986). The drug was found to be easily administered, having good oral bioavailability (about 60%), and virus inhibitory levels could be obtained in patients. The half-life of the drug was about one-hour, and the chief route of drug clearance was via a inactive metabolite.

Importantly, the drug was efficiently transported across the blood-brain barrier and would thus be expected to inhibit virus in clinical cases of AIDS virus brain infection.

The drug was found, in the phase 1 study, to bring about improvement in several parameters (both clinical and immunological), whilst having haematological toxicity problems which could be tolerated. Thus a phase 2 study was initiated with 281 patients. Initially, this was a randomized double-blind placebo-controlled study, but on examination of the preliminary results the trial was opened, and patients receiving placebo were placed on the drug. The chief reason for this was that only 1 patient receiving Retrovir (AZT) had died, whilst 19 in the placebo group had done so. Not only did the drug reduce mortality, but it also significantly reduced the incidence of opportunistic infection. Positive indications were also seen in measuring the quality of the patient's life, patient's weight gain, T_4 cell counts, DTH skin test response, and virologically in P24 antigen levels.

Retrovir clearly has adverse effects, producing neutropenia, leucopenia, and anaemia. These effects were most pronouned in AIDS patients with low T_4 counts on entry into the study. 50% of patients have tolerated the full recommended dose, and most patients have had a tolerable dose identified even with toxicity problems. Further studies are under way both in Europe and the USA to evaluate the drug completely.

6.3.4 SUMMARY

Existing antiviral drugs have been found either with excellent properties, enabling their safe and effective use (e.g. Acyclovir), or with tolerable toxicity, allowing their limited but valuable application (e.g. Azidothymidine). These drugs were developed through random screening or semi-rational approaches to drug design. The next part of this paper discusses (1) how a more deliberate approach is being made to the discovery of new antiviral agents, and (2) the AIDS virus reverse transcriptase as an example of how future work might proceed.

6.3.5 RATIONAL DRUG DESIGN

At Wellcome we have decided that the success of AZT establishes the HIV reverse transcriptase as an ideal target for the design of antiviral drugs. Such drug design requires work on the target, examining its biochemistry, structure/function, and three-dimensional structure. The last part of this paper reports our progress in this direction.

6.3.5.1 Production of reverse transcriptase *in vitro*

The HIV particle contains the enzyme (RT), albeit in very small amounts. Purification of the enzyme from this source has allowed limited characterization of the HIV enzyme, but could not produce enough enzyme for crystallographic studies. In order to do these studies large amounts of enzyme would be required, and this could only be obtained by gene cloning. Our first step was to acquire part of the AIDS genome as cloned material from Dr Malcolm Martin at NIH. The first task was to 'tailor' these genes to allow expression of the RT. The virus 'pol' gene encodes 3 proteins a protease, the reverse transcriptase and an endonuclease which are made as a polyprotein in virus-infected cells. Cleavage of the polyprotein by proteases yields each gene product (Muesing *et al.* 1985, Ratner *et al.* 1985, Sanchez-Pescador *et al.* 1985, Wain-Hobson *et al.* 1985). We wanted to express the RT gene in the absence of the other products. Thus from the original clone a construct was made in the M13 phage system (which allows easy genetic manipulation) by directly cloning the BglII-EcoRI-fragment containing the protease and RT encoding portions and part of the endonuclease into mptac18, a specially constructed cloning vector (B. Larder, unpublished information) designed to contain the RT gene behind the strongly inducible *tac* promoter (see Fig. 1). We next removed the extraneous material by a

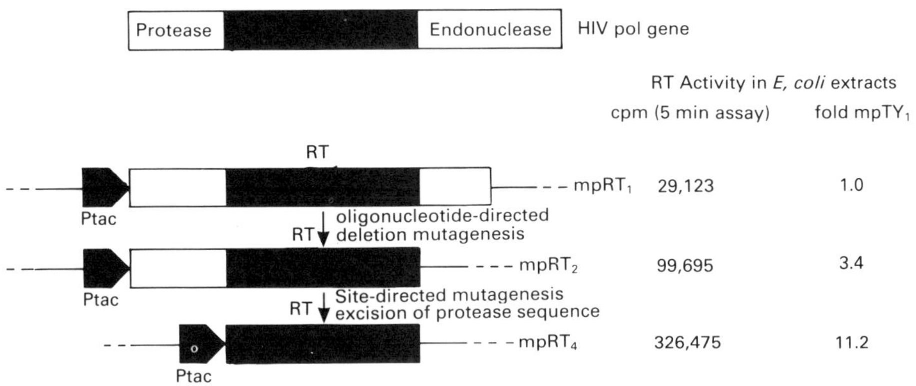

Fig. 1.—Cloning and expression for the HIV RT activity in *E. coli*. The upper map indicates the relative positions of protease and endonuclease coding sequences to those encoding RT (black box). The BglII, EcoRI fragment containing the protease. RT and part of the endonuclease coding sequence (boxed area) is shown inserted into mptacl8 in the second map, and each subsequent map illustrates the steps in refining the RT expressing constructs. To the right of the map of each construct is shown the activity induced in *E. coli* with infection by the phase

series of specific deletions. Firstly the endonuclease remnants were removed by oligonucleotide directed mutagenesis using a single 'deletion' oligonucleotide with 15 nucleotides complementary to the C terminal portion of the RT and 15 complementary to the 5′end of the lacZ gene in mptac 18. The protease region was removed from the resulting clone by first inserting an $EcoR_1$ restriction enzyme site just upstream from the RT start by site-directed mutagenesis, then removing the DNA from between the pair of EcoR1 sites thus created forming the phage mpRT4. The RT produced by each of these clones was examined and each reduction in the material superfluous to the reverse transcriptase was found to improve the level of RT activity (Fig. 1).

These manipulations had given us levels of RT activity which were useful and would allow detailed biochemical study, but to get sufficient protein for crystallization purposes still higher levels of enzyme were required. These levels were achieved by removing the 'casette' we had created from mpRT4 and inserting it into the high-level expression plasmid pKK 233-2. This resulted in the plasmid pRT1 which on insertion into *E. coli* produced the RT polypeptide at the level of about 10% of the *E. coli* total cell protein: this level of protein production was mirrored by enzyme activity and represented authentic enzyme as judged by reaction with AIDS patient sera, thus allowing purification of the RT in quantity (Larder *et al.* 1987b). Thus far we have used combinations of affinity- and ion-exchange chromatography to produce more than 100 mg of purified HIV reverse transcriptase. Using this material, crystallization of the RT has been achieved. X-ray crystallographic studies of the pure enzyme are now beginning.

The 3-D structure of the enzyme will not of course reveal the importance of individual amino acids in the active sites of the enzyme. To begin to come to terms with this difficulty we have looked at sequence similarities between the HIV reverse transcriptase gene and that of closely related polymerase genes revealed by Johnson *et al.* (1986). We have then mutated each of these regions of the gene to produce site-specific mutants in the conserved areas (Fig. 2). I shall not go into this study

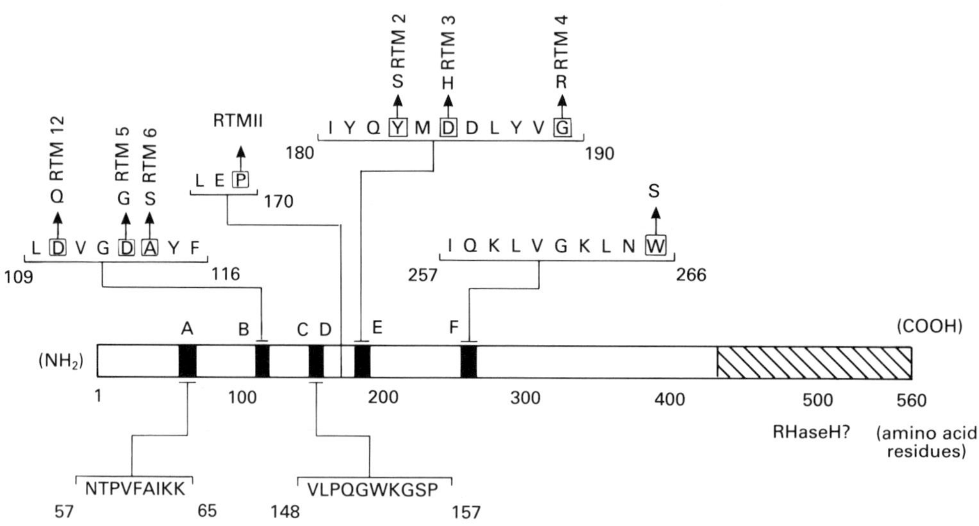

Fig. 2.—Position of conserved regions and mutations in HIV RT. The diagram is a linear map of the amino acid sequence of the HIV RT. Each black box indicates a conserved region (lettered A to F). Each conserved amino acid sequence is shown in single letter code, and mutations made in the region are indicated by boxes and arrows indicating the changes made. The position of the putative RNAse H encoding sequence is indicated at the carboxy-terminus of the polypeptide (cross-hatched) (Johnson *et al.* 1986)

(Larder *et al.* 1987a) in detail, but just point out how interesting the results can be. Firstly, to convince you that the result of any mutation is not always interesting, the change from pro-leu in mutant RTM11 in conserved region D had no effect on the enzyme. Further mutants show much more interesting effects; for example, in region E changing one of a pair of conserved aspartates to histidine totally abolished activity, thus identifying a region of great interest in the enzyme's activity. Two other mutants in this region, RTM2 and RTM4, also reduced enzyme activity, confirming this result. Secondly, two mutants in region B RTM5 and RTM6 drastically altered the enzyme—it was less active than the wild type and was markedly less sensitive to inhibition by AZT-triphosphate and phosphonoformic acid. These changes are most interesting, indicating both where the triphosphate binding site of the enzyme might be located and also raising the possibility of alterations in sensitivity of AIDS virus to drugs by alteration of the reverse transcriptase (of course we do not know if a virus carrying such a mutation would be viable or if it were able to induce full-blown AIDS).

It is not appropriate to go into this series of experiments at great deapth here, but they indicate the promise of these molecular approaches to antiviral drug design.

ACKNOWLEDGEMENTS

The authors would like to thank C. Bradley, S. Kemp, P. Ertl, V. Parmar, and S. Court for their technical help, and P. Ward for her help with the manuscript. Fig. 1 is redrawn from a figure in a *Nature* article (Larder *et al.* 1987a) and Fig. 2 from an article in the *EMBO Journal* (Larder *et al.* 1987b).

REFERENCES

Barré-Sinoussi, F., Cherman, J. C., Rey, F., Nugeybe, M. T., Charmaret, S., Gruest, J., Dauguet, C., Axler-Blin, C., Vézinet-Brun, F. Rouzioux, C., Rozenbaum, W., & Montagnier, L. (1983). Isolation of a T-lymphotropic retrovirus from a patient at risk of acquired immune deficiency syndrome (AIDS). *Science* **220,** 868–870.

Elion, G. (1986). History, mechanism of action, spectrum and selectivity of nucleoside analogs. In: *Antiviral chemotherapy: new directions for clinical applications and research* (eds Mills, J. & Corey, L.). Elsevier, New York, pp. 118–137.

Furman, P. A., St. Clair, M. H., Fyfe, J. A., Rideout, J. L., Keller, P. M., & Elion, G. (1979). Inhibition of herpes simplex virus induced DNA Polymerase and viral DNA replication by 9-(2-hydroxyethoxymethyl)guanine and its triphosphate. *J. Virol.* **32,**72–77.

Furman, P. A., St. Clair, M. H., & Spector, T. (1984). Acyclovir triphosphate is a suicide inactivator of the herpes simplex virus DNA polymerase. *J. Biol. Chem.* **259,** 9575–9579.

Furman, P. A., Fyfe, J. A., St. Clair, M. H., Weinhold, K., Rideout, J. L., Freeman, G. A., Lehrman, S. N., Bolognesi, D. P., Broder, S., Mitsuya, H., & Barry, D. W. (1986). Phosphorylation of 3′-azido-3′-deoxythymidine and selective interaction of the 5′-triphosphate with human immunodeficiency virus reverse transcriptase. *Proc. Natl. Acad. Sci. USA* **83,** 8333–8337.

Fyfe, J. A., Keller, P. A., Furman, P. A., Miller, R. L., & Elion, G. B. (1978). Thymidine kinase from herpes simplex virus phosphorylates the new antiviral compound 9-(2-hydroxyethoxymethoxy)-guanine. *J. Biol. Chem.* **253,** 8721–8727.

Galasso, G. (1981). An assessment of antiviral drugs for the management of infectious diseases in humans. *Antiviral Research* **1,** 73–96.

Johnson, M. S., McLure, M. A., Feng, D.-F., Gray, J., & Doolittle, R. F. (1986). Computer analysis of retroviral pol genes: assignment of enzymatic functions to specific sequences and homologies with non-viral enzymes. *Proc. Natl. Acad. Sci. USA* **83,** 7648–7652.

Kaufman, H. E., Nesburh, A. B., & Maloney, E. (1962). IDU therapy of herpes simplex. *Arch. Opthamol.* **67,** 583–591.

Keller, P. M., McKee, S. A., & Fyfe, J. A. (1985). Cytoplasmic 5′-nucleotidase catalyzes Acyclovir phosphorylation. *J. Biol. Chem.* **260,** 8664–8667.

Larder, B. A. & Darby, G. K. (1984). Virus drug-resistance: mechanisms and consequences. *Antiviral Research* **4,** 1–42.

Larder, B. A., Purifoy, D. J. M., Powell, K. L., & Darby, G. K. (1987a). Site-specific mutagenesis of AIDS virus reverse transcriptase. *Nature* **327,** 716–717.

Larder, B. A., Purifoy, D. J. M., Powell, K. L., & Darby, G. (1987b). AIDS virus reverse transcriptase defined by high level expression in *E. coli*. *E.M.B.O. J.* **6,** 3133–3137.

Miller, W. H. & Miller, R. L. (1980). Phosphorylation of acyclovir monophosphate by GMP Kinase. *J. Biol. Chem.* **253,** 7204–7207.

Miller, W. H. & Miller, R. L. (1982). Phosphorylation of acyclovir diphosphase by cellular enzymes. *Biochem. Pharm.* **31,** 3879–3884.

Mitsuya, H., Weinhold, K. J., Furman, P. A., St. Clair, M., Lehrman, S. N., Gallo, R. C., Bolognesi, D., Barry, D. M., & Broder, S. (1985). 3′Azido-3′deoxythymidine (BW A509U): an antiviral agent that inhibits the infectivity and cytopathic effect of human T-lymphotropic virus type III/lymphoadenopathy-associated virus *in vitro*. *Proc. Natl. Acad. Sci. USA* **82,** 7096–7100.

Muesing, M. A., Smith, D. H., Cabradilla, C. D., Benton, C. V., Lasky, L. A., & Capon, D. J. (1985). Nucleic acid structure and expression of the human AIDS/lymphoadenopathy retrovirus. *Nature* **313,** 450—458.

Ratner, L., Haseltine, W., Patarca, R., Livak, K. J., Starchich, B. Josephs, S. F., Doran, E. R., Rafalski, J. A., Whitehorn, E. A., Baumeister, K., Ivanoff, L., Petteway, S. R., Pearson, M. L., Lautenberger, J. A., Papas, T. S., Ghrayeb, J., Chang, N. T., Gallo, R. C., & Wong-staal (1985). Complete nucleotide sequence of the AIDS virus, HTLV-III. *Nature* **313,** 277–284.

Sanchez-Pescador, R., Power, M. D., Barr, P. J., Steimer, K. S., Stempien, M. M., Brown-Shimer, S. L., Gee, W. W., Renard, A., Randolph, A., Levy, J. A., Dina, D., & Luciw, P. A. (1985). Nucleotide sequence and expression of an AIDS-associated retrovirus (ARV-2) *Science* **227,** 484–492.

Wain-Hobson, S., Sonigo, P., Danos, O., Cole, S., & Alizon, M. (1985). Nucleotide sequence of the AIDS virus, LAV. *Cell* **40,** 9–17.

Yarchoan, R., Weinhold, K. J., Lyerly, H. K., Gelmann, E., Blum, R. M., Shearer, G. M., Mitsuya, H., Collins, J. M., Myers, C. E., Klecker, R. W., Markham, P. D., Durack, D. T., Lehrman, S. N., Barry, D. W., Fischl, M. A., Gallo, R. C., Bolognesi, D. P., & Broder, S. (1986). Administration of 3′-Azido-3′-deoxythymidine, an inhibitor of HTLV/III/LAV replication, to patients with AIDS or AIDS-related complex. *Lancet* **1,** 575–590.

6.4 Effect of alkyl-phospholipids on mammalian cell permeability

A. Kotyk†, J. Kára‡, M. Baudyšová†, A. Knotková†, & Z. Drahota†

(1) Alkyl-phospholipids carrying one alkyl chain and one or two acyl chains are known to be cancerostatic both *in vitro* toward tissue culture cells and *in vivo* toward different types of tumours.
(2) A major two-acyl one-alkyl phospholipid has been isolated from highly active embryonated chicken egg extract.
(3) This phospholipid, as well as others, some of them synthetic analogues, were found to increase the passive permeability of a tumour cell line, leaving control fibroblasts intact even at much higher concentrations.

6.4.1 ALKYL-PHOSPHOLIPIDS

The group of substances known generically as alkyl-phospholipids have been recognized for some time as potential anticancer drugs (e.g., Runge *et al.* 1980, Berdel 1982, Berdel *et al.* 1984). Their toxicity for neoplastic cells and tissues appears to exceed by at least one order of magnitude any detrimental effect on normal tissue cells (e.g., Andreesen *et al.* 1978, Scott *et al.* 1979), and several mechanisms of their selective action have been proposed, most of them gravitating toward the view that phospholipid metabolism and/or incorporation of phospholipids into cell membranes are disturbed (Modolell *et al.* 1979).

Alkyl-phospholipids that have been used therapeutically are almost exclusively synthetic derivatives of phosphatidic acid, with an *O*-alkyl at C_1 of the glycerol backbone and an *O*-acyl at C_2. They resemble plasmalogens where the *O*-alkyl is obligatorily alk-1-enyl, and the platelet-activating factor which carries a saturated alkyl at C_1 but obligatorily an acetyl group at C_2 (cf. Hoffman *et al.* 1984).

6.4.2 ACTIVE AGENTS FROM EMBRYONATED CHICKEN EGGS

Potentially therapeutically useful substances have been isolated from rat brain myelin (Kino *et al.* 1982) as well as from egg yolk and some vegetable oils (Ganley *et al.* 1958), but only recently has a complete purification been achieved of the major

† Institute of Physiology, Czechoslovak Academy of Sciences, Vídeňská 1083, 142 20 Prague, Czechoslovakia
‡ Laboratory of Evolutionary Biology, Czechoslovak Academy of Sciences Na, Folimance 5, 120 00 Prague, Czechoslovakia

constituent of a highly active preparation of embryonated chicken egg (Kára *et al.* 1986). This constituent is 1-*O*-octadecyl-2-oleoyl-*syn*-glycero-3-phospho-(*N*-palmitoyl)-ethanolamine

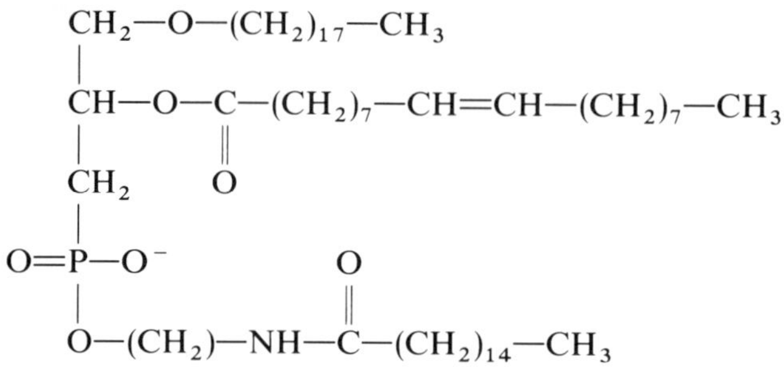

A similar compound is known to exist in bovine erythrocytes (Matsumoto & Miwa 1973), in mammalian epidermis (Gray 1976), and in infarcted myocardium (Epps *et al.* 1979). The extract from which it had been isolated (CAPL) was shown to be cytostatic toward cancer cells and relatively innocuous toward normal cells (Kára *et al.* 1984).

6.4.3 EFFECTS OF CAPL AND ITS CONSTITUENTS ON MEMBRANE PERMEABILITY

The general effect on membrane permeability of the crude alkyl phospholipid isolated according to Kára *et al.* (1984), as well as of some synthetic analogues and homologues of its main constituent, was demonstrated by using human embryonal pulmonary fibroblasts (HEPF) as a control and MNB E7 cells as typical neoplastic cells. Both types of cell were grown by a standard tissue-culture procedure in 5 ml medium. Growth reached saturation after 12 and 7 days, respectively, whereupon 0.2 ml 1 mM ^{3}H-labelled 2-deoxy-D-glucose (2-dglc) was added. This sugar is readily phosphorylated in all animal cells by a hexokinase, but further metabolism stops, and the 2-deoxy-D-glucose-6-phosphate formed is trapped in cells as sugar phosphates which show a very low diffusional permeability (Pasternak 1985, Kotyk *et al.* 1987).

After a three-hour incubation with the labelled sugar, the medium was replaced with a fresh one containing either its normal constituents or, in addition, the alkyl-phospholipid tested, in amounts ranging from 0.5 to 50 μg per 5 ml. Samples

Table 1—Exit of radioactivity, due to [^{3}H]2-deoxy-D-glucose-6-phosphate, from tissue culture fibroblasts (HEPF) and neoplastic cells (MNB E7) upon the application of CAPL (0, 0.1, 1.0 and 10 μg/ml)

Time after medium replacement (h)	Radioactivity in external medium, in cpm							
	HEPF				MNB E7			
	0	0.1	1.0	10	0	0.1	1.0	10
0	650	645	627	648	564	641	697	712
2	2046	2010	2037	1785	1626	2239	2485	2996
18	3224	3373	3850	3613	2382	4006	4286	5981
24	4955	4617	4584	4811	3601	5195	6410	6817

were then withdrawn from the medium over a period of 24 h, and their radioactivity was measured.

The release of radioactivity from cells was influenced by some of the compounds tested, both by those of the embryonated egg extract and by those synthesized in a novel, stereospecific, way (Smrčina & Kotyk 1987). An example is shown in Table 1.

On the whole, several of the compounds tested show a distinct avidity for neoplastic cells as compared with normal cells grown in tissue culture. This might indicate that the observed and previously described cancerostatic effects of alkyl-phospholipids have to do with increasing passive membrane permeability, so that the cell contents of ions and small molecules leak out uncontrollably from neoplastic cells, and those cells perish.

REFERENCES

Andreesen, R., Modolell, M., Weltzien, H. U., Eibl, H., Common, H. H., Löhr, G. W., & Munder, P. G. (1978). Selective destruction of human leukemic cells by alkyl-phospholipids, *Cancer Res.* **33,** 3894–3899.

Berdel, W. E. (1982). Antineoplastic activity of synthetic lysophospholipid analogs, *Blut* **44,** 71–78.

Berdel, W. E., Greiner, E., Fink, U., Zänker, K. S., Stavrou, D., Trappe, A., Fahlbusch, R., Reichert, A., & Rastetter, R. (1984). Cytotoxic effects of alkyl phospholipids in human brain tumor cells, *Oncology* **41,** 140–145.

Epps, D. E., Schmid, P. C., Natarajan, V., & Schmid, H. H. O. (1979). N-Acyl-ethanolamine accumulation in infarcted mycoardium, *Biochem. Biophys. Res. Commun.* **90,** 628–633.

Ganley, O. H., Graessle, O. E., & Robison, H. J. (1958). Anti-inflammatory activity of N-acyl-ethanolamines: anti-inflammatory activity of compounds obtained from egg yoke, peanut oil and soybean lecithin, *J. Lab. Clin. Med.* **51,** 709–714.

Gray, G. M. (1976). Phosphatidyl-(N-acyl)-ethanolamine, a lipid component of mammalian epidermis, *Biochim. Biophys. Acta* **431,** 1–8.

Hoffman, D. R., Hajdu, J., & Snyder, F. (1984). Cytotoxicity of platelet activating factor and related alkyl-phospholipid analogs in human leukemia cells, polymorphonuclear neutrophils, and skin fibroblasts, *Blood* **63,** 545–552.

Kára, J., Borovička, M., & Liebl, V. (1984). Alkyl-phospholipid with a selective anticancer effect and mode of its preparation, Czechoslovak Patent PV-07132-84, Prague.

Kára, J., Borovička, M., Liebl, V., Smolíková, A., & Ubik, K. (1986). A novel nontoxic alkyl-phospholipid with selective antitumor activity, plasmanyl-(N-acyl)-ethanolamine (PNAE), isolated from degenerating chick embryonal tissues and from an anticancer biopreparation CAPL, *Neoplasma* **33,** 187–205.

Kino, M., Matsumura, T., Gamo, M., & Saito, K. (1982). Studies on molecular species of choline and ethanolamine glycerophospholipids obtained from rat brain myelin and synaptosomes by gas-liquid chromatography/mass spectrometry, *Biomed. Mass Spectrometry* **9,** 363–369.

Kotyk, A., Janáček, K., & Koryta, J. (1987). *Biophysical chemistry of membrane functions*, John Wiley, Chichester, UK.

Modolell, M., Andreesen, R., Pahlke, W., Brugger, U., & Munder, P. G. (1979). Disturbance of phospholipid metabolism during the selective destruction of tumor cells induced by alkyl-lysophospholipids, *Cancer Res.* **39,** 4681–4686.

Runge, M. H., Andreesen, R., Pfleiderer, A., & Munder, P. G. (1980). Destruction of human solid tumors by alkyl-lysophospholipids. *J. Nat. Cancer Inst.* **64,** 1301–1306.

Scott, C. G., Heckman, C. A., Nettesheim, P., & Snyder, F. (1979). Metabolism of ether-linked glycerolipids in cultures of normal and neoplastic rat respiratory tract epithelium. *Cancer Res.* **39,** 207–214.

Smrčina, M. & Kotyk, A. (1987). Stereospecific synthesis of cancerostatic alkyl-phospholipids. Czechoslovak patent pending.

Part 7

Molecular mechanisms of toxicity

7.1 The role of drug metabolism in initiating drug toxicity

J. W. Gorrod & A. Raman†

(1) Pharmacologically desirable interactions between drugs and cellular macromolecules are usually reversible.
(2) Toxic effects may manifest if cellular macromolecules gain or lose activity as a result of irreversible covalent binding to drugs or reactive drug metabolites.
(3) Examples of the metabolic generation of toxic species from drugs containing arylamine, arylamide, quinone, hydrazine, furan, haloalkane, thione, or hydropyridine functionalities are described.

7.1.1 INTRODUCTION

In order for a drug or any xenobiotic to exert an effect in a biological system there clearly has to be an interaction between the compound and the system. It is now recognized that these interactions can be of several types and may involve different classes of cellular macromolecules. Pharmacologically desirable interactions are in general reversible, and are often mediated via electrostatic or Van der Waal's bonds. This allows dissociation of the drug–macromolecule complex and thus termination of pharmacological activity. Conversely, toxication reactions often occur when cellular macromolcules form stable, irreversibly bound adducts with foreign chemicals, via covalent bonds (Gorrod 1981).

Drugs are, in general, chemically stable moieties, and prior biochemical activation, or metabolism, to reactive species is usually required for covalent binding to macromolecules to occur (Gorrod 1979). These metabolic processes (Testa & Jenner 1976) may be oxidative, reductive, or hydrolytic (Phase I metabolism) or involve conjugation with small endogenous molecules (Phase II metabolism). Such reactions occur predominantly in the liver, but are also present to varying extents in virtually all organs (Gorrod 1978). The metabolism of drugs generally leads to more polar, and hence more easily excretable compounds, and comprises a detoxication mechanism. However, in some cases the metabolites or intermediates in their formation are highly reactive, and their interaction with macromolecules in the body leads to the observed toxic effects of the drug. As both detoxication and toxication pathways will be influenced by a variety of physiological and pharmacological factors,

† Chelsea Department of Pharmacy, Kings College, University of London, Chelsea Campus, Manresa Road, London SW3 6LX, UK

the interrelationship between the two pathways is not always clearly apparent. In some cases, the toxication processes can be considered as aberrant pathways which only occur as an alternative to the predominant detoxication pathway. In other cases, they may be the major pathway but only express their toxic potential because of other factors e.g. drug overdose, failure of a conjugation pathway, or failure of an excretory mechanism.

Reactive species which bind covalently to macromolecules are usually electrophilic in nature. These include epoxides, carbonium ions, quinones, quinoneimines, and free radicals. Examples of drugs giving rise to such species by metabolic processes are described in the following sections. The electrophiles bind covalently with nucleophilic centres on macromolecules such as proteins, lipids, polysaccharides, and nucleic acids.

It is apparent that 'covalent binding' *per se* is not responsible for initiating a toxic response to a drug. The drug–macromolecule adduct must have either gained or lost biological activity or function. Reaction with a protein, for example, could block enzyme activity, or cause the protein to become antigenic. Binding to polysaccharides could also cause immunological effects. Reaction with a nucleic acid could block the transfer of genetic information, and interfere with protein synthesis. Alternatively, mutagenesis or carcinogenesis could occur. Cell membranes may be disrupted as a result of covalent binding to lipids or lipoproteins. It is important to note that a particular electrophile may react with a variety of macromolecules or even different sites within a macromolecule and need not produce the same effect in every case.

The generation of reactive and therefore potentially toxic metabolic products is fairly widespread. However, in the majority of cases, toxic effects are not manifest, owing to the presence of natural protective mechanisms. Thus small nucleophiles, such as water and thiols, are often responsible for 'neutralizing' the toxic intermediates. Epoxides may be converted to dihydrodiols by the action of epoxide hydrolases, and radicals and other electrophiles may react with endogenous glutathione to form innocuous thioethers. This latter reaction is usually, but not always, mediated by glutathione-S-transferases in cell cytosol. Cellular defence mechanisms against reactive metabolites have been reviewed by Reed (1985). Normally, these protective mechanisms are sufficient to protect the cell from the onslaught of reactive compounds. However, as already mentioned, in cases of drug overdose or the failure of a particular metabolic pathway, toxic effects may be experienced.

7.1.2 METABOLIC ACTIVATION OF SOME FUNCTIONAL GROUPS ENCOUNTERED IN DRUG MOLECULES

7.1.2.1 Aromatic amines and amides

The metabolic activation of aromatic amines and amides to carcinogenic and mutagenic species is well documented (Gorrod & Manson 1986). The toxicity arises as a result of metabolic N-hydroxylation of these compounds to arylhydroxylamines or aryl-hydroxamic acids respectively. Most compounds undergoing such activation are environmental or industrial chemicals rather than drugs. A second form of toxicity mediated by aryl hydroxylamines is the oxidation of ferrohaemoglobin to ferri-haemoglobin (Kiese 1974). When ferrihaemoglobin is further oxidized, it leads to the precipitation of haemoglobin. This becomes attached to red cell membranes, causing deformities (Heinz bodies) in the cell and thereby stimulating their destruction by

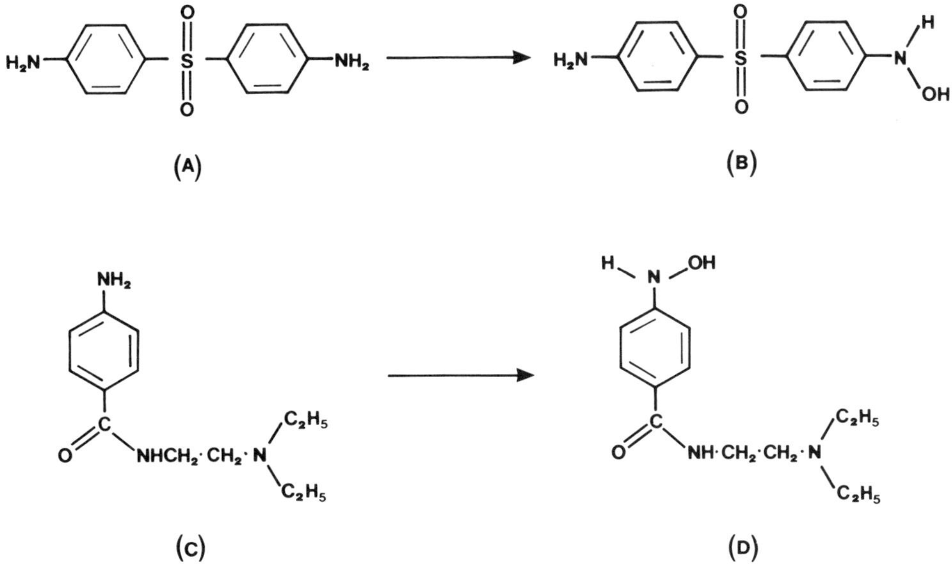

Fig. 1.—The metabolic conversion of dapsone (A) and procainamide (B) to N-hydroxy derivatives.

the reticulo-endothelial systems (Allen & Jandel 1961). Ferrihaemoglobinaemia and Heinz body production in red blood cells has been shown to occasionally arise following administration of dapsone (Fig. 1, A). Dapsone is an antimicrobial compound, which is used in the treatment of leprosy and dermatitis herpetiformis. The formation of a hydroxylamine metabolite (Fig. 1, B) of dapsone has been demonstrated both *in vitro* and *in vivo* (Tabarelli & Uehleke 1971).

Procainamide (Fig. 1, C) is an antihysrhythmic drug which, on chronic therapy, can induce a syndrome similar to lupus erythematosus, and the production of antinuclear antibodies. One metabolic route of this compound is the acetylation of the aromatic amino function. Studies by Woosley *et al.* (1978) demonstrated that the duration of therapy required to induce antibodies was shorter in patients of the slow acetylator phenotype than in rapid acetylators. This implied that N-acetylation was not the metabolic activation step initiating the toxic effects, and that either the parent compound or another metabolite was responsible. In further studies (Freeman *et al.* 1981), it was discovered that covalent binding of procainamide (or a derivative) to hepatic protein was increased *in vivo* when animals were pretreated with mono-oxygenase inducers (phenobarbitone and 3-methylcholanthrene), and reduced *in vitro* in the presence of glutathione or the monooxygenase inhibitor SKF 525A. These studies showed that metabolic activation was required for covalent binding. The formation of a hydroxylamine metabolite (Fig. 1, D) of the drug by rat and human microsomes has since been demonstrated (Uetrecht *et al.* 1984), and this or the nitroso derivative is believed to be the reactive metabolite responsible for covalent binding of procainamide to cellular macromolecules (Uetrecht 1985).

The substitution of a hydroxyl group onto the ring of an aromatic amine or amide can result in new possibilities for reactive intermediates. The analgesic drug paracetamol (acetaminophen, Fig. 2, A) is an example of a phenolic arylamide with

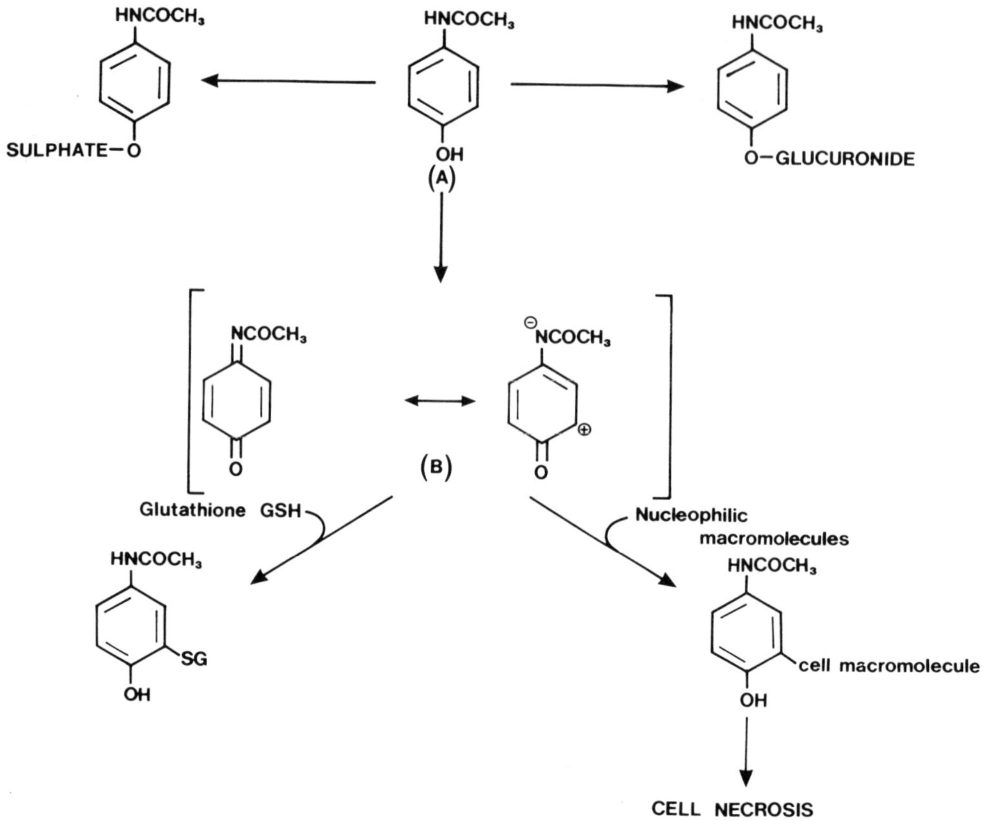

Fig. 2.—The metabolism of paracetamol.

well documented toxic effects. These effects manifest in cases of paracetamol overdosage, when normal defence mechanisms are overwhelmed. The main features of paracetamol toxicity are hepatic necrosis (following acute overdosage) and kidney damage (in chronic abuse). The detoxication and intoxication pathways of paracetamol metabolism are shown in Fig. 2. Glucuronidation and sulphation represent detoxication pathways. However, oxidative metabolism by hepatic cytochrome P-450 can result in the generation of a reactive metabolite. At normal dosage levels, this is inactivated by binding to glutathione, but in overdose, glutathione levels are depleted and the metabolite can bind covalently to cellular macromolecules. The occurrence and degree of hepatic necrosis correlates quantitatively with covalent binding to liver proteins in experimental animals (Gillete 1974).

The reactive intermediate involved in paracetamol toxicity is believed to be an imidoquinone (Fig. 2, B) which can exist in a number of canonical forms. Two of these are shown in Fig. 2 in order to explain the electrophilicity of the species. The imidoquinone could arise from the simple dehydration of N-hydroxyparacetamol (Hinson *et al.* 1975) or by one-electron oxidations at the amide nitrogen and phenol oxygen (Nelson 1985). Prostaglandin synthetase catalysed hydrogen abstraction to give an imidoquinone may be implicated in the renal toxicity of paracetamol (Ormstad & Moldeus 1985).

7.1.2.2 Quinones

Quinones are diketo derivatives of aromatic systems; hydroquinones are the reduced form of quinones. Both quinones and hydroquinones can give rise to semiquinone radicals by enzymatic reduction or oxidation respectively. The anthraquinone class of cytotoxic agents are associated with considerable cardiotoxicity, related to the peroxidation of cell membrane lipids (Olsen *et al.* 1981). With this class of compound, redox cycling (Fig. 3) between the anthraquinone and anthrasemiquinone radical forms of the compound can occur. It is believed that NADPH cytochrome P-450

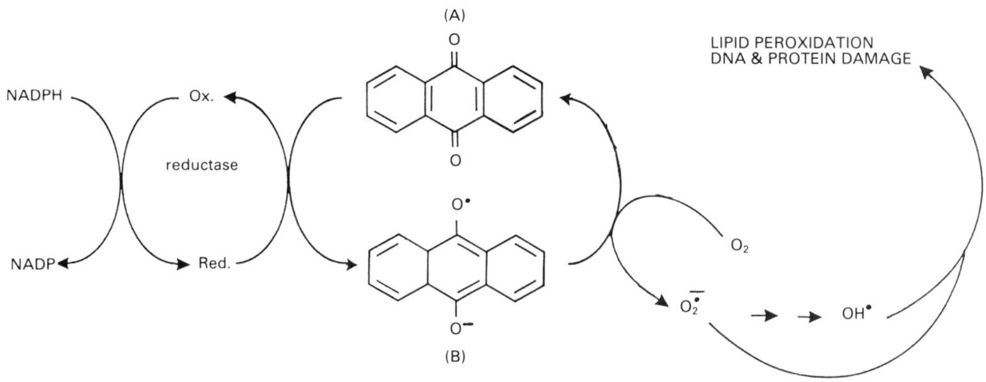

Fig. 3.—The formation of an anthrasemiquinone radical (B) from anthraquinone (A).

reductase reduces the quinone (Fig. 3, A) to a semiquinone radical (Fig. 3, B) (Bachur *et al.* 1979). This interacts with molecular oxygen to generate superoxide anion radicals and returns to the quinone form (Fig. 3). Thus radicals derived both from the drug, and from oxygen, are generated. Toxic consequences of this process include lipid peroxidation, protein covalent binding, and DNA damage (Trush *et al.* 1982). It has been shown (Basra *et al.* 1985) that human liver mediated free-radical formation and superoxide generation from doxorubicin (adriamycin, Fig. 4) is much greater than from mitoxantrone (Fig. 4). This latter drug appears less cardiotoxic than doxorubicin.

7.1.2.3 Hydrazines

The hydrazine moiety is incorporated into the structure of a number of drugs (Fig. 5) e.g. isoniazid (A), iproniazid (B), procarbazine (C) and hydralazine (C) which are currently used in clinical practice, and in a number of compounds of industrial importance. Hydrazines can be up to tetrasubstituted and symmetrical or unsymmetrical. The metabolism of hydrazines has been extensively studied, and the products differ markedly depending upon the degree and nature of substitution (Prough & Moloney 1985).

Hydrazines are toxic, and some types of toxicity may be due to the inherent ability of this structure to react with carbonyl compounds and thereby disorganize carbohydrate and amino acid metabolism. In other cases, oxidative metabolic activation of the hydrazine appears to be a prerequisite for initiating a toxic response.

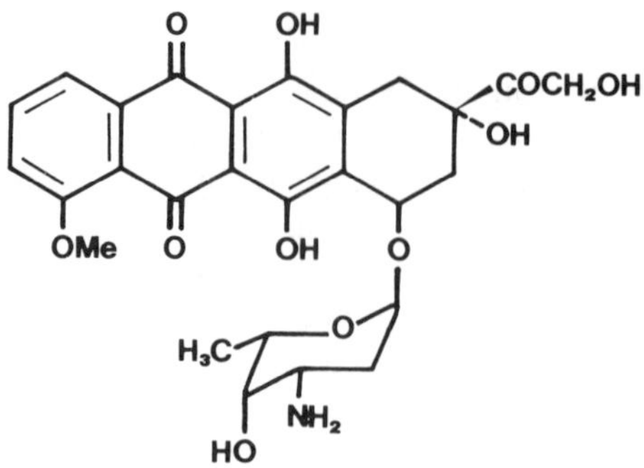

Adriamycin (A)

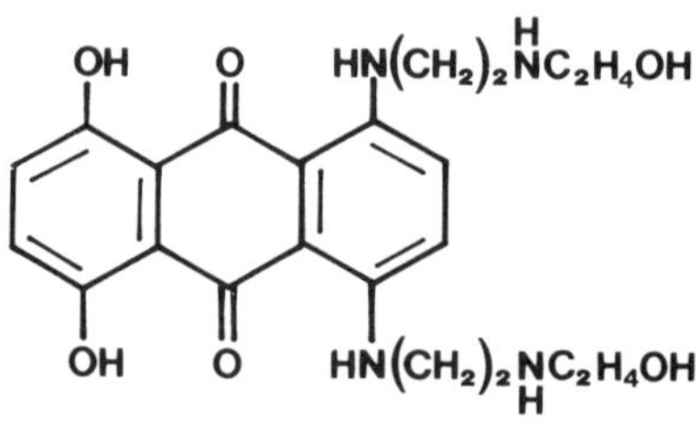

Mitoxantrone (B)

Fig. 4.—The structures of adriamycin (A) and mitoxantrone (B).

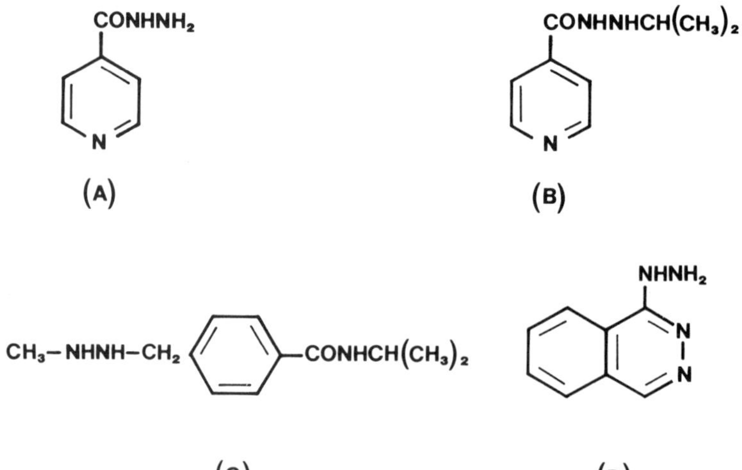

Fig. 5.—The structures of isoniazid (A), iproniazid (B), procarbazine (C) and hydralazine (D).

The nature of the primary metabolites derived from hydrazines are presently not known, owing to their instability, and these probably vary according to the structure of the parent hydrazine. From a consideration of the products formed during metabolism, Cummings & Prough (1983) have suggested that both mono and 1,1-disubstituted hydrazines are oxidized to form unstable diazines. These can undergo further reactions to produce either molecular nitrogen and a hydrocarbon,

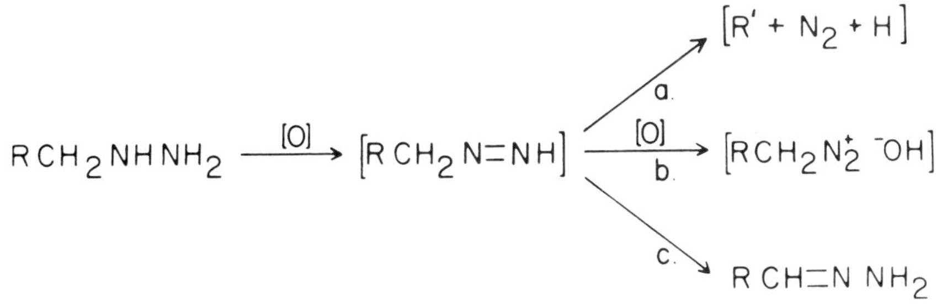

Fig. 6.—The metabolism of hydrazines to reactive intermediates.

or be oxidized to a diazo alkane or form a hydrazone (Fig. 6). The formation of an intermediate diazine would also account for the generation of carbon centred radicals, which is probably the mechanism by which haemoglobin (Ortiz de Montellano & Kunze 1981) and proteins (Prough *et al.* 1981) are alkylated by hydrazine. 2,2′-Disubstituted hydrazines are converted into azo compounds (Fig. 7); Dunn *et al.* 1979, Fiala *et al.* 1976) which are further oxidized to azoxy compounds (Fiala 1977, Dunn *et al.* 1979, Wiebkin & Prough 1980, Koh & Gorrod 1988a,b).

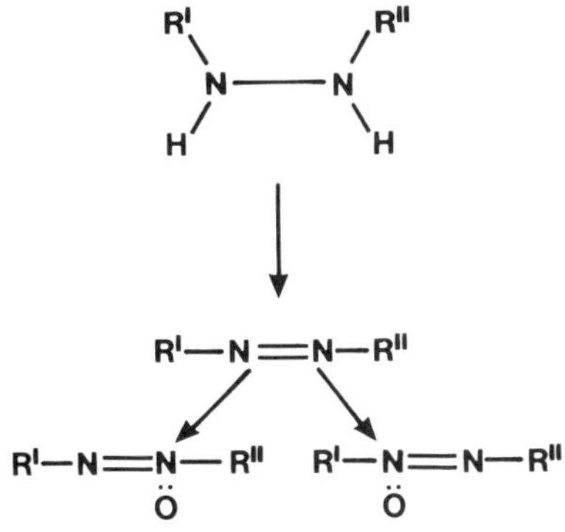

Fig. 7.—The metabolic oxidation of hydrazines to azo and azoxy compounds.

The widely used antibiotic drug isoniazid is associated with a number of untoward side effects, including peripheral neuritis and hepatic damage (Nelson *et al.* 1978). It has long been known that isoniazid undergoes acetylation which is under genetic control (Weber 1987). Acetylisoniazid can then yield acetylhydrazine by hydrolysis of the amide bond adjacent to the pyridyl group. Acetylhydrazine can in turn be metabolized to yield a diazine which decomposes to a radical (Fig. 8). In this case, diazine formation has been proposed to proceed via initial N-hydroxylation involving cytochrome P-450. The acetyl radical released by the unstable diazine reacts with hepatic protein, and this is thought to initiate hepatotoxicity (Timbrell *et al.* 1980). An analogous series of reactions has been proposed for isopropylhydrazine released from iproniazid (Nelson *et al.* 1976).

The antihypertensive drug hydralazine causes a lupus erythematosus-like syndrome which is thought to be immunologically mediated (Lunde *et al.* 1977). This

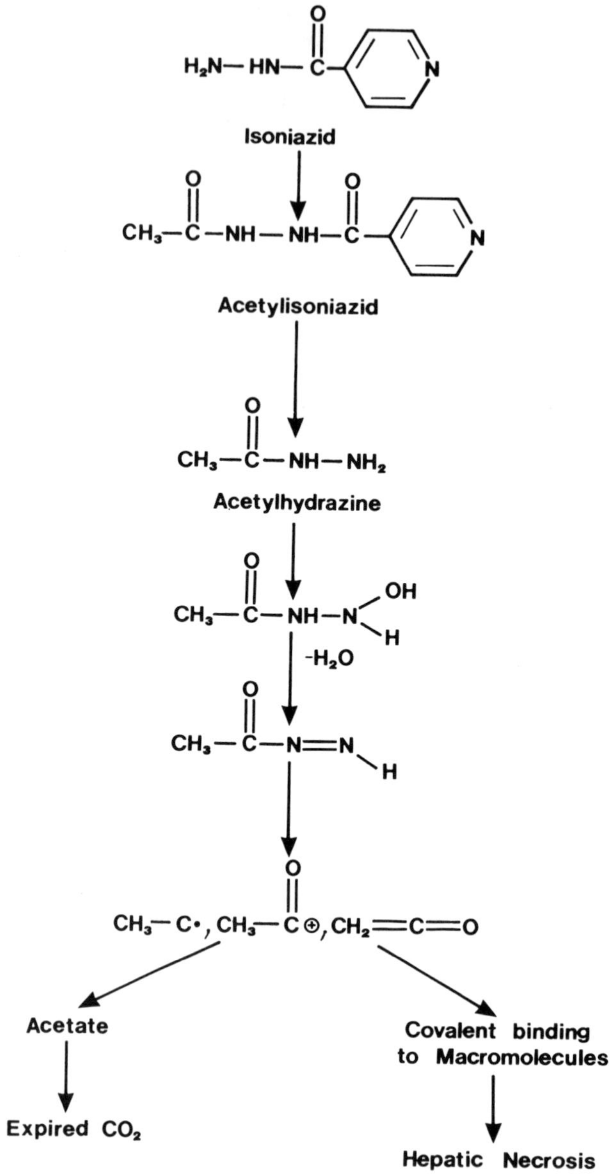

Fig. 8.—The proposed metabolic activation of isoniazid.

drug is also metabolized to a reactive compound that has the ability to react with proteins (Streeter & Timbrell 1983). Whilst, again, the reactive intermediate(s) has not been characterized, a metabolic pathway involving N-hydroxylation → diazine → radical is consistent with the experimental data (Streeter & Timbrell 1985).

7.1.2.4 Furans

Furan-containing compounds are widely distributed in nature. Drugs incorporating a furan ring include the diuretic frusemide (Fig. 9) and the antibacterial compound

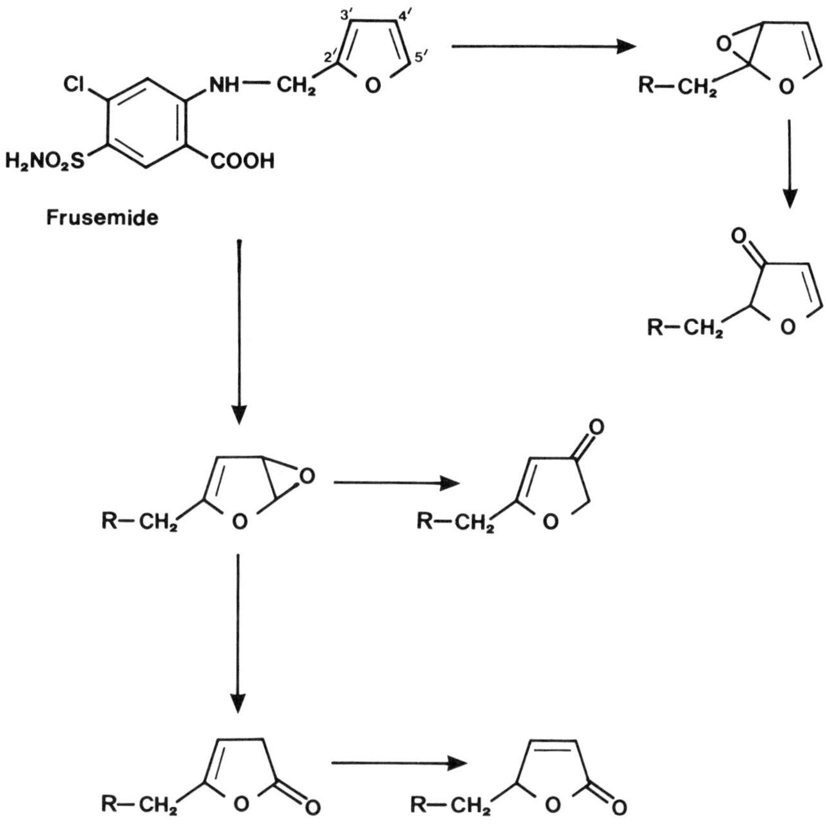

Fig. 9.—Epoxidation as a postulated metabolic activation process for frusemide.

nitrofurantoin (Fig. 10). A feature of frusemide toxicity is liver necrosis. This drug is known to be activated to a hepatotoxic species by a cytochrome P-450-dependent metabolic reaction (Mitchell *et al.* 1976). Studies by these authors, using radio-labelled drug, indicated that the furan ring was the functionality involved in initiating toxicity. Indirect evidence (Wirth *et al.* 1975) for the epoxidation of frusemide (Fig. 9) came from the observation that the addition of 1,2-epoxy-3,3,3-trichloropropane (ETC) to mouse liver microsomal incubation mixtures resulted in a marked increase in the extent of covalent binding of the frusemide metabolite. This was attributed to the inhibition of epoxide hydrolase by ETC, resulting in higher concentrations of the active frusemide metabolite in incubates.

By contrast, the bioactivation of nitrofurans, e.g. nitrofurantoin, is believed to involve the metabolic reduction of the ring nitro group (Swaminathan & Lower 1978). A nitroso derivative is formed which is further reduced via a hydroxylamine derivative and ring opening to a cyano derivative (Fig. 10). The highly reactive nitroso and hydroxylamine derivatives are believed to be responsible for interaction with biological molecules such as protein and DNA. Nitrofurantoin and other 5-nitrofurans have been shown to have cytotoxic, mutagenic, and carcinogenic effects (Bryan 1978).

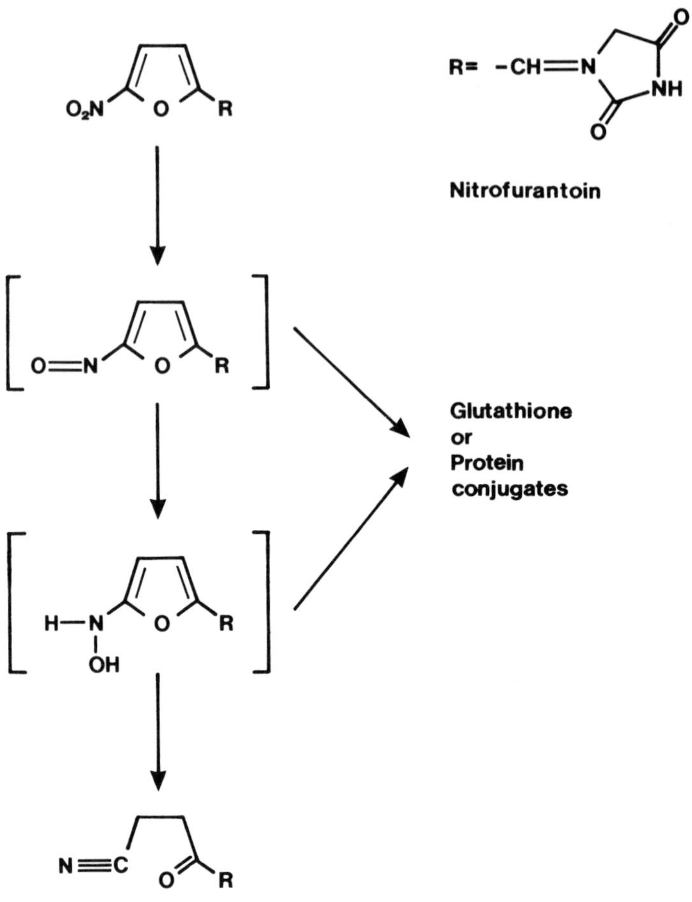

Fig. 10.—Metabolic activation and ring opening in nitrofurantoin metabolism.

7.1.2.5 Halogenoalkanes

Halogen-contaning compounds may be metabolized by a number of mechanisms. These include oxidative dehalogenation, oxygenation of halocarbon radicals, cytochrome P-450-dependent reduction reactions, and gluthathione-dependent metabolism. These mechanisms have been reviewed elsewhere (Anders & Pohl 1985). Halogen-containing drugs associated with covalent binding reactions include the antibacterial agent chloramphenicol (Fig. 11, A) and the general anaesthetic gas halothane (2-bromo-2-chloro-1,1,1-trifluoroethane, Fig. 11, B).

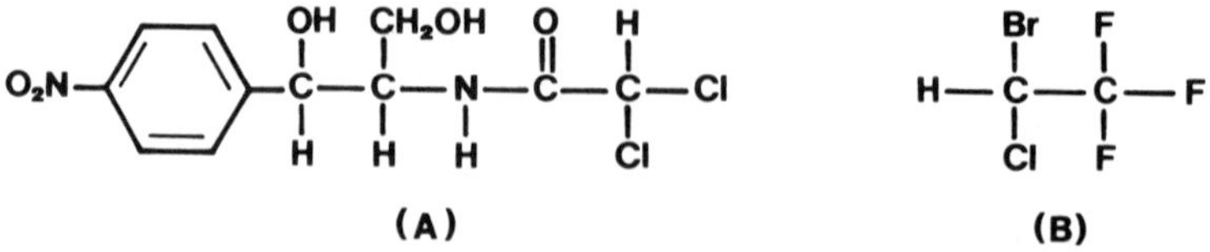

Fig. 11.—Two clinically used halogen-containing drugs—chloramphenicol (A) and halothane (B).

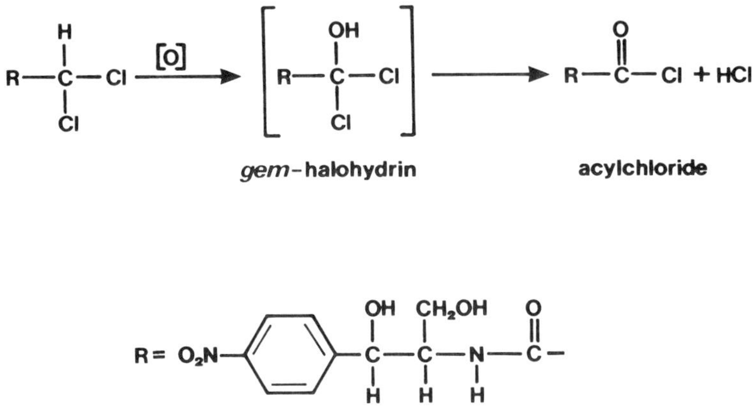

Fig. 12.—Metabolic activation of chloramphenicol to toxic species.

Chloramphenicol toxicity appears to be mediated by an oxidative dehalogenation mechanism (Pohl & Krishna 1978, Pohl *et al.* 1978). The initial metabolic step is cytochrome P-450-mediated oxidation at the halogen-carrying carbon to form a gem halohydrin (Fig. 12). This spontaneously eliminates hydrochloric acid to form a carbonyl derivative, in this case an acyl chloride (Fig. 12). The acyl chloride may be hydrolysed by water to form the corresponding acid. Alternatively, this reactive metabolite may selectively and irreversibly acylate the cytochrome P-450 molecule that catalysed its formation, thus acting as a suicide inactivator of the enzyme. The major site of acylation is a lysine residue on the enzyme (Halpert 1981).

Halothane is associated with hepatotoxicity. Evidence for the mechanism of metabolic activation of halothane (Fig. 13) has been reviewed by Anders & Pohl (1985). The process is believed to be initiated by cytochrome P-450-catalysed one-electron reduction of the compound to a radical anion. Loss of a bromide ion then results in the generation of a 2-chloro-1,1,1-trifluoroethane radical which appears to be the species bound to lipids (Wood *et al.* 1976). This radical may also be responsible for the ability of halothane to destroy cytochrome P-450 *in vivo* (Reynolds & Moslen 1974) and *in vitro* (Kreiter & Van Dyke 1983).

7.1.2.6 Thiones

Sulphur occurs in drugs and xenobiotics in a wide range of chemical environments (Fig. 14). In most cases oxidation of constituent sulphur produces sulphoxides or sulphones—compounds that are generally not associated with enhanced toxicity compared to the parent compound.

Compounds possessing sulphur as a thione moiety must be considered potential toxicants (Neal 1985) as these can undergo metabolic desuphuration to yield the oxygen analogue (Fig. 15) and release a particularly reactive form of elemental sulphur. The desulphuration of thiones occurs in the endoplasmic reticulum and is a cytochrome P-450 mediated process (De Matteis 1974). Initial metabolic attack on the C=S or P=S bond produces oxygenated intermediates that rearrange to generate elemental sulphur (Fig. 16). This sulphur reacts with the immediate environment of

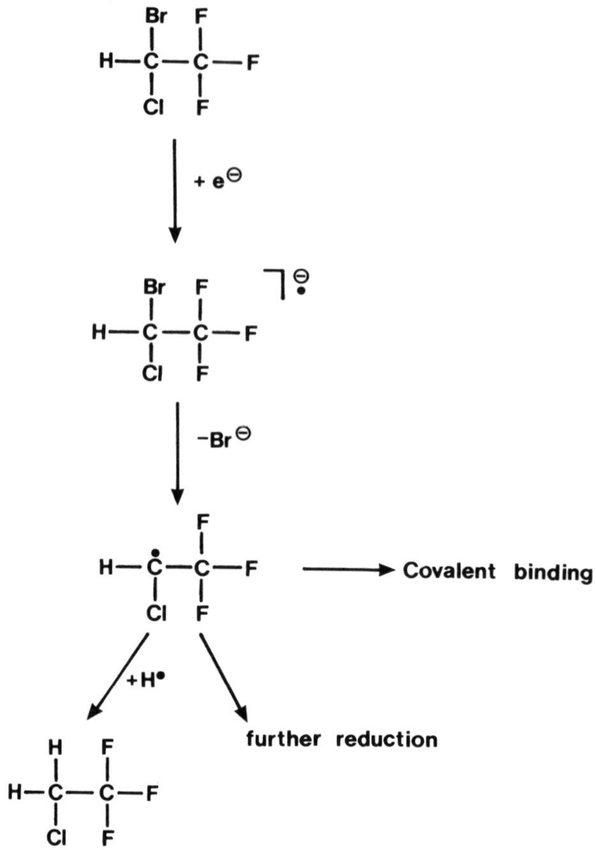

Fig. 13.—Metabolic activation of halothane to toxic species.

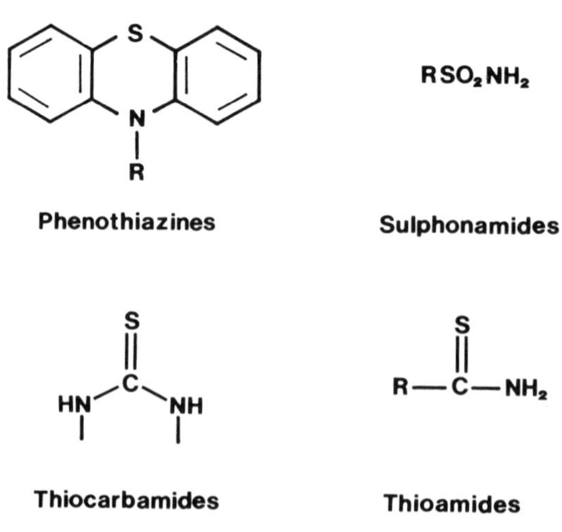

Fig. 14.—Sulphur containing functional groups occurring in drugs.

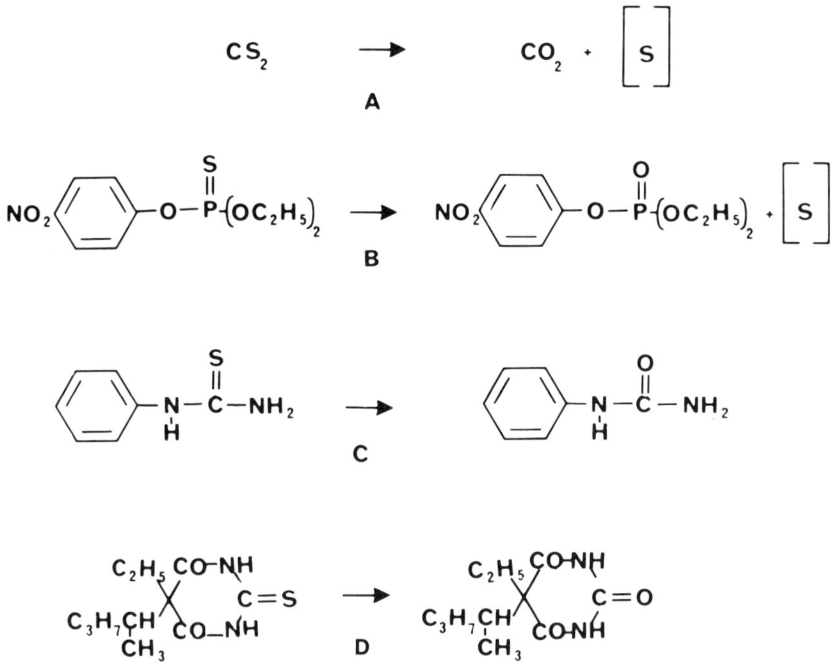

Fig. 15.—Thiones undergoing desulphuration.

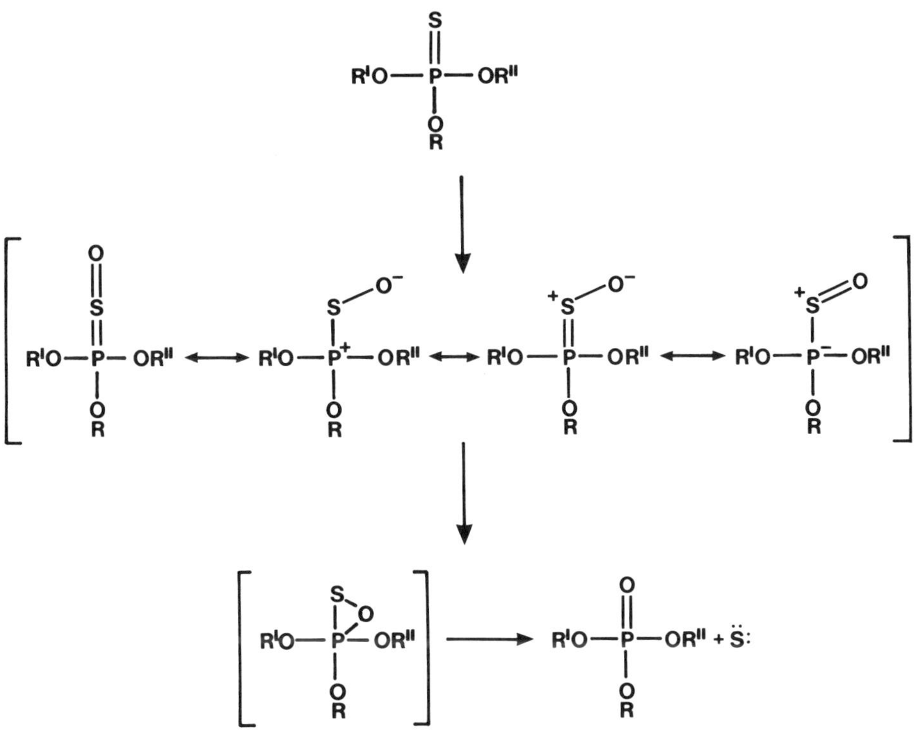

Fig. 16.—Mechanism of metabolic desulphuration of parathion.

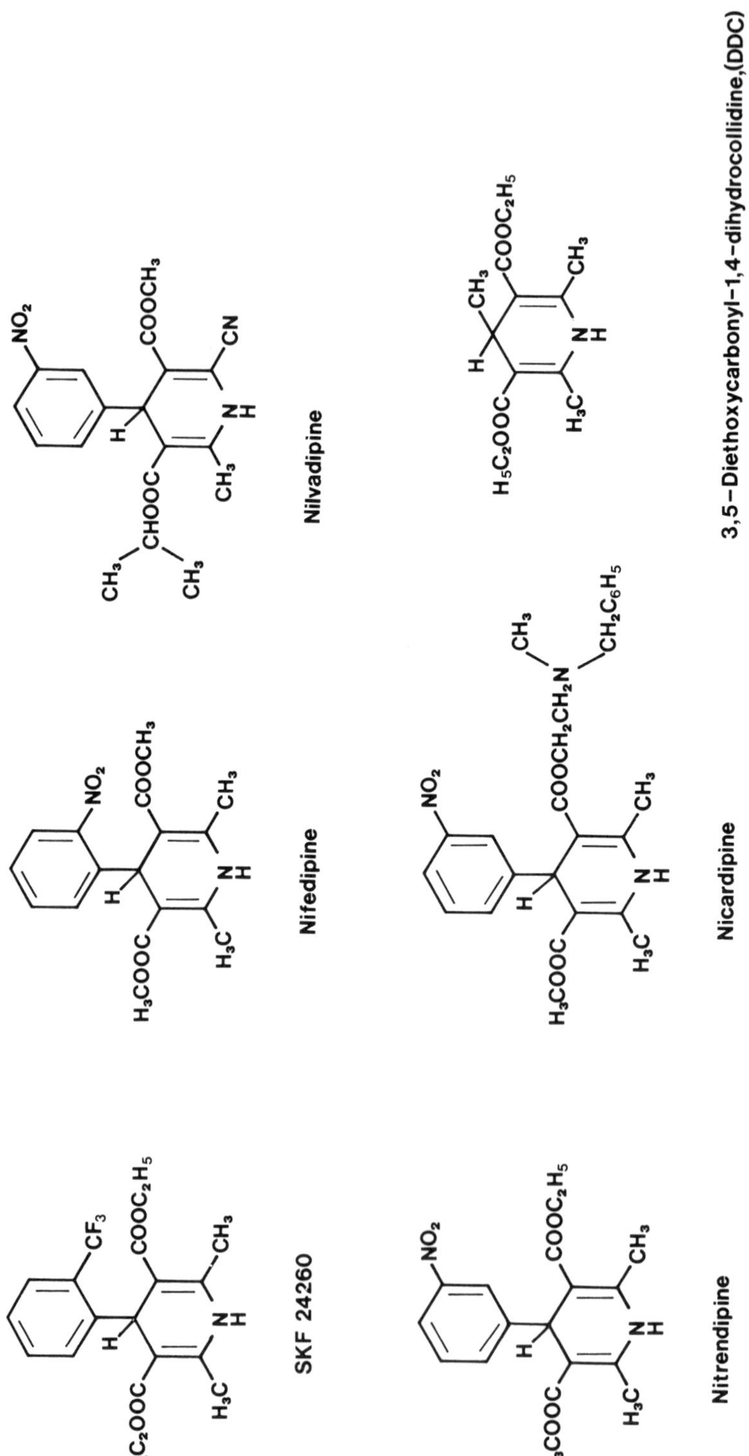

Fig. 17.—The structures of some pharmacologically active dihydropyridines.

its formation and thus acts as a suicide inhibitor of cytochrome P-450-mediated reactions by the conversion of protein thiols to hydrodisulphides (Ptashne *et al.* 1971, Kamataki *et al.* 1976).

7.1.2.7 Hydropyridines

The hydropyridines are a group of substances in which the aromaticity of the pyridine ring is eliminated by full or partial reduction. These structures are now frequently incorporated into drugs (Fig. 17) which act by blocking calcium ion channels. These drugs are structurally related to 3,5-diethoxycarbonyl-1,4-dihydrocollidine (DDC, Fig. 17), a toxic compound having the ability to produce hepatic porphyria in experimental animals (De Matteis 1987). More recently, a chance observation involving a contaminant of 'home-produced' 1-methyl-4-phenyl-4-propionoxypiperidine (MPPP, Fig. 18, A), which was being used as a heroin substitute by young

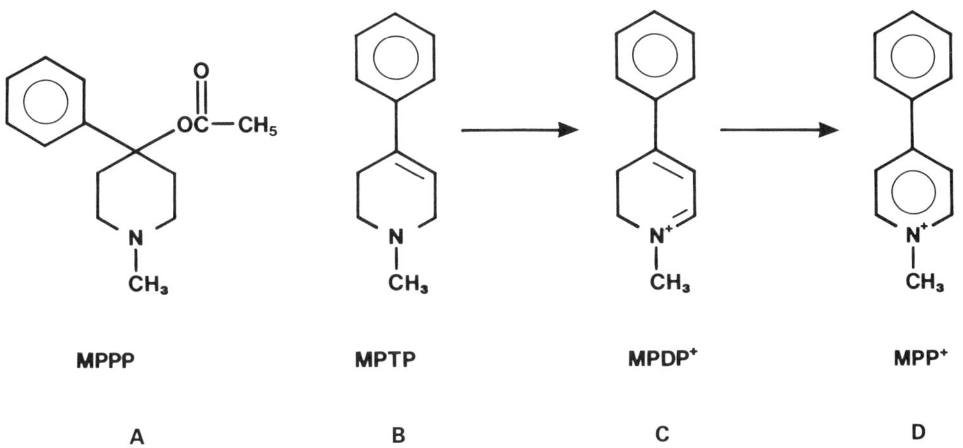

Fig. 18.—The structure of MPPP and the metabolism of MPTP.

addicts has indicated that this group of compounds must be thoroughly tested for toxicological phenomena before being utilized in the clinic.

The contaminant self-administered by the addicts was 1-methyl-4-phenyl-1,2,3,6-tetrahydropyridine (MPTP, Fig. 1, B) which produced a toxicological syndrome virtually identical to idiopathic Parkinson's disease (Jenner & Marsden 1987). MPTP-induced Parkinsonism is reversed by dopamine agonists and precursors. Distribution studies on MPTP showed that it rapidly disappeared from most tissues to be replaced by the oxidation product 1-methyl-4-phenylpyridinium ion (MPP^+, Fig. 18, D). This highly polar compound appears to be uniquely persistent in the brain of those species sensitive to the toxic action of MPTP. The compound is present for between 48 and 100 hours in primates, and is rapidly eliminated in those species relatively resistant to neurotoxicity by this agent, i.e. mice (4 hours) (Irwin 1986).

The metabolism of MPTP has been studied *in vivo* and *in vitro*, and differences have been observed depending upon the tissue and subcellular organelle used. In hepatic microsomal prparations, MPTP is metabolized by N-demethylation and

N-oxidation, whereas in brain preparations it is converted to MPP^+ by the mitochondrial fraction. This latter oxidation is carried out by monoamine oxidases and proceeds via the intermediate $MPDP^+$ (Fig. 18, C). Whilst oxidation by both monoamine oxidase A and B can occur, inhibitor studies indicate that form B is the important enzyme *in vivo* (Chiba *et al.* 1985). The result is supported by the protective effect offered to monkeys against MPTP toxicity when they coincidentally received either pargyline or deprenyl (Langston *et al.* 1984).

At the present time, it seems that MPTP is oxidized to MPP^+ in certain cells of the CNS. This leads to specific toxicity of the dopaminergic cells, and hence dopamine depletion related to persistence of MPP^+ in the body. The actual mechanism by which toxicity is initiated still remains to be unequivocally established, and either $MPDP^+$ or MPP^+ are candidates for the ultimate toxicant. The formation of a pyridinium ion is reminiscent of the structure of paraquat, which is also toxic under certain circumstances and is thought to act by generation of superoxide anions or other radicals (Bus *et al.* 1974). This mechanism could also be applicable to MPP^+. An alternative mechanism has been elucidated for DDC toxicity, where it has been shown that an intermediate is produced capable of alkylating the haem moiety of haemoglobin (De Matteis *et al.* 1981).

Conversely, it has been shown that a high correlation occurs between covalent binding of a compound to cellular macromolecules in an organ and the expression of a toxic phenomenon in that organ (Gorrod 1981). The metabolism of MPTP to a reactive intermediate, presumably the iminium ion, $MPDP^+$, has been observed and implicated in MPTP toxicity (Chiba *et al.* 1985). However, much further work needs to be done to establish the mechanism by which MPTP is able to elicit such a specific neurotoxic effect.

If a partially reduced pyridine is involved, then other compounds of this type also having neurotoxic properties might be expected to emerge; similar arguments apply to substrates capable of being biotransformed into pyridines, iminium ions or N-methylpyridinium ions, all now well established metabolic reactions (Baarnhielm *et al.* 1984, Midgley *et al.* 1985, Niwa *et al.* 1988, Lindeke & Cho 1982, Murphy 1973; Gorrod 1979, Hoag *et al.* 1987, 1988, Caldwell 1982).

7.1.3 CONCLUSIONS

Whilst the above examples are by no means exhausitive, it can be seen that many xenobiotics are converted by metabolic processes to reactive species capable of reacting with cellular constituents and thereby eliciting deleterious effects on cells. The wide variety of these processes and the diverse nature of the functional groups within drugs that can be activated obviously should cause concern to all involved in drug design and use. However, despite the above, the incidence of toxicity caused by medication normally remains very low, indicating that the mammalian system either possesses efficient protective and/or repair mechanisms or that the activated drug species does not get to a site (molecule) within the cell that would allow toxicity to be initiated.

At the present time the nature of the molecules critical for a particular type of cellular damage have not been established, and even in the case of carcinogens, where it is generally thought that they or their metabolites have to react with genetic material, exceptions are known. Indeed, it is clear that toxicants may also act by indirect mechanisms whereby an initial insult to an organelle may trigger the release of a signal in the form of a protein (enzyme) or other molecules including metal ions, which in turn initiate toxicity.

The continuing search for molecular mechanisms of drug toxicity including metabolism to reactive species and cellular defence and repair mechanisms should ultimately allow the development of medications devoid of deleterious effects.

REFERENCES

Anders, M. W. and Pohl, L. R. (1985), Halogenated alkanes. In: *Bioactivation of foreign compounds* (ed. Anders, M. W.), Academic Press Inc., Orlando, Florida, 283–315.

Allen, D. W. & Jandel, J. H. (1961), Oxidative hemolysis and precipitation of hemoglobin. II. Role of thiols in oxidant drug action, *Journal of Clinical Investigation* **40,**454–475.

Baarnhielm, C., Skanberg, I., & Borg, K. O. (1984), Cytochrome P-450-dependent oxidation of felodipine—a 1,4-dihydropyridine—to the corresponding pyridine, *Xenobiotica* **14,** 719–726.

Bachur, N. R., Gordon, S. L., Gee, M. V., & Kon, H. (1979), NADPH cytochrome P-450 reductase activation of quinone anticancer agents to free radicals, *Proc. Nat. Acad. Sci. USA* **76,** 954–957.

Basra, J., Wolf, C. R., Brown, J. R., & Patterson, L. H. (1985), Evidence for human liver mediated free-radical formation by doxorubicin and mitozanthrone, *Anticancer Drug Design* **1,** 45–52.

Bryan, G. T. (1978), Carcinogenesis, a comprehensive survey. In: *Carcinogenesis,* Vol. 4, *Nitrofurans* (ed. Bryan, G. T.), Raven Press, New York, p. 1–11.

Bus, J. S., Aust, S. D., & Gibson, J. E. (1974), Superoxide and singlet oxygen-catalysed lipid peroxidation as a possible mechanism for paraquat (methyl viologen) toxicity, *Biochemical and Biophysical Research Communications* **58,** 749–755.

Caldwell, J. (1982), Conjugation reactions of nitrogen centres. In: *Metabolic basis of detoxication* (eds Jakoby, W. B., Bend, J. R., & Caldwell, J.), Academic Press, New York, USA, p. 292–306.

Chiba, K., Peterson, L. A., Castagnoli, K. P., Trevor, A. J., & Castagnoli, N. (1985), Studies on the molecular mechanism of bioactivation of the selective nigrostriatal toxin 1-methyl-4-phenyl-1,2,3,6-tetrahydropyridine, *Drug Metabolism and Disposition* **13,** 342–347.

Cummings, S. W. & Prough, R. A. (1983), Metabolic formation of toxic metabolites. In: *Biological basis of detoxication* (eds Caldwell, J. & Jakoby, W. B.), Academic Press, New York, USA, p. 1–30.

De Matteis, F. (1974), Covalent binding of sulfur to microsomes and loss of cytochrome P-450 during the oxidative desulfuration of several chemicals, *Molecular Pharmacology* **10,** 849–854.

De Matteis, F. (1987), Drugs as suicide substrates. In: *Selectivity and molecular mechanisms of toxicity* (eds De Matteis, F. & Lock, E. A.), Macmillan Press, Basingstoke, UK, p. 183–210.

De Matteis, F. Gibbs, A. H., Farmer, P. B., & Lamb, J. H. (1981), Liver production of N-alkylated porphyrins caused in mice by treatment with substituted dihydropyridines. Evidence that the alkyl group on the pyrrole nitrogen atom originates from the drug, *FEBS Letters* **129,** 328–331.

Dunn, D. L., Lubet, R. A., & Prough, R. A. (1979), Oxidative metabolism of N-isopropyl-α-(2-methylhydrazine)-p-toluamide hydrochloride (procarbazine) by rat liver microsomes, *Cancer Research* **39,** 4555–4563.

Fiala, E. S. (1977), Investigations into the metabolism and mode of action of the colon carcinogen, 1,2-dimethylhydrazine and azomethane, *Cancer* **40,** 2436–2445.

Fiala, E. S., Kulakis, C., Bobotis, G., & Weisburger, J. H. (1976), Detection and estimation of azomethane in expired air of 1,2-dimethylhydrazine-treated rats, *Journal of the National Cancer Institute* (*US*) **56,**1271–1273.

Freeman, R. W., Uetrecht, J. P., Woosley, R. L., Oates, J. A., & Harbison, R. D. (1981), Covalent binding of procainamide *in vitro* and *in vivo* to hepatic protein in mice, *Drug Metabolism and Disposition* **9,** 188–192.

Gillete, J. R. (1974), A perspective on the role of chemically reactive metabolites of foreign compounds in toxicity—1. Correlation of changes in covalent binding of reactive metabolites with changes in the incidence and severity of toxicity, *Biochemical Pharmacology* **23,** 2785–2794.

Gorrod, J. W. (1978), Extrahepatic metabolism of drugs. In: *Drug metabolism in man* (eds Gorrod, J. W. & Beckett, A. H.), Taylor and Francis Ltd, London, 157–174.

Gorrod, J. W. (1979), Toxic products produced during metabolism of drugs and foreign compounds. In: *Drug toxicity* (ed. Gorrod, J. W.), Taylor and Francis Ltd, Basingstoke, UK, 1–24.

Gorrod, J. W. (1981), Covalent binding as an indicator of drug toxicity. In: *Testing for toxicity* (ed. Gorrod, J. W.), Taylor and Francis Ltd, Basingstoke, UK, 77–93.

Gorrod, J. W. & Manson, D. (1986), The metabolism of aromatic amines, *Xenobiotica* **16,** 933–955.

Halpert, J. (1981), Covalent modification of lysine during the suicide inactivation of rat liver cytochrome P-450 by chloramphenicol, *Biochemical Pharmacology* **30,** 875–881.

Hinson, J. A., Mitchell, J. R., & Jollow, D. J. (1975), Microsomal N-hydroxylation of p-chloroacetanilide, *Molecular Pharmacology* **11,**462–469.

Hoag, M. K. P., Trevor, A. J., Kalir, A., & Castagnoli, Jr., N. (1987), Phencyclidine iminium ion—NADPH-dependent metabolism, covalent binding to macromolecules, and inactivation of cytochrome(s) P-450, *Drug Metabolism and Disposition* **15,** 485–490.

Hoag, M. K. P., Schmidt-Peetz, M., Lampen, P., Trevor, A., & Castagnoli Jr., N. (1988), Metabolic studies on phencyclidine: Characterisation of a phencyclidine iminium ion metabolite, *Chemical Research in Toxicology* **1,** 128–131.

Irwin, I. (1986), The neurotoxin 1-methyl-4-phenyl-1,2,3,6-tetrahydropyridine (MPTP): A key to Parkinsons disease, *Pharmaceutical Research* **3,** 7–11.

Jenner, P. & Marsden, C. D. (1987), Parkinsonian syndrome caused by 1-methyl-4-phenyl-1,2,3,6-tetrahydropyridine in man and animals. In: *Selectivity and molecular mechanisms of toxicity* (eds De Matteis, F. & Lock, E. A.), Macmillan Press, Basingstoke, UK, p. 213–248.

Kamataki, T., Lee Lin, M. C. M., Belcher, D. H., & Neal, R. S. (1976), Studies of the metabolism of parathion with an apparently homogenous preparation of rabbit liver cytochrome P-450, *Drug Metabolism and Disposition* **4,** 180–189.

Kiese, M. (1974) In: *Methaemogloinaemia: a comprehensive treatise*, CRC Press, Cleveland, Ohio.

Koh, M. H. & Gorrod, J. W. (1988a), Metabolic N-oxidation of azo compounds. I. Evidence for formation of azo N-oxides (azoxy compounds), *Drug Metabolism and Drug Interactions* (submitted).

Koh, M. H. & Gorrod, J. W. (1988b), Metabolic N-oxidation of azo compounds. II. Some factors influencing N-oxidaton, *Drug Metabolism and Drug Interactions* (submitted).

Kreiter, P. A. & Van Dyke, R. A. (1983), Cytochrome P-450 and halothane metabolism. Decrease in rat liver microsomal P-450 *in vitro*, *Chemico-Biological Interactions* **44,** 219–235.

Langston, J. W., Irwin, I., Langston, E. B., & Forno, L. S. (1984), Pargyline prevents MPTP-induced parkinsonism in primates, *Science* **225,** 1480–1482.

Lindeke, B. & Cho, A. K. (1982), N-dealkylation and deamination. In: *Metabolic basis of detoxication* (eds Jakoby, W. B., Bend, J. R., & Caldwell, J.), Academic Press, New York, USA, p. 105–206.

Lunde, P. K. M., Frislid, K., & Hansteen, V. (1977), Disease and acetylation polymorphism, *Clinical Pharmacokinetics* **2,** 182–197.

Midgley, I., Chasseaud, L. F., Taylor, I. W., Walmsley, L. M., Fowkes, A. G., Darragh, A., Lambe, R. F., & Bonn, R. (1985), Metabolism and pharmacokinetics of the dihydropyridine calcium antagonist, rysodine, in man, *Xenobiotica* **15,** 965–977.

Mitchell, J. R., Nelson, W. L., Potter, W. Z., Sasame, H. A., & Jollow, D. J. (1976), Metabolic activation of furosemide to a chemically reactive, hepatotoxic metabolite, *The Journal of Pharmacology and Experimental Therapeutics* **199,** 41–52.

Murphy, P. J. (1973), Enzymatic oxidation of nicotine to an iminium ion, *Journal of Biological Chemistry* **248,** 2796–2800.

Neal, R. A. (1985), Thiono-sulphur compounds. In: *Bioactivation of foreign compounds* (ed. Anders, M. W.), Academic Press, New York, p. 519–540.

Nelson, S. D. (1985), Arylamines and arylamides: oxidation mechanisms. In: *Bioactivation of foreign compounds* (ed. Anders, M. W.), Academic Press Inc., Orlando, Florida, p. 359.

Nelson, S. D., Mitchell, J. R., Snodgras, W. R., & Timbrell, J. A. (1978), Hepatotoxicity and metabolism of iproniazid and hydrazine, *The Journal of Pharmacology and Experimental Therapeutics* **206,** 574–585.

Nelson, S. D., Mitchell, J. R., Timbrell, J. A., Snodgras, W. R., & Corcoran III, G. B. (1976), Isoniazid and iproniazid: activation of metabolites to toxic intermediates in man and rat, *Science* **193,** 901–903.

Niwa, T., Tokuma, Y., & Noguchi, H. (1988), Oxidaton of nilvadipine, a new dihydropyridine calcium antagonist, to the correspondig pyridine by rat liver microsomes, *Xenobiotica* **18,** 217–224.

Olsen, R. D., Boerth, R. C., Gerber, J. G., & Nies, A. S. (1981), Mechanism of adriamycin cardiotoxicity: evidence for oxidative stress, *Life Sciences* **29,** 1393–1401.

Ormstad, K. & Moldeus, P. (185), The role of metabolic activation in drug toxicity, *Chemioterapia* **IV,** 343–348.

Ortiz de Montellano, P. R. & Kunze, K. L. (1981), Formation of N-phenylheme in the hemolytic reaction of phenylhydrazine with hemoglobin, *Journal of the American Chemical Society* **103,** 6534–6536.

Pohl, L. R. & Krishna, G. (1978), Study of the mechanism of metabolic activation of chloramphenicol by rat liver microsomes, *Biochemical Pharmacology* **27,** 335–341.

Pohl, L. R., Nelson, S. D., & Krishna, G. (1978), Investigation of the mechanism of the metabolic activation of chloramphenicol by rat liver microsomes. Identification of a new metabolite, *Biochemical Pharmacology* **27,** 491–496.

Prough, R. A., Cummings, S. W., Coomes, M. W., Wiebkin, P., & Moloney, S. J. (1981), Evaluation of possible reactive intermediates formed from the antitumour agent, procarbazine, *Proc. American Association of Cancer Research* **22,** 0395.

Prough, R. A. & Moloney, S. J. (1985), Hydrazines. In: *Bioactivation of foreign compounds* (ed. Anders, M. W.), Academic Press Inc., Orlando, Florida, p. 433–449.

Ptashne, K. A., Wolcott, R. M., & Neal, R. A. (1971), Oxygen-18 studies on the chemical mechanisms of the mixed-function oxidase-catalysed desulfuration and dearylation reactions of parathion, *The Journal of Pharmacology and Experimental Therapeutics* **179,** 380–385.

Reed, D. J. (1985), Cellular defense mechanisms. In: *Bioactivation of foreign compounds* (ed. Anders, M. W.), Academic Press Inc., Orlando, Florida, p. 71–108.

Reynolds, E. S. & Moslen, M. T. (1974), Liver injury following halothane anesthesia in phenobarbital pre-treated rats, *Biochemical Pharmacology* **23,** 189–195.

Streeter, A. J. & Timbrell, J. A. (1983), Enzyme mediated covalent binding of hydralazine to rat liver microsomes, *Drug Metabolism and Disposition* **11,** 179–183.

Streeter, A. J. & Timbrell, J. A. (1985), The *in vitro* metabolism of hydralazine, *Drug Metabolism and Disposition* **13,** 255–259.

Swaminathan, S. & Lower, G. M. (1978), Biotransformations and excretions of nitrofurans. In: *Carcinogenesis*, Volume 4, *Nitrofurans* (ed. Bryan, G. T.), Raven Press, New York.

Tabarelli, S. & Uehleke, H. (1971), N-hydroxlation of 4,4′-diaminodiphenylsulphone in liver microsomes and *in vivo*, *Xenobiotica* **1,** 501–502.

Testa, B. & Jenner, P. (1976). In: *Drug metabolism: chemical and biochemical aspects*, Marcel Dekker, Inc., New York and Basle.

Timbrell, J. A., Mitchell, J. R., Snodgras, W. R., & Nelson, S. D. (1980), Isoniazid hepatotoxicity: The relationship between covalent binding and metabolism *in vivo*, *The Journal of Pharmacology and Experimental Therapeutics* **213,** 364–369.

Trush, M. A., Mimnaugh, E. G., & Gram, T. E. (1982), Activation of pharmacological agents to radical intermediates. Implications for the role of free radicals in drug action and toxicity, *Biochemical Pharmacology* **31,** 3335–3346.

Uetrecht, J. P. (1985), Reactivity and possible significance of hydroxylamine and nitroso metabolites of procainamide, *The Journal of Pharmacology and Experimental Therapeutics* **232,** 420–425.

Uetrecht, J. P., Sweetman, B. J., Woosley, R. L., & Oates, J. A. (1984), Metabolism of procainamide to a hydroxylamine by rat and human hepatic microsomes, *Drug Metabolism and Disposition* **12,** 77–81.

Weber, W. W. (1987), *The acetylator genes and drug response*, Oxford University Press, New York, USA, p. 1–247.

Wiebkin, P. & Prough, R. A. (1980), Oxidative metabolism of N-isopropyl-α-(2-methylazo)-*p*-toluamide (azoprocarbazine) by rodent liver microsomes, *Cancer Research* **40,**3524–3529.

Wirth, P. J., Bettis, C. J., & Nelson, W. L. (1975), Microsomal metabolism of furosemide: evidence for the nature of the reactive intermediate involved in covalent binding, *Molecular Pharmacology* **12,** 759–768.

Wood, C. L., Gandolfi, A. J., & Van Dyke, R. A. (1976), Lipid binding of a halothane metabolite, *Drug Metabolism and Disposition* **4,** 305–313.

Woosley, R. L., Drayer, D. E., Reidenberg, M. M., Nies, A. S., Carr, K., & Oates, J. A. (1978), Effect of acetylator phenotype on the rate at which procainamide induces antinuclear antibodies and the lupus syndrome, *New England Journal of Medicine* **298,** 1157–1159.

7.2 Molecular mechanisms of cell toxicity

Sten Orrenius, Hjördis Thor, David McConkey, Pierluigi Nicotera, & Giorgio Bellomo†

Molecular mechanisms involved in the development of lethal cell injury have attracted increased interest in recent years. In particular, the possible existence of a final common pathway in toxic cell killing has been addressed in a number of studies. This presentation summarizes recent work from our laboratory, suggesting that a disruption of intracellular thiol and calcium ion homeostasis may represent a common step in the development of toxic damage to hepatocytes, and that the activation of Ca^{2+}-dependent degradative processes due to a sustained increase in cytosolic free Ca^{2+} concentration may be responsible for cell killing by agents which cause intracellular Ca^{2+} accumulation.

Tissue necrosis has long been known to be associated with the accumulation of large amounts of calcium in the necrotic tissue, and it has been proposed that the calcium ion may play a critical role in the development of lethal alterations of cell structure and function (Campbell 1983). Although the generality of this hypothesis has been questioned (Starke *et al.* 1986), the involvement of Ca^{2+} in the development of lethal cell injury is now supported by a large number of observations. For example, Shanne *et al.* (1979) found that removal of Ca^{2+} from the medium exerted a protective effect against the toxicity of a number of agents in cultured hepatocytes. This and similar observations led to the proposal that an influx of extracellular Ca^{2+} could play a predominant role in the development of irreversible cell damage (Farber 1981). However, subsequent studies have shown that an influx of extracellular Ca^{2+} is not necessarily required for cytotoxicity, and that a disruption of intracellular Ca^{2+} homeostasis may also result in irreversible cell damage.

Studies in this and other laboratories have demonstrated that oxidative stress in hepatocytes is associated with the inhibition of Ca^{2+} translocases involved in the maintenance of intracellular Ca^{2+} homeostasis (Orrenius & Bellomo 1986). This may lead to a sustained elevation of cytosolic Ca^{2+} concentration which, in turn, can cause the activation of various Ca^{2+}-dependent degradative enzymes, including phospholipases, proteases, and endonucleases, whose activities may combine to cause irreversible damage (Fig. 1). The following sections will be concerned with the mechanisms by which a perturbation of intracellular Ca^{2+} homeostasis can cause cytotoxicity and cell death.

† Department of Toxicology, Karolinska Institutet, S-104 01 Stockholm, Sweden

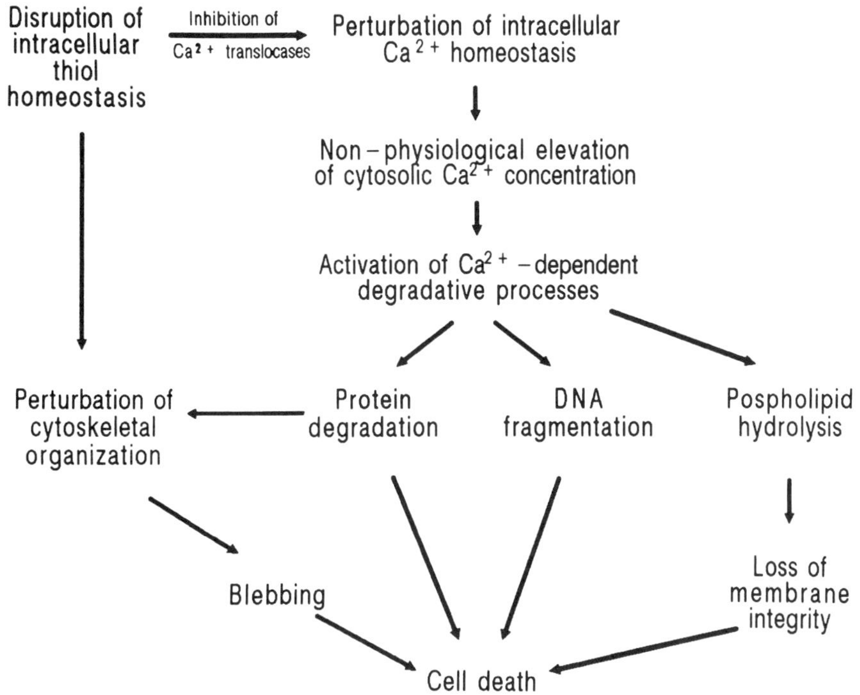

Fig. 1.—Schematic illustration of the thiol/calcium hypothesis of toxic cell injury

7.2.1 CALCIUM COMPARTMENTATION IN HEPATOCYTES

The low resting concentration of Ca^{2+} in the cytosol of hepatocytes (~0.1 μM) is maintained by active compartmentation processes. The mitochondria and the endoplasmic reticulum represent the predominant sites of intracellular Ca^{2+} sequestration, whereas the plasma membrane Ca^{2+} translocase plays a major role in the maintenance of the concentration gradient existing between the extra- and intra-cellular environments by actively extruding Ca^{2+} from the cell.

Mitochondrial Ca^{2+} homeostasis is regulated by a cyclic mechanism, involving Ca^{2+} uptake by an energy-dependent pathway, and Ca^{2+} release which, in the liver, is probably mediated by a Ca^{2+}/H^+ antiporter. The latter appears to be regulated by the redox level of intramitochondrial pyridine nucleotides (Lehninger *et al.* 1978), although membrane-bound protein thiols may also be important in modulating mitochondrial Ca^{2+} fluxes. The active transport of calcium ions through the endoplasmic reticular and plasma membranes is mediated by Ca^{2+}-stimulated, Mg^{2+}-dependent ATPases which appear to be dependent on free sulfhydryl groups for their activity (Moore *et al.* 1975, Bellomo *et al.* 1983).

Thus, it seems that the major mechanisms responsible for Ca^{2+} transport across cellular membranes are all dependent on protein thiol groups. It is therefore conceivable that oxidation and/or arylation of these critical thiol groups may result in the inactivation of the translocases involved in the regulation of intracellular Ca^{2+} compartmentation, leading to an alteration of the level of cytosolic Ca^{2+}.

7.2.2 ROLE OF GLUTATHIONE AND PROTEIN THIOL MODIFICATION IN TOXICITY

Damage to biological systems caused by generation of active oxygen species is often referred to as 'oxidative stress' (Sies 1986). Since aerobic cells possess antioxidant systems to trap and/or inactivate such reactive species, oxidative stress is the result of an imbalance between the generation of active oxygen species and their inactivation by the protective systems. Glutathione (GSH) plays a unique role in cellular defence against reactive intermediates, inasmuch as it functions as a reductant in the metabolism of hydrogen peroxide and organic hydroperoxides and can also bind electrophilic metabolites (Orrenius & Moldéus 1984). During the glutathione peroxidase-catalysed metabolism of hydroperoxides, GSH serves as an electron donor, and the glutathione disulfide (GSSG) formed in the reaction is subsequently reduced back to GSH by glutathione reductase at the expense of NADPH. Under conditions of oxidative stress, when the cell must cope with large amounts of H_2O_2 and/or organic hydroperoxides, the glutathione reductase is unable to match the rate of glutathione oxidation, and GSSG accumulates. In an apparent effort to avoid the detrimental effects of increased intracellular levels of GSSG, e.g. formation of mixed disulfides with protein thiols, the cell actively excretes the disulfide, which can lead to a depletion of the intracellular glutathione pool.

Other thiol groups of toxicological significance are those present in cellular proteins. In general, sulfhydryl groups are highly reactive and can participate in several different types of reactions, such as arylation, oxidation, and thiol-disulfide exchange. All of these reactions may be involved in the modification of protein thiols as a consequence of their interaction with reactive intermediates formed during the metabolism of toxic chemicals. Such modifications of protein thiols may be particularly important during oxidative stress (Di Monte *et al.* 1984).

7.2.3 MENADIONE-INDUCED OXIDATIVE STRESS

For several years our laboratory has been actively engaged in the study of possible mechanisms of cell killing by oxidative stress. A model compound extensively used in our studies is menadione (2-methyl-1,4-naphthoquinone). In liver cells menadione metabolism involves both one- and two-electron reduction pathways which differ in their contribution to cytotoxicity (Thor *et al.* 1982). One-electron reduction of quinones results in the formation of semiquinone radicals which can rapidly reduce dioxygen, forming the superoxide anion radical ($O_2^{\cdot-}$), and regenerating the parent quinone. Dismutation of $O_2^{\cdot-}$ to hydrogen peroxide, and the production of other highly reactive species, quickly lead to a condition of oxidative stress as redox cycling of the quinone continues.

Exposure of hepatocytes to toxic concentrations of menadione results in the extensive formation of $O_2^{\cdot-}$ and H_2O_2 and the oxidation of GSH and pyridine nucleotides. Following GSH depletion, a dose- and time-dependent loss of protein thiols precedes cell death in hepatocytes exposed to menadione (Di Monte *et al.* 1984). Although a general decrease in protein thiols has been observed in cells exposed to cytotoxic levels of menadione, this does not imply that all protein thiols are equally important for cell survival. It appears that the fraction of critical thiols may be quite small. As mentioned above, the proper functioning of intracellular Ca^{2+} translocases is dependent on thiol groups in specific proteins, and the disruption of Ca^{2+} homeostasis resulting from their modification appears to be ultimately related to the onset of cytotoxicity. Other critical thiols affected by menadione metabolism are located on microfilament proteins, whose modification may result in the disruption of the structural integrity of the plasma membrane and the onset of widespread bleb formation.

7.2.4 APPEARANCE OF SURFACE BLEBS IN HEPATOCYTES EXPOSED TO TOXIC AGENTS

Incubation of hepatocytes with menadione results in an alteration of surface morphology characterized by a loss of microvilli and the appearance of multiple blebs on the surface of the hepatocytes (Thor *et al.* 1982). Many other toxic agents cause similar alterations in surface structure, indicating that plasma membrane blebbing is a common event in the progression of toxic injury (Jewell *et al.* 1982). Blebs usually appear before any sign of increased plasma membrane permeability is observed, and seem to be initially reversible, i.e. they often disappear when the toxic agent is removed from the incubation.

Cell surface morphology is thought to be determined by the organization of cortical microfilaments associated with the plasma membrane. This assumption is supported by the finding that two classes of compounds, the cytochalasins and phalloidins which disrupt cortical microfilament structure, cause bleb formation on the surface of hepatocytes similar to that observed with other toxic agents.

As will be discussed below, during oxidative stress a perturbation of intracellular Ca^{2+} homeostasis is intimately related to a modification of the intracellular thiol status. Disruption of intracellular thiol and Ca^{2+} homeostasis may both result in alterations of cytoskeletal structure. Thiol oxidaton can perturb microfilament organization through S–S-cross-linking of actin molecules (Mirabelli *et al.* 1987). A change in intracellular Ca^{2+} distribution can affect cytoskeletal structure because the calcium ion and its associated binding proteins play a pivotal role in regulating the cytoskeletal network (Cheung 1980). Alternatively, Ca^{2+}-activated catabolic enzymes, such as cytosolic proteases, can cleave cytoskeletally-associated proteins and thus cause alteration of the microfilament network and blebbing (Collier & Wang 1982, Nicotera *et al.* 1986a,b). It is therefore conceivable that both thiol modification and Ca^{2+}-dependent processes may combine to produce cytoskeletal alterations during oxidative stress.

7.2.5 DISRUPTION OF INTRACELLULAR CALCIUM HOMEOSTASIS DURING OXIDATIVE STRESS

In studies with isolated hepatocytes we have been able to demonstrate that menadione-induced oxidative stress causes the mobilization of Ca^{2+} from both the mitochondria and the endoplasmic reticulum (Thor *et al.* 1982). Further studies with isolated subcellular fractions have shown that menadione metabolism impairs the ability of mitochondria to take up and retain Ca^{2+} by causing the oxidation of pyridine nucleotides (Moore *et al.* 1986). Menadione also inhibits Ca^{2+} uptake by rat liver microsomes through a mechanism which seems to involve oxidation/arylation of thiol group(s) required for Ca^{2+}-ATPase activity (Thor *et al.* 1985). The incubaton of hepatocytes with menadione therefore causes the release into the cytosol of Ca^{2+} which cannot be resequestered. Normally, this would result in only a transient rise in the cytosolic Ca^{2+} concentration, because the plasma membrane Ca^{2+}-ATPase would remove this Ca^{2+} from the cell, and the Ca^{2+} concentration would return to its usual, very low level. However, recent studies in our laboratory have shown that the hepatic plasma membrane Ca^{2+}-ATPase is inhibited by agents, including menadione, which oxidize membrane protein thiols (Nicotera *et al.* 1985). The redox cycling of menadione can therefore inhibit the Ca^{2+} translocases present in the mitochondria, endoplasmic reticulum, and plasma membrane of hepatocytes, leading to a sustained rise in cytosolic Ca^{2+}.

Under physiological conditions the cytosolic Ca^{2+} concentration in hepatocytes is modulated by various hormones and other Ca^{2+}-mobilizing agents. To investigate the difference between physiological and toxicological fluctuations in cytosolic Ca^{2+} level, we have recently compared the effects of an alpha-adrenergic agonist, phenylephrine, with those of both non-toxic and toxic concentrations of menadione in Quin-2-loaded hepatocytes. Our study has shown that both the extent and the duration of the rise in cytosolic Ca^{2+} differ between non-toxic and toxic conditions. Toxic concentrations of menadione caused a sustained elevation of cytosolic Ca^{2+}, which reached micromolar concentrations and fully saturated the binding capacity of the entrapped dye. Furthermore, in view of the ability of reducing agents to prevent protein thiol modification and to protect hepatocytes from menadione toxicity, we investigated the effect of dithiothreitol on the increase in cytosolic Ca^{2+} caused by menadione. Treatment of hepatocytes with dithiothreitol prevented both the increase in cytosolic Ca^{2+} and the onset of cytotoxicity in hepatocytes exposed to menadione.

7.2.6 MECHANISMS OF CALCIUM-MEDIATED CYTOTOXICITY

The discovery of a relationship between a sustained increase in cytosolic Ca^{2+} concentration and the toxicity of menadione and several other agents in hepatocytes has led to a search for mechanism(s) by which the increased cytosolic Ca^{2+} could trigger cytotoxicity. It has been proposed that a sustained increase in Ca^{2+} concentration may cause abnormal stimulation of physiological functions, including various Ca^{2+}-dependent degradative processes.

Ca^{2+}-activated phospholipases are widely distributed in mammalian cells, and it has been suggested that an enhanced rate of phospholipid hydrolysis may result in irreversible cell damage. This assumption is supported by the observation that inhibitors of phospholipase activity can prevent ischemic cell death in liver and heart, and by the finding that phospholipid breakdown is enhanced during tissue injury (Chien *et al.* 1979). We have recently investigated whether phospholipase activation may contribute to the toxicity of the reactive disulfide cystamine in hepatocytes (Nicotera *et al.* 1986a). Indeed, exposure to cystamine did increase the rate of phospholipid hydrolysis, and this effect followed the elevation of cytosolic Ca^{2+} and preceded loss of cell viability. However, in our study, phospholipase inhibitors failed to prevent cystamine toxicity.

Intracellular protein degradation is also known to be stimulated by a rise in cytosolic Ca^{2+}, and a group of cytosolic, thiol proteases, whose activity depends on micromolar concentrations of Ca^{2+}, seems to be involved in this process (Murachi

1983). These proteases function in the cleavage of membrane receptors, cytoskeletal proteins, and protein kinase C. Exposure of hepatocytes to toxic levels of cystamine resulted in enhanced proteolytic activity which was prevented by inhibitors of the Ca^{2+}-dependent proteases; the same inhibitors also protected the cells from cystamine toxicity.

A third catabolic process found to be sensitive to a non-physiological elevaton of cytosolic Ca^{2+} concentration is that of an endogenous endonuclease, whose activity has been associated with 'apoptosis', or programmed cell death (Wyllie 1980). Thus, both glucocorticoid hormones and the calcium ionophore A23187 stimulate apoptosis in isolated mouse thymocytes (Cohen & Duke 1984, Wyllie *et al.* 1984). Characteristic morphological changes accompany this process, including plasma membrane blebbing and extensive chromatin condensation.

As noted above, we have found that plasma membrane blebbing can often be linked to a disruption of Ca^{2+} homeostasis, and that the blebbing observed in hepatocytes treated with ionophore A23187 is associated with the activation of Ca^{2+}-dependent proteases (Nicotera *et al.* 1986b). The appearance of blebs on apoptotic cells could therefore be an indication that a perturbation of Ca^{2+} homeostasis accompanies this process. Since menadione metabolism creates such a disruption, we have recently studied its effects on endogenous endonuclease activity in hepatocytes (McConkey *et al.* 1987). In the presence of moderately toxic concentrations of menadione, endonuclease activation was apparent after about 2 hours; maximal DNA cleavage was seen with 100 μM menadione after 4 hours of incubation. Moreover, activation of the endonuclease preceded cell death by an appreciable period, and was associated with the appearance of plasma membrane blebbing, characteristic of menadione-induced oxidative stress.

Interestingly, morphological alterations associated with menadione treatment of hepatocytes follow those observed with apoptotic thymocytes quite closely. The formation of surface blebs has already been mentioned, but chromatin condensation is also seen, and a close similarity exists between DNA cleavage products isolated from apoptotic thymocytes and from menadione-treated hepatocytes. Gel electrophoresis of these products has shown that host chromatin is preferentially cleaved into oligonucleosome-length fragments by the endonuclease in each case (Wyllie 1980, McConkey *et al.* 1987). Thus, it appears that endonuclease activation is not only a critical step in the sequence of events involved in programmed cell death, but can also occur during the development of oxidative injury in hepatocytes.

7.2.7 CONCLUDING REMARKS

A series of potentially toxic mechanisms are activated when a cell is exposed to agents which cause oxidative stress. They include a perturbation of the normal redox balance, thiol depletion, and disruption of intracellular Ca^{2+} homeostasis. The pathways through which a perturbation of intracellular Ca^{2+} homeostasis may cause irreversible damage appear to involve the activation of degradative enzymes such as phospholipases, proteases, and endonucleases. Although additional mechanisms may contribute to cell killing, our findings suggest that a disruption of Ca^{2+} homeostasis is a critical event in the development of lethal cell injury.

REFERENCES

Bellomo, G., Mirabelli, F., Richelmi, P., & Orrenius, S. (1983), Critical role of sulfhydryl group(s) in the ATP-dependent Ca^{2+}-sequestration by the plasma membrane fraction from rat liver, *FEBS Letters* **163,** 136–139.

Campbell, A. K. (1983), *Intracellular calcium: its universal role as regulator*, Wiley and Sons, Chichester, UK.

Cheung, W. Y. (1980), Calmodulin plays a pivotal role in cellular regulation, *Science* **217,** 1257–1259.

Chien, K. R., Pfau, R. G., & Farber, J. L. (1979), Ischemic myocardial cell injury. Prevention by chlorpromazine of an accelerated phospholipid degradation and associated membrane dysfunction, *Am. J. Pathol.* **97,** 505–530.

Cohen, J. J. & Duke, R. L. (1984), Glucocorticoid-activation of a calcium-dependent endonuclease in thymocyte nuclei leads to cell death, *J. Immunol.* **132,** 38–42.

Collier, N. L. & Wang, K. (1982), Purification and properties of human platelets P235, *J. Biol. Chem.* **257,** 6937–6943.

Di Monte, D., Bellomo, G., Thor, H., Nicotera, P., & Orrenius, S. (1984), Menadione-induced cytotoxicity is associated with protein thiol oxidation and alteraton in intracellular Ca^{2+} homeostasis, *Arch. Biochem. Biophys.* **235,** 343–350.

Farber, J. L. (1981), The role of Ca^{2+} in cell death, *Life Sciences* **29,** 1289–1295.

Jewell, S. A., Bellomo, G., Thor, H., Orrenius, S., & Smith, M. T. (1982), Bleb formation in hepatocytes during drug metabolism is caused by disturbances in thiol and calcium ion homeostasis, *Science* **214,** 1257–1259.

Lehninger, A. L., Vercesi, A., & Bababunmi, E. (1978), Regulation of Ca^{2+} release from mitochondria by the oxidation-reduction state of pyridine nucleotides, *Proc. Natl. Acad. Sci. USA* **75,** 1690–1694.

McConkey, D., Hartzell, P., Nicotera, P., Wyllie, A. H., & Orrenius, S. (1988), Menadione activation of the endogenous endonuclease involved in programmed cell death is associated with an increase in cytosolic Ca^{2+} concentration. *Toxicol. Letters* **42,** 123–130.

Mirabelli, F., Salis, A., Marinoni, V. Finardi, G., Bellomo, G., Thor, H., & Orrenius, S. (1988), Menadione-induced bleb formation in hepatocytes is associated with the oxidation of thiol groups in actin, *Arch. Biochem. Biophys.* **264**, 261–269.

Moore, L., Chen, T., Knapp, H. R., & Landon, E. (1975), Energy-dependent Ca^{2+} sequestration activity in rat liver microsomes, *J. Biol. Chem.* **250**, 4562–4568.

Moore, G. A., O'Brien, J. P., & Orrenius, S. (1986), Menadione (2-methyl-1,4-naphthoquinone)-induced Ca^{2+} release from rat-liver mitochondria is caused by NAD(P)H ioxidation, *Xenobiotica* **16,** 873–882.

Murachi, T. (1983), Intracellular Ca^{2+} proteases and its inhibitor protein: Calpain and Calpastatin. In: *Calcium and cell function*, Vol. IV (ed. Cheung, W. Y.), Academic Pres, Orlando, FA, pp. 376–410.

Nicotera, P., Hartzell, P., Baldi, C., Svensson, S. Å., Bellomo, G., & Orrenius, S. (1986a). Cystamine induces toxicity in hepatocytes through the elevation of cytosolic Ca^{2+} and the stimulation of a non-lysosomal proteolytic system, *J. Biol. Chem.* **261,** 14628–14635.

Nicotera, P., Hartzell, P., Davis, G., & Orrenius, S. (1986b). The formation of plasma membrane blebs in hepatocytes exposed to agents that increase cytosolic Ca^{2+} is mediated by the activation of a non-lysosomal proteolytic system, *FEBS Letters* **209,** 139–144.

Nicotera, P., Moore, M., Mirabelli, F., Bellomo, G., & Orrenius, S. (1985), Inhibition of hepatocyte plasma membrane Ca^{2+}-ATPase activity by menadione metabolism and its restoration by thiols, *FEBS Letters* **181,** 149–153.

Orrenius, S. & Bellomo, G. (1986). Toxicological implications of perturbation of Ca^{2+} homeostasis in hepatocytes In: *Calcium and cell function*, Vol. VI (ed. Cheung, W. Y.), Academic Press, Orlando, FA, pp. 186–204.

Orrenius, S. & Moldéus, P. (1984), The multiple roles of glutathione in drug metabolism. *Trends Pharmacol. Sci.* **5,** 432–435.

Shanne, F. A., Kane, A. B., Young, E. E., & Farber, J. L. (1979), Calcium dependence of toxic cell death: a final common pathway, *Science* **206,** 700–702.

Sies, H. (1986), Biochemistry of oxidative stress, *Angewandte Chemie International Editions English* **25,**1058–1071.

Starke, P. E., Hoek, J. B., & Farber, J. L. (1986), Calcium-dependent and calcium-independent mechanisms of irreversible cell injury in cultured hepatocytes *J. Biol. Chem.* **261,** 3006–3012.

Thor, H., Hartzell, P., Svensson, S. Å., Orrenius, S., Mirabelli, F., Marinoni, V., & Bellomo, G. (1985), On the role of thiol groups in the inhibition of liver microsomal Ca^{2+}-sequestration by toxic agents, *Biochem. Pharmacol.* **34,** 3717–3723.

Thor, H., Smith, M. T., Hartzell, P. Bellomo, G., Jewell, S. A., & Orrenius, S. (1982), The metabolism of menadione (2-methyl-1,4-naphthoquinone) by isolated hepatocytes—A study of implications of oxidative stress i intact cells, *J. Biol. Chem.* **257,** 12419–12424.

Wyllie, A. H. (1980), Glucocorticoid-induced thymocyte apoptosis is associated with endogenous endonuclease activation, *Nature* **284,** 555–556.

Wyllie, A. H., Morris, R. G., Smith, A. C., & Dunlop, D. (1984), Chromatin cleavage in apoptosis: association with condensed chromatin morphology and dependence on macromolcular synthesis, *J. Pathol.* **14,** 67–77.

7.3 Inducible cellular responses to X-rays and chemical agents in cancer therapy

Carmia Borek† & Michael Lambert‡

As an approach to identifying specific cellular markers for the cytotoxic action of X-rays and chemotherapeutic drugs in mammalian cells we have used the QUEST system of high-resolution two-dimensional protein gel electrophoresis and computer-based protein database development to score quantitative and qualitative changes in patterns of protein synthesis. We measured the responses elicited after treatment of normal and oncogene-transformed rodent fibroblast lines with either X-rays or bleomycin. Specifically, we compared acute responses seen in the normal REF52 cell and two oncogene-transformed REF52 lines containing E1a or E1a plus the activated Harvey c-ras T24 allele. The two oncogene transformants differed substantially in the patterns of changes in protein synthesis seen immediately after DNA damage. Further, we have identified a specific subset of growth-regulated cellular polypeptides which are related to the observed increase in X-ray induced cell killing seen in the two oncogene transformants. This set includes PCNA (Proliferating Cell Nuclear Antigen) a cell cycle specific DNA polymerase delta auxiliary factor. PCNA synthesis was rapidly suppressed by X-ray only in normal REF52 cells. The inability of PCNA to be suppressed in the two transformed lines correlated with the increased susceptibility to X-ray-induced cell killings, suggesting that cellular processes which underlie regulation of DNA damage-induced growth arrest at the level of replicative elongation play an important role in determining the survival of X-ray-damaged cells.

7.3.1 INTRODUCTION

Radiation is a fact of life. It occurs in nature and pervades the environment. Radiation acts as a 'double-edged sword'. It is a ubiquitous environmental carcinogen, probably the most precisely studied of all known carcinogens, and it is also an agent used in cancer therapy.

The development of cell culture systems has made it possible to study the cellular and molecular mechanisms involved in radiation action under defined conditions devoid of host-mediated homeostatic modulating factors. These *in vitro* systems allow qualitative and quantitiative assessments of underlying mechanisms. They afford the opportunity to study dose-related and time-dependent interactions of radiation with single cells. They allow allow us to identify factors and conditions which modulate

† Radiological Research Laboratory, Department of Radiation Oncology, College of Physicians and Surgeons, Columbia University New York, New York, 10032 (Corresponding author)
‡ Cold Spring Harbor Laboratory, Cold Spring Harbor, New York 10032

radiogenic transformation (Borek & Sachs 1966, Borek & Hall 1973, Borek *et al.* 1987) and radiogenic cytotoxicity (Borek 185, Borek & Hall 1982).

In earlier work we focused on the carcinogenic effects of radiation at a cellular and molecular level (Borek & Sachs 1966, 1967, Borek 1985, Borek *et al.* 1987). The present studies were undertaken to investigate molecular mechanisms underlying radiation cytotoxicity in its action as a cancer therapy agent (Borek & Hall 1982).

The molecular and cellular mechanisms which underlie the increased susceptibility of many types of neoplastic cells to killing by ionizing radiation and chemotherapeutic drugs is poorly understood (Borek *et al.* 1987, Friedberg 1985). One possibility is that transformed cells differ from normal cells in their ability to undergo a regulated process of DNA damage-induced growth arrest. An inability to rapidly suppress DNA synthesis would be expected to increase the probability of cell killing by reducing the overall effectiveness of cellular DNA repair processes before progression of the cell cycle through following rounds of DNA synthesis and cell division. Further, the regulation of those cellular processes which underlie DNA damage-induced growth arrest could occur at the level of either DNA replication initiation or replicative elongation. To address these questions, we have studied the effects of X-ray-induced DNA damage on the behaviour of several known growth-regulated and DNA replication associated polypeptides in both normal and transformed rodent cell lines.

Specifically, we have compared the changes in patterns of protein synthesis observed after X-ray-induced DNA damage in a well characterized normal rat cell line REF52 (Franza & Garrels 1984, McClure *et al.* 1982) and two oncogenically-transformed isogenic variants derived by transfection with specific combinations of oncogenes, including E1a or E1a plus the mutated c-Harvey ras T24 allele. To characterize both the quantitative and qualitative patterns of changes in cellular protein expression we have utilized the QUEST system of high-resolution two-dimensional protein gel electrophoresis, quantitative analysis, and computer-based protein database development (Garrels *et al.* 1984).

The QUEST system provides tools for quantitative evaluation of standardized high resolution 2D protein gel patterns and for the systematic comparison of the regulatory behaviour of sets of polypeptides in multiple biological contexts. In the current study, we first created a protein database to evaluate changes in the patterns of protein synthesis seen immediately after treatment of normal and oncogene-transformed REF52 lines with X-rays or chemical agents. We then addressed the question of how specific growth-related polypeptides, which have been identified in protein database studies of proliferation control in REF52 cells, behave during the X-ray-induced DNA damage stress response in either the normal or oncogene transformed REF52 lines.

7.3.2 METHODS AND MATERIALS

7.3.2.1. Cell culture and cell treatments

REF52 cells (McClure *et al.* 1982), E1a-REF52 cells, and E1a-T24ras-REF52 cl. 7 cells (R. Franza, unpublished studies) were maintained in DMEM supplemented with 10% fetal calf serum (Flow) and streptomycin (100 μg/ml) and penicillin (100 units/ml) (Gibso) in 5% CO_2 at 37°C. In metabolic labelling studies, cells were plated 24 hours

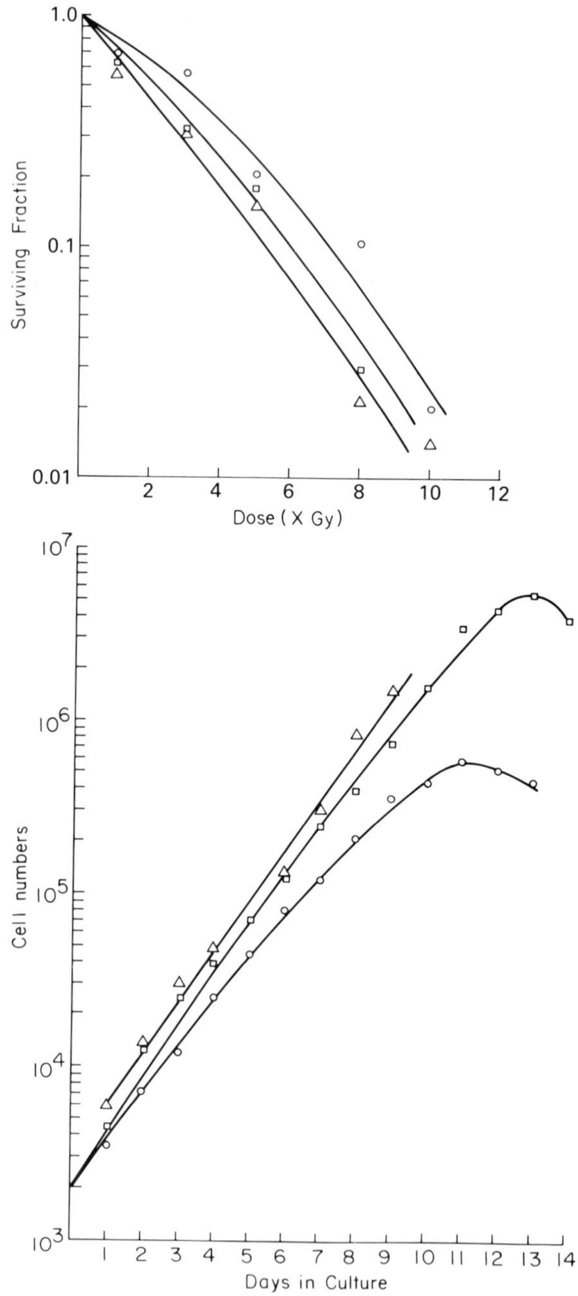

Fig. 1.

A. Effects of X-rays on survival of normal and transformed REF52 cells
Symbols: ○ REF52; □ E1a–REF52; △ E1a–T24ras–REF52. Cells were plated 24 h before treatment in 60 mm dishes at 5×10^2 cells/dish for controls and for treatment with 1 and 3 Gy, and at 1×10^3 per dish for cells irradiated with 5, 8, and 10 Gy. The cells were grown for 10 days with one medium change, after which they were stained and counted.

B. Growth curves of normal and transformed REF52 cells
Symbols: See legend to Fig. 1A. Cells were plated in 60 mm dishes at 1.2×10^3 cells/dish and grown for 14 days with medium change every two days. Cells were counted daily with a Coulter counter, and each point plotted represents the average of 3 independent dishes.

before irradiation or drug treatment at 1×10^5 in 35 mm dishes. Cells for cell survival and growth curve studies were plated as indicated in the legend to Fig. 1.

Cells were irradiated in complete medium using a Caesium 137 source at a dose rate of 1.36 Gy/min. MNNG was obtained from Aldwich Pharmaceutical, and bleomycin sulfate was a gift from the Bristol–Meyers Company. A stock solution of MNNG (1 mg/ml) was freshly prepared in dmso. The final concentraton of dmso in the culture fluid was not greater than 0.1%. Cells were exposed for 2 hours to MNNG (1 μg/ml) in DMEM without serum, followed by replenishment with age-matched conditioned complete media. Bleomycin sulfate was dissolved in sterile water at a final concentration of 10 mg/ml, and REF52 cells were exposed for 2 hours (10 μg/ml) in complete media, followed by replenishment with age-matched conditioned complete media.

7.3.2.2 Metabolic cell labelling and sample preparation

At various times after exposure, cells were labelled for 2 hours with 500 μCi of high specific activity S^{35}-methionine (> 1200 Ci/mmol) (Amersham Product #SJ235) in complete media. After aspiration of labelling medium and three rinses with ice-cold PBS, cell lysates were prepared by addition to 100 μl 100°C dSDS lysis solution (0.3% SDS; 1% BME; 0 05M Tris, pH 8.0) and 10 μl Dnase/Rnase solution (1 mg/ml Dnase I; 0.5 mg/ml Rnase A; 0.5 M Tris; 0.05 M Mg Cl_2; pH 7.0) and quick freezing in liquid N_2, all as previously described (Garrels 1979). Samples were lyophilized, resuspended in sample buffer (Garrels 1979), and TCA-precipitable counts were determined.

7.3.2.3 Two-dimensional protein gels

Gels were run at the Cold Spring Harbor QUEST Laboratory. Equal counts were loaded per gel (average; 300 000 dpms) on Type H, broad range ampholyte (pH 3–10) first dimension isoelectric focusing, 10% acrylamide second dimension slab gels, all is previously described (Garrels 1979). Gels were fluorographed and exposed to XAR film at −70°C. On average, three autoradiographic exposures of varying durations were obtained of each fluorograph, as calculated by the QUEST algorithm.

7.3.2.4 QUEST analysis

Quantitative analysis and protein database analysis were carried out with the Cold Spring Harbor version of QUEST (Garrels *et al.* 1984) operated on a MASSCOMP work station. The QUEST software is licensed for commercial development to Protein Databases Inc. (Huntington Station, New York). On average, over 1500 individual polypeptides were computer matched within each experiment (designated MATCHSETS), and the entire series of MATCHSETS was linked to form a protein database by computer matching of the standard reference gels from each experiment.

7.3.3 RESULTS

7.3.3.1 Normal and oncogene-transformed REF52 cells differ in their susceptibility to X-ray-induced cell killing

Initially, we compared the effects of X-ray on cell survival in REF52 and the two isogenic REF52 variants. As shown in Fig. 1a, both the E1a and E1a-T24 c-ras transformants were more sensitive than REF52 cells to the killing effects of X-ray starting at 1 Gy, as measured by colony forming ability. The increased susceptibility to X-ray-induced cell killing in the two transformants was also directly proportional to the increased growth rates and saturation densities observed in the two oncogene transfectants (compare Fig. 1a and Fig. 1b).

7.3.3.2 Expression of growth-regulated polypeptides after X-ray in normal and transformed REF52 cells

We next examined changes in patterns of protein synthesis after X-ray damage in the three cells lines by use of standardized two-dimensional protein gels (Garrels 1979). Treated cultures were pulse labelled for 2 h with high specific activity S-35 methionine at intervals up to 24 h after exposure, and the radiolabelled proteins resolved on broad range ampholyte (pH 3–10) first dimension, 10% acrylamide slab gel second dimension gels. Sets of autoradiographic images from individual experiments were quantitated and matched, using the QUEST algorithm, and the entire series was then linked to form a protein database in which the behaviour of any single or set of polypeptides from any experiment could be easily studied and compared.

We initially selected a set of protein spots which are suppressed by 4–6 h after either X-ray treatment in REF52 cells. This set was derived by selecting from among over 2000 matched spots the set of proteins suppressed by 2-fold or greater after 5 Gy rads of X-ray treatment and then restricting this set to those which were also suppressed within the same time frame and to at least an equal degree by 10 Gy. This set was found to include the protein PCNA (Prliferating Cell Nuclear Antigen or Cyclin), a nuclear, cell cycle-specific phosphoprotein (36 kd, I.E.F. pH 5.0) (Mathews *et al.* 1984) which has been shown to be serum-inducible (MacDonald-Bravo & Bravo 1985) and an auxliary protein to DNA polymerase delta (Bravo *et al.* 1987, Prelich *et al.* 1987).

We then compared this PCNA and co-regulated set of early suppressed proteins from X-ray-treated REF52 cells with a set of 16 PCNA co-regulated polypeptides originally identified in the Cold Spring Harbor Rat Protein Database as being growth-regulated. This set, which includes several nuclear proteins, represents a set of proteins which are suppressed during confluence in normal REF52 cells and are also over-expressed in virally-transformed REF52, as seen in studies of several independently derived adenovirus-transformed REF52 lines. Among the known proteins in this set, in addition to PCNA, are a 85K co-regulated polypeptide and nuclear Lamin. The 85K co-regulated protein is a nuclear protein that displays tight coordinate regulation with PCNA in both rat and human cells during either serum or growth factor-induced proliferation and during both viral and chemical transformation (M. Lambert, M. Quinlan, T. Grodzicker, & J. Garrels, manuscript in preparation). When these two sets were compared, 5 of the 16 growth-related polypeptides were found to be contained in the set of proteins from X-ray-damaged REF52 cells which were decreased by at least 2-fold by 4–6 h at doses of 5 Gy or higher, and an additional 9 members of this set were also found to be decreased by less than 2-fold.

The relative expression of this set of 14 polypeptides is shown in Table 1 for all three cell lines tested. The behaviour of these polypeptides in the two transformants

Table 1—Relative expression of PCNA and growth co-regulated polypeptides 4 h after X-ray (5 Gy) induced DNA damage†

	Protein‡	Cell line: REF52	E1a–REF52	E1a–T24 REF52
		(Fold change relative to untreated cells)		
1	PCNA	0.49	1.22	0.97
2	85K	0.96	1.01	2.30
3	Lamin	0.47	0.57	1.59
4	Spot n	0.53	0.73	0.86
5	Spot p	0.82	0.82	1.20
6	Spot q	0.59	1.48	0.59
7	Spot s	0.88	1.18	n.d.
8	Spot t	0.40	0.75	0.74
9	Spot u	0.96	2.20	0.91
10	Spot v	0.76	0.75	0.89
11	Spot w	0.51	0.68	1.08
12	Spot x	0.74	0.76	0.86
13	Spot y	0.50	1.00	0.59
14	Spot z	0.47	0.63	1.01
	Average ratio:	0.65	0.98	1.04

† Expressed as the ratio of ppm values (parts per million counts loaded per gel) for each protein relative to untreated, control cells from the same experiment. Quantitation was carried out by use of the QUEST algorithm.
‡ Proteins designated as Spots n through z refers to the set of PCNA co-regulated polypeptides designated in the Cold Spring Harbor Rat Protein Database.
N.D., not detected.

differs substantially from that seen in REF52 cells. On average, the ratio of treated to non-treated cells is 0.65 in REF52 cells, whereas the two transformants, on average, show no change from treated to untreated cultures (0.98 and 1.04 for the E1a and E1a-T24 REF52 lines, respectively). From these data we conclude that the two transformed REF52 lines are deficient relative to nomal REF52 cells in their ability to rapidly suppress the expression of a discrete family of known growth-related polypeptides including PCNA, following exposure to single doses (5 Gy) of X-rays.

To extend these studies to other classes of DNA-damaging agents, we compared the behaviour of this set of growth-related polypeptides after exposure of REF52 cells to either the mono-functional alkylating agent N-methyl-N″-nitro-N-nitroso-guanidine (MNNG) or bleomycin sulfate, which induces primilarly single-stranded DNA lesions. As shown in Fig. 2, bleomycin, like X-rays, induces a striking suppression in the expression of members of this set, including PCNA, 85K, Lamin, and Spots V, T, and O, by 24 h after treatment, starting at 1 Gy. MNNG, by contrast, induced elevated expression of PCNA at 8 h and PCNA synthesis remains elevated above basal levels at 24 h. Lack of suppression of this set of growth-related polypeptides at 24 h after MNNG exposure of REF52 cells is a distinguishing property of this type of alkylation damage (Lambert & Garrels, manuscript in preparation). The difference in sensitivity to suppression of these growth-related polypeptides after bleomycin and MNNG treatment is being investigated.

In summary, the present investigation has shown that there are quantitative similarities to the patterns of change in gene expression seen during DNA damage-induced growth arrest and during confluency-induced inhibition of growth, and these similarities extend to nuclear replication associated polypeptides of known cellular function, including the DNA polymerase delta auxiliary protein, PCNA.

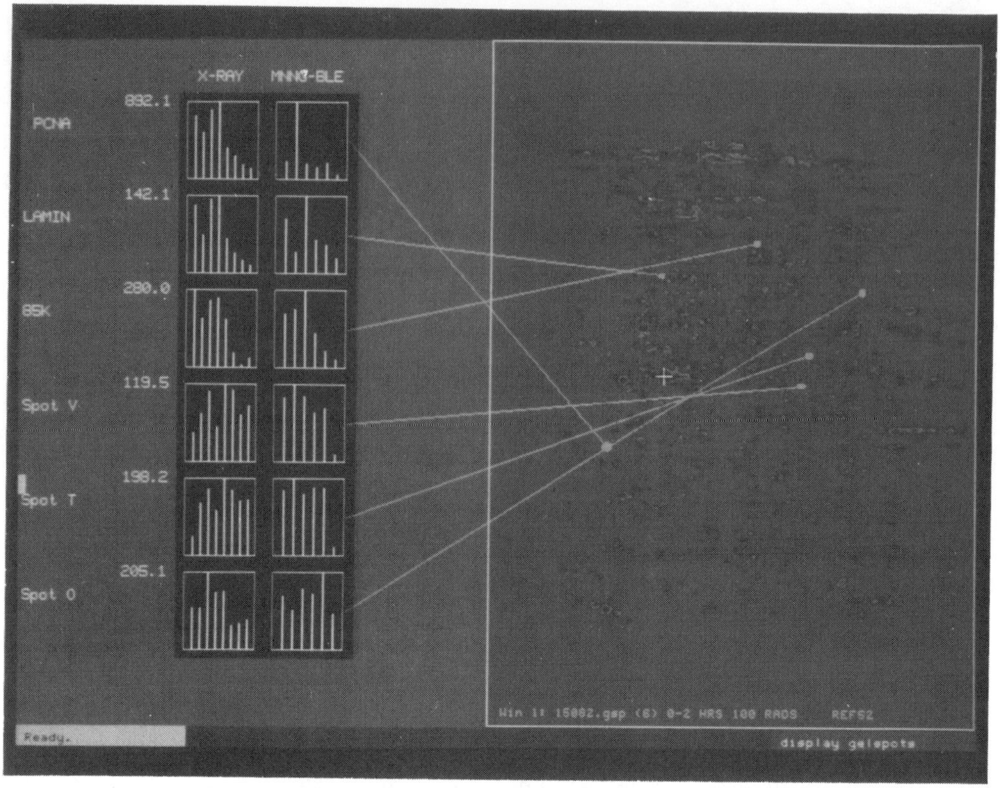

Fig. 2.
Expression of PCNA and co-regulated growth related polypeptides after X-ray or bleomycin induced DNA damage in REF52 cells

For the proteins listed at the left, quantitative data are plotted on the right. Each bar represents a gel, and the gels compared in each matchset are listed below. The maximum ppm (parts per million counts loaded per gel) detected for a polypeptide for the entire series of samples is displayed on the left. The height of each bar is scaled within each individual graph to the maximum detected value (shown as full scale). The synthetic image shown on the right is of a broad range ampholyte (pH 3–10), first dimension, 10% acrylamide slab gel, second dimension gel. Basic proteins are to the right, acidic to the left. The crosshatch is shown displayed on Actin. For additional experimental details see Methods and Materials.

Graph 1 XRAY: X-Ray-treated REF52 cells (left to right) A. Control cells labelled at 0–2 h. B. X-ray (1 Gy)-treated cells labelled at 0–2 h. C. X-ray (5 Gy)-treated cells labelled at 0–2 h. D. X-ray (10 Gy)-treated cells labelled at 0–2 h. E through H: same order as A–D, labelled at 22–24 h after exposure.

Graph 2 MNNG–BLEO: MNNG or bleomycin-treated REF52 cell (left to right) A. Control cells labelled at 4–8 h. B. MNNG-treated cells (1 μg/ml) labelled at 4–8 h. C. Bleomyin-treated cells (10 μg/ml) labelled at 4–8 h. D through F: same order as A–C, labelled at 20–24 h after exposure.

7.3.4 DISCUSSION

We have used the QUEST system of protein database analysis to reveal highly discrete sets of co-regulated cellular polypeptides, selected by quantitative criteria, which are synthesized at altered levels in response to several types of DNA-damaging agents, and then compared the responses between normal and transformed isogenic lines.

We examined the behaviour of a set of growth-related polypeptides, identified from studies of confluency-associated changes in protein expression in REF52 cells, and found that a number of these polypeptides are differentially regulated in two oncogene-derived transformants of REF52 after X-ray-induced DNA damage. Specifically, we found that the inability to effectively and rapidly suppress the expression of members of this set correlates directly with the observed increased sensitivity to cell killing. This set was found to include PCNA, a co-regulated polypeptide 85K, and nuclear Lamin, and this set was also sensitive to suppression of synthesis after damage by another DNA-damaging agent, bleomycin sulfate.

This set of proteins may play a central role in the highly regulated process of DNA damage-induced growth arrest. The triggering signal for the onset of DNA damage-induced growth arrest is itself not known, though the burden of regulation could be expected to fall, in part, on either DNA replication proteins associated with initiation or elongation, or both. The rapid suppression of PCNA synthesis seen with certain regimens suggests that at least one regulatory component in the process of induced growth arrest is at the level of synthesis of a known DNA polymerase auxiliary protein.

These data indicate that suppression of PCNA synthesis after exposure to ionizing radiation is a predictive marker of X-ray-induced cell killing in certain transformed cells. The use of oncogene-transfected, isogenic transformants provide a valuable model system for controlled study of the action of specific oncogene products on both abrogation of proliferation control (Borek *et al.* 1987) as well as abrogation of the molecular and cellular mechanisms which control the ordered cellular responses elicited by DNA damage (Lambert *et al.* 1986).

Overall, these studies demonstrate that X-ray and chemical agent-induced stress responses can be defined in a highly precise and quantitative manner in terms of inducible changes in patterns of protein synthesis. The overall complexity of the changes observed presumably reflects the pleiotropic effects of DNA damage on induction of distinct DNA repair pathways (Friedberg 1985), cellular transformation (Borek & Hall 1973, 1982, Borek 1985), and the highly-regulated process of induced growth arrest.

ACKNOWLEDGEMENTS

We are grateful to R. Franza for providing the two REF52 oncogene transformants, to J. Garrels for use of the QUEST facility, and to H. Mason and C. Chang and P. Myers for technical assistance. This work was supported by grant CA12536 to C.B. and a contract from the National Foundation for Cancer Research to C.B.

REFERENCES

Borek, C. & Sachs, L. (1966) *In vitro* cell transformation by X-irradiation, *Nature* **210,** 276–278.

Borek, C. & Sachs, L. (1967) Cell susceptibility to transformation by X-irradiation and fixation of the transformed state, *Proc. Natl. Acad. Sci. USA* **57,** 1522–1527.

Borek, C. & Hall, E. J. (1973) Transformation of mammalian cells *in vitro* by low doses of X-rays, *Nature* **243,** 450–453.

Borek, C. & Hall, E. J. (1982) Oncogenic transformation produced by agents and modalities used in cancer therapy and its modulation, *Ann. N.Y. Acad. Sci. USA* **397,** 193–219.

Borek, C. (1985) The induction and control of radiogenic transformation *in vitro*; cellular and molecular mechanisms. *Pharmacol. Ther.* **27,**99–142.

Borek, C., Ong, A., & Mason, H. (1987) Distinctive transforming genes in X-ray transformed mammalian cells. *Proc. Natl. Acad. Sci. USA* **84,** 794–798.

Bravo, R., Frank, R., Blundell, P. A., & Macdonald-Bravo H. (1987) Cyclin/PCNA is the auxiliary protein of DNA polymerase delta, *Nature* **326,** 515–517.

Franza, B. R. & Garrels, J. I. (1984) Transformation sensitive proteins of REF52 cells detected by computer analyzed two-dimensional gel electrophoresis. In: *Cancer cell I: the transformed phenotype* (eds Levine, A, Woude, G. F. Vande, Topp, W. C., & Watson, J. D.), Cold Spring Harbor Laboratory, Cold Spring Harbor, New York, pp. 137–145.

Friedberg, E. (1985) *DNA repair*. W.H. Freeman and Co., San Francisco, New York.

Garrels, J. I. (1979) Two dimensional gel electrophoresis and computer analysis of proteins synthesized by clonal cell lines. *J. Biol. Chem.* **254,** 7961.

Garrels, J. I., Farrar, J. T., & Burwell, C. B. (1984) The QUEST system for computer analyzed two dimensional electrophoresis of proteins. In: *Two dimensional gel electrophoresis of proteins: methods and applications* (eds Celis, J. E. & Bravo, R.), Academic Press, New York, pp. 37–91.

Lambert, M. E., Garrels, J. I., McDonald, J., & Weinstein, I. B. (1986) Inducible cellular responses to DNA damage in mammalian cells. In: *Antimutagenesis and anticarcinogenesis mechanisms* (eds Shankel, D. M., Hartman, P. E., Kada, T., & Hollaender, A.), Plenum Press, New York, pp. 291–311.

Mathews, M. B., Bernstein, R. M., Franza, B. R., & Garrels, J. I. (1984) Identity of the proliferating cell nuclear antigen and cyclin, *Nature* **309,** 374–376.

MacDonald-Bravo, H. & Bravo, R. (1985) Induction of protein cyclin in serum stimulated quiescent 3T3 cells is independent of DNA synthesis, *Exp. Cell. Res.* **156,** 455–461

McClure, D. B., Hightower, M. J., & Topp, W. C. (1982) Effect of SV40 transformation on the growth factor requirements of the rat embryo cell line REF52 in serum free medium, *Cold Spring Harbor Conf. Cell Proliferation* **9,** 345.

Prelich, G., Tan, C. K., Kostura M., Mathews, M. B., So, A. G., Downey, K. M., & Stillman, B. (1987) Functional identity of proliferating cell nuclear antigen and a DNA polymerase delta auxiliary protein, *Nature* **326,** 517–520.

7.4 Perspectives in the molecular mechanism of tricyclic antidepressives on peripheral nerve fibres

D. Mitolo-Chieppa & M. R. Carratú

(1) The effects of the antidepressant imipramine and amitriptyline upon the node of Ranvier of frog isolated nerve fibres were investigated under current and voltage clamp conditions.
(2) Imipramine (5 μM) or amitriptyline (2 μM) reversibly decreased the amplitude of the action potential.
(3) Both Na and K currents were decreased without any change in kinetic or shape of current–voltage relationships.
(4) Acid pH (6) or high Ca^{2+} (18 mM)-Ringer failed to influence the effects of both antidepressives in contrast to the relieving effects on procaine (500 μM)- and chlorpromazine (20 μM)-induced block.
(5) We conclude that both antidepressives act on the nodal membrane with a mechanism different from that of local anaesthetics, an alteration of membrane surface charge properties being involved.

7.4.1 INTRODUCTION

Tricyclic antidepressives are reported to have inhibitory effects on axonal conduction and on the electrical activity of cardiac Purkinje fibres and striated muscle (Chang & Chuang 1972, Rawling & Fozzard 1979, Schauf *et al.* 1975). This suggests direct membrane actions, in addition to the well-known modulatory effects on neurotransmission of these drugs. The present study is focused on the possible interaction of imipramine and amitriptyline with ionic channels of peripheral nerve membrane; their mode of action is compared with that of other drugs (procaine, chlorpromazine) also affecting ionic conductances.

7.4.2 METHODS

The experiments were carried out on sensory and motor myelinated nerve fibres isolated from the sciatic nerve of the frog, *Rana esculenta*. The action potential and membrane currents were recorded under current and voltage clamp conditions using the method of Nonner (1969). The normal resting potential of fibres (−70 mV) was defined as the potential at which fast Na inactivation occurred by 30%. Na and K

† Institute of Pharmacology, Medical Faculty, University of Bari, I-70124 Bari, Italy

currents were monitored with a conventional two pulses protocol and calculated assuming an axoplasmic resistance of 10 MΩ. Linear leakage and capacity currents were analogically subtracted from the total current. The series resistance was not compensated for (Chiu 1977).

7.4.3 RESULTS AND DISCUSSION

External application of imipramine (5 μM) or amitriptyline (2 μM) reduced the amplitude of action potential by 30% within 2 minutes; the effect was reversed about 5 minutes after washing out the drug (Fig. 1). Both initial sodium and delayed potassium currents were decreased by imipramine (5 μM) or amitriptyline (2 μM) without significant changes either in their time course or in the shape of current–voltage relationships (Fig. 2). The reversal potential for the sodium current was not affected, implying that the relative permeabilities of the node to Na^+ and K^+ ions

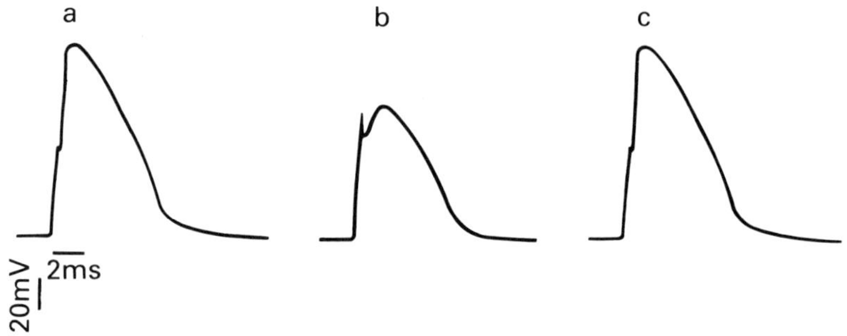

Fig. 1.—Effect of imipramine on action potential recorded from a single myelinated nerve fibre. (a) Control action potentials in Ringer solution. (b) Action potential recorded 2 min after the addition of 5 μM imipramine. (c) Action potential recorded about 5 min after washout of the drug with Ringer solution.

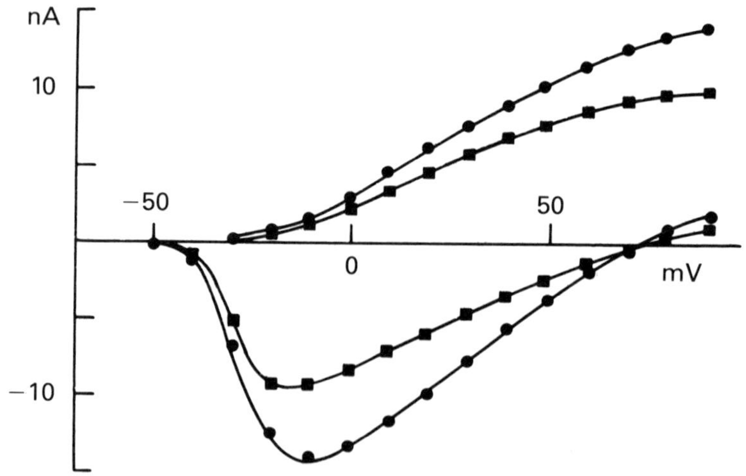

Fig. 2.—Effects of imipramine on Na and K currents. Current–voltage relationship of the steady-state K current (upper trace) and peak Na current (lower trace). The current were measured at the end of a 18 ms period of depolarization of various amplitudes preceded by 50 ms hyperpolarization to −120 mV under control condition (●) and in the presence of 5 μM imipramine (■). Temperature 15°C.

Table 1—Influence of $[Ca^{++}]_0$ and pH modifications on the effects of amitriptyline, imipramine, chlorpromazine, and procaine on action potential amplitude (AP) and peak Na current (I_{Na})

Drugs	**ED_{30} (μM)	AP (mV)			I_{Na} (nA)			Number of fibres
		1.8 mM $[Ca^{++}]_0$ pH 7.4	1.8 pH 6	18 mM $[Ca^{++}]_0$ pH 7.4	1.8 mM $[Ca^{++}]_0$ pH 7.4	1.8 mM $[Ca^{++}]_0$ pH 6	18 mM $[Ca^{++}]_0$ pH 7.4	
Amitriptyline	2	99.8 ± 0.69	99.8 ± 0.69	99.8 ± 0.69	9.7 ± 0.19	9.7 ± 0.19	9.7 ± 0.19	7
Imiprmaine	5	99.4 ± 0.73	99.4 ± 0.73	99.4 ± 0.73	9.5 ± 0.06	9.5 ± 0.06	9.5 ± 0.06	7
Chlorpromazine	20	99.8 ± 0.46	*126.8 ± 1.06	*139.5 ± 0.22	9.7 ± 0.14	*12.2 ± 0.06	*13.9 ± 0.12	9
Procaine	500	99.5 ± 0.26	*127.1 ± 0.62	*139.4 ± 0.28	9.3 ± 0.06	*12.3 ± 0.04	*14 ± 0.02	9

* Significant level: $P < 0.01$
** Concentration which reduces by 30% amplitude of the action potential and peak Na current

were not altered (Hille 1971). The above described effects were observed in normal Ca^{++} (1.8 mM)-Ringer at physiological pH (7.4). To check whether modifications of the Ca^{++} concentration or pH in the medium could have modified the responses of the node to the tested drugs, experiments were carried out by superfusing the node either with high Ca^{++}-Ringer at normal pH or with normal Ca^{++}-Ringer at acid pH (6). A comparison of the effects of antidepressant imipramine and amitriptyline—as influenced by Ca^{++} concentration and pH—was made with those of a typical local anaesthetic, procaine (500 μM) and with those of a neuroleptic, chlorpromazine (20 μM). Acid pH and high Ca^{++} concentration affected the degree of inhibition of action potential and membrane currents produced by procaine and chlorpromazine, whereas no influence was observed on the effects produced by imipramine and amitriptyline (Table 1).

Our data show that the potency of activity of the tested antidepressives is by one order of magnitude greater than that of chlorpromazine and by two orders than that of procaine.

Modification of pH failed to influence the effects of both antidepressives; but we should remark that these molecules are cations at all reasonable pH values, so that, as for the cationic quaternary anaesthetics, their rate of actions would be pH-independent. It is well known that raised external Ca^{++} concentration relieves the blocking effects of local anaesthetics; this is explained by assuming that the anaesthetic receptor is strongly coupled to the sodium inactivation mechanism which is in turn sensitive to the membrane potential changes induced by external Ca^{++} ions (Hille 1977). The effects of tricyclic antidepressives are not influenced by raising the Ca^{++}, so that we could conclude that the mechanism of action does not involve the sodium inactivation system but rather an aspecific alteration of membrane surface charge properties.

REFERENCES

Chang, C. C. & Chuang, S. T. (1972). Effects of desipramine and imipramine on the nerve, muscle and synaptic transmission of rat diaphrams. *Neuropharmacology* **11,** 777–788.

Chiu, S. Y. (1977). Inactivation of sodium channels: second order kinetics in myelinated nerve. *J. Physiol.* **273,** 573–596.

Hille, B. (1971). The permeability of the sodium channel to organic cations in myelinated nerve. *J. gen. Physiol.* **58,** 599–619.

Hille, B. (1977). Local anaesthetics: hydrophilic and hydrophobic pathways for the drug-receptor reaction. *J. gen. Physiol.* **69,** 497–515.

Nonner, W. (1969). A new voltage clamp method for Ranvier nodes. *Pflügers Arch.* **309,** 116–192.

Rawling, D. A. & Fozzard, H. A. (1979). Effects of imipramine on cellular electrphysiological properties of cardiac Purkinje fibers. *J. Pharm. exp. Ther.* **209,** 371–375.

Schauf, C. L., Davis, F. A., & Kesler, R. L. (1975). Actions of the antidepressant drug imipramine on the voltage-clamped myxicola giant axon. *J. Pharm. exp. Ther.* **193,** 669–675.

7.5 Developmental neurotoxicity of psychotropic drugs: neurochemical and behavioural markers

V. Cuomo, R. Cagiano, G. Ianieri, C. Lacomba, & G. Renna†

(1) Interactions with specific mechanisms of central neurotransmission during development alter the course of neural development in rodents.
(2) Prenatal and/or early postnatal exposure to some psychotropic drugs produces both short- and long-term neurochemical and behavioural alterations in rats.
(3) Compensatory mechanisms occurring in response to a chronic treatment with some neuroleptic and antidepressant agents during development seem to be markedly different from those occurring in response to a prolonged administration in adult animals.

7.5.1 INTRODUCTION

In recent years a large number of studies have been devoted to the investigation of neurochemical mechanisms underlying the neurotoxic effects produced by exposure to various chemical agents. In particular, several experiments have been carried out to correlate behavioural alterations with changes in neuronal function, and neurochemical findings have provided one way of understanding target sites for neurotoxicity (DeHaven & Mailman 1986). An increasing amount of evidence suggests that neurochemical variables could be considered as markers of neurotoxicity of some psychotropic drugs and environmental toxicants.

The developing nervous system is extremely susceptible to various chemicals; the blood–brain barrier is absent or incomplete in the neonate, so that animals prenatally or neonatally treated with chemical agents seem to be at greatest risk from substances which have potential neurotoxic effects. Interactions with specific mechanisms of neurotransmission during development alter the course of neural development and may induce short- and long-term neurochemical and behavioural alterations (Leonard 1983, Zbinden *et al.* 1983, Riley & Vorhees 1986).

In the present paper, examples of neurochemical and behavioural changes produced by the developmental administration of some psychotropic drugs affecting central catecholaminergic neurotransmission are reported. In particular, the results of experiments carried out on our laboratory on the neurochemical and behavioural consequences of prenatal and/or neonatal exposure to some neuroleptic and antidepressant agents are discussed.

† Institute of Pharmacology, University of Bari, Policlinico, Piazza G. Cesare, I-70124 Bari, Italy

7.5.2 DEVELOPMENTAL EXPOSURE TO NEUROLEPTICS

The prolonged administration of haloperidol during gestation markedly affects the behavioral responsiveness of adult rats to a dopamine receptor agonist such as apomorphine. The effects of apomorphine in the dose range (1–2 mg/kg) used in these experiments seem to be due to the stimulation of postsynaptic dopamine receptors. The intensity of stereotyped behaviour as well as the effects on locomotor activity induced by apomorphine in haloperidol-pretreated rats were significantly reduced with respect to controls. These data parallel neurochemical results, showing a significant decrease in the number of dopamine receptors in the striatum of animals exposed to haloperidol during prenatal life (Cuomo *et al.* 1985, Rosengarten & Friedhoff 1979). On the contrary, the prolonged exposure to this neuroleptic during the first three weeks of postnatal life, which seem to be vulnerable periods for the functional maturation of the central dopaminergic system in the rat, produces an opposite response pattern: behavioural supersensitivity to apomorphine which correlates with neurochemical results showing an increased number of striatal dopamine receptors. Moreover, the administration of a challenge dose of haloperidol produced smaller increases in dopamine turnover (striatal levels of HVA and DOPAC) of adult rats treated with this neuroleptic during early postnatal life (Cuomo *et al.* 1981). Even though dopamine receptor supersensitivity to apomorphine as well as an attenuated response to a challenge of haloperidol on dopamine turnover after prolonged haloperidol administration in adult rats has been shown, there is no evidence that these effects persist up to 40 days after haloperidol withdrawal (Cuomo *et al.* 1983a). It is of interest that the developmental exposure to a non-cataleptogenic neuroleptic, such as clozapine, produces neurochemical and behavioural changes which markedly differ from those elicited by a cataleptogenic neuroleptic, such as haloperidol. In particular, early postnatal exposure to clozapine modified neither apomorphine-induced stereotypes nor the effect of apomorphine of locomotor activity in adult rats. Moreover, neurochemical data indicate that even if an acute challenge dose of clozapine (10 mg/kg) shows a certain degree of tolerance, a single dose of 20 mg/kg of this neuroleptic is still able to increase striatal HVA levels in adult rats postnatally treated with clozapine (Cuomo *et al.* 1983b).

7.5.3 DEVELOPMENTAL EXPOSURE TO ANTIDEPRESSANTS

We carried out a comparative evaluation of neurochemical and behavioural changes produced by early postnatal and adult administration of antidepressants influencing central noradrenergic transmission with different profiles of action. In particular, the experiments reported here were performed to investigate in rats the effects of desipramine (an antidepressant preferentially blocking norepinephrine reuptake) and mianserin (an antidepressant influencing noradrenergic system through the blocking of central presynaptic α2-adrenoceptors) on the following parameters: (1) cortical levels of normetanephrine, the O-methylated norepinephrine metabolite; (2) clonidine-induced inhibition of locomotion, which represents a functional response to the activation of α2-adrenoreceptors. Our data show that chronic administration of both antidepressants to adult rats significantly decreased normetanephrine levels in cerebral cortex, and reduced the effects of clonidine on cortical concentrations of this norepinephrine metabolite. Moreover, the prolonged exposure to desipramine and mianserin during adulthood significantly attenuated the inhibition of locomotor activity elicited by a challenge dose of clonidine (Racagni *et al.* 1982). Conversely, the prolonged exposure to these two antidepressants during early postnatal life produced different neurochemical and behavioural changes. In particular, cortical normetaneprhine levels were significantly increased by postnatal treatment with desipramine, whereas they were not affected by mianserin administration. Furthermore, early postnatal exposure to desipramine did not influence the effects of a challenge dose of clonidine on normetanephrine concentrations, whereas this α2-adrenoreceptors agonist was ineffective in mianserin-pretreated animals. Finally, clonidine-induced inhibition of locomotion was significantly reduced only in rats exposed to desipramine during postnatal life (Racagni *et al.* 1983). Moreover, unlike the prolonged treatment with desipramine and mianserin in adult rats, the prolonged administration of these antidepressants either during gestation or during early postnatal life produces long-lasting behavioural alterations (Racagni *et al.* 1983, Cuomo *et al.* 1984).

7.5.4 CONCLUSIONS

These data indicate that the particular period of exposure to psychotropic drugs affecting catecholaminergic system has a critical role in causing both short- and long-term neurochemical and behavioural changes in rats. It seems that compensatory mechanisms occurring in response to a prolonged developmental administration of some neuroleptic and antidepressant agents are markedly different from those occurring in response to a chronic exposure in mature animals. These findings may have implications for the exposure of the human foetus or neonate to psychotropic drugs. On the other hand, clinical studies have already shown that behavioural alterations have occurred in newborns of women treated with various psychotropic drugs either during pregnancy or during lactation. Finally, the data reported here further confirm that an integrated approach, based on neurochemical and behavioural determinations, may be useful for identifying biological markers for neurotoxicity.

ACKNOWLEDGEMENTS

This paper was partly supported by a grant of M.P.I.

REFERENCES

Cuomo, V., Cagiano, R., Coen, E., Mocchetti, I., Cattabeni, F., & Racagni, G. (1981) Enduring behavioural and biochemical effects in the adult rat after prolonged postnatal administration of haloperidol, *Psychopharmacology* **74,** 166–169.

Cuomo, V., Cagiano, R., Mocchetti, I., Coen, E., Cattabeni, F., & Racagni, G. (1983a) Biochemical and behavioural effects after early postnatal administration of neuroleptics in rats. In: *Application of behavioural pharmacology in toxicology* (eds Zbinden, G., Cuomo, V., Racagni, G., & Weiss, B.), Raven Press, N.Y., 173–185.

Cuomo, V., Cagiano, R., Mocchetti, I., Coen, E., Cattabeni, F., & Racagni, G. (1983b) Behavioural and biochemical effects in the adult rat after prolonged postnatal administration of clozapine, *Psychopharmacology* **81,** 239–243.

Cuomo, V., Cortese, I., Cagiano, R., Renna, G., & Racagni, G. (1984) Behavioural changes in rats after prenatal administration of typical and atypical antidepressants, *Arch. Toxicol., Suppl.* **7,** 504–507.

Cuomo, V., Cagiano, R., Renna, G., Serinelli, A., Brunello, N., & Racagni, G. (1985) Comparative evaluation of the behavioural consequences of prenatal and early postnatal exposure to haloperidol in rats, *Neurobehav. Toxicol. Teratol.* **7,** 489–492.

DeHaven, D. L. & Mailman, R. B. (1986) The interactions of behavior and neurochemistry. In: *Neurobehavioral toxicology* (ed. Annau, Z.), The Johns Hopkins University Press, Baltimore, Maryland, 214–243.

Leonard, B. E. (1983) In: *Preclinical psychopharmacology* (eds Grahame-Smith, D. G. & Cowen, P. J.), Excerpta Medica, 248–299.

Racagni, G., Mocchetti, I., Renna, G., & Cuomo, V. (1982) *In vivo* studies on central noradrenergic synaptic mechanisms after acute and chronic antidepressant drug treatment: biochemical and behavioural comparison. *J. Pharmacol. Exp. Ther.* **223,** 227–234.

Racagni, G., Mocchetti, I., Brunello, N., Renna, G., & Cuomo, V. (1983) Early biochemical and behavioural changes after prolonged postnatal exposure to antidepressant drugs. In: *Application of behavioural pharmacology in toxicology* (eds Zbinden, G., Cuomo, V., Racagni, G., & Weiss, B.), Raven Press, N.Y., 161–172.

Riley, E. P. & Vorhees, C. V. (eds) (1986) *Handbook of behavioral teratology*, Plenum Press, N.Y.

Rosengarten, H. & Friedhoff, A. J. (1979) Enduring changes in dopamine receptor cells of pups from drug administration to pregnant and nursing rats, *Science* **203,** 1133–1135.

Zbinden, G., Cuomo, V., Racagni, G., & Weiss, B. (eds) (1983) *Application of behavioural pharmacology in toxicology*, Raven Press, N.Y.

7.6 Distribution of sodium and potassium channels in mammalian myelinated nerve fibres

Jürgen R. Schwarz†

(1) Membrane currents and action potentials were recorded from single myelinated nerve fibres isolated from the rat sciatic nerve.
(2) The ionic currents of a normal node of Ranvier consisted of sodium currents and unspecific leakage currents. In addition, there were potassium channels (K_1) which were in the open state at the resting potential.
(3) The time- and voltage-dependent parameters of the sodium currents were evaluated. They sufficed to compute action potentials which agreed with those measured.
(4) Acute paranodal and internodal demyelination uncovered potassium channels which were closed at the resting potential and were activated by a depolarization. At least three different populations of potassium channels were distinguished (K_{2-4}).

7.6.1 INTRODUCTION

Myelinated nerve fibres are designed to transmit action potentials from their site of origin at a receptor or a neuron to their target cells. Normal functioning of the nervous system presumes that this transmission of action potentials is performed with high reliability. This property is lost in nerve fibre diseases. Functional and structural changes of the myelin and/or the axolemma may lead to symptoms either caused by hyperexcitability or by a decrease or loss of excitability. To understand these pathophysiological conditions the physiology of mammalian nerve fibres has to be investigated.

Our understanding of the biophysical mechanisms underlying the generation of the action potential and its propagation along nerve fibres is based on the now classical experiments performed by Hodgkin & Huxley (1952) on the unmyelinated giant axon of the squid. In myelinated nerve fibres action potentials are generated only every 1–2 mm at the nodes of Ranvier (Tasaki 1953), and their conduction along the fibre is saltatory (Huxley & Stämpfli 1949). Voltage clamp experiments in frog myelinated nerve fibres showed that the ionic hypothesis of Hodgkin & Huxley (1952) is also valid to explain the generation of the action potential in these fibres (Frankenhaeuser & Huxley 1964). According to this hypothesis the upstroke of the

† Physiologisches Institut, UKE, Universität Hamburg, Martinistraße 52, D-2000 Hamburg 20, W. Germany

action potential is brought about by an autoregenerative opening of sodium channels, whereas repolarization is due to the closing of sodium channels and the opening of potassium channels. Until recently it was generally believed that the same ionic mechanisms were also responsible for repolarization of action potential in mammalian nerve fibres.

This was questioned by the results of voltage clamp experiments in rat (Brismar 1980) and rabbit (Chiu *et al.* 1979), which showed that in the mammalian node of Ranvier there were almost no voltage-dependent potassium channels. Furthermore, experiments with acute internodal demyelination (Chiu & Ritchie 1981) and with diabetic rats (Brismar 1979) demonstrated that voltage-dependent potassium channels of large amplitude are also present in mammalian nerve fibres but they normally occur only in the paranodal and internodal axolemma. Thus, in mammalian myelinated nerve fibres there is a segregation of ionic channels in correlation to myelination, sodium channels being confined to the nodal axolemma and the voltage-dependent potassium channels to the para- and internode.

7.6.2 IONIC CHANNELS

7.6.2.1 Nodal axolemma

Voltage and current clamp experiments were performed in single myelinated nerve fibres which had been isolated from the rat sciatic nerve (Nonner 1969). Fig. 1 compares two myelinated nerve fibres isolated from a rat (above) and a frog (below) nerve. Obviously, in rat the nodal gap is barely visible in contrast to that in the frog.

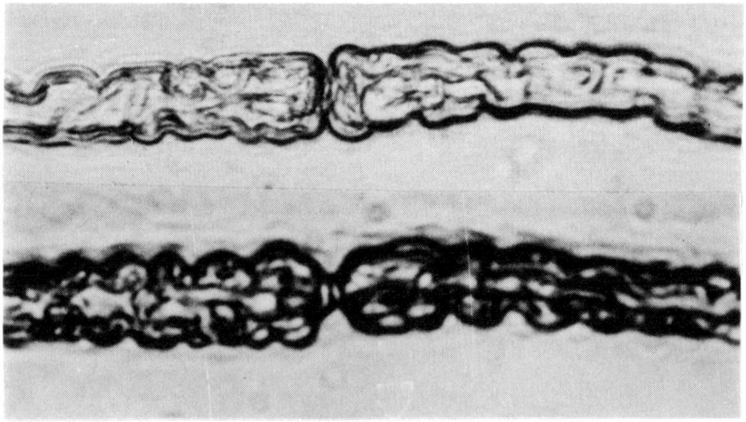

Fig. 1.—Single myelinated nerve fibres isolated from the sciatic nerve of a rat (above) and a frog (below). Note the narrow gap in the rat compared to that in the frog.

Fig. 2 shows a family of superimposed membrane currents. Each current trace was elicited by a depolarizing potential step and consisted of an initial short (about 20 μs) capacity current followed by a transient sodium current. The macroscopic sodium current, I_{Na}, can be described by the equation:

$$I_{Na} = m^3 h \cdot N \cdot \gamma_{Na}(V - V_{Na}),$$

where N denotes the number of the nodal sodium channels (about 20 000 in the rat

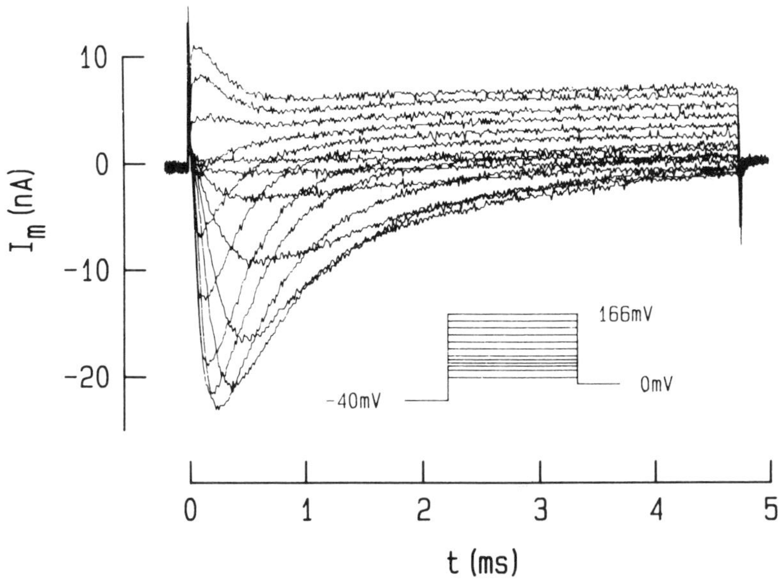

Fig. 2.—Membrane currents elicited by depolarizing potential steps of increasing amplitude. The depolarizing pulses were preceded by a 50 ms hyperpolarizing pulse of 40 mV to remove the resting sodium inactivation. No correction for capacity and leakage currents had been made. Temperature 20°C.

node (Neumcke & Stämpfli 1982) and Na the conductance of a single channel. $V - V_{Na}$is the driving force, given by the difference between the test potential V and the sodium equilibrium potential V_{Na}. The Hodgkin–Huxley expression m^3h denotes the probability for one channel to be in the open state, with m, activation and h, inactivation of the sodium channels. The exponent 3 allows for the delay in sodium current activation which is clearly visible in Fig. 2. A comparative study has shown that there are almost no differences in the activation and inactivation parameters of the macroscopic sodium currents of frog and rat nodes (Neumcke *et al.* 1987).

The sodium channel is a membrane-spanning protein, which now has been sequenced by deduction from the cDNA sequence of sodium channels from eel electroplax (Noda *et al.* 1984) and rat brain (Noda *et al.* 1986). The sodium channel protein can be in either of two states, open or closed. The probability (m^3h) to be in the open state is dependent on time and voltage. This is reflected by the time- and voltage-dependent macroscopic sodium currents. The sodium current is inwardly directed at $V < V_{Na}$ and reverses direction when the testpulse amplitude V exceeds the sodium equilibrium potential. The steady-state outward currents shown in Fig. 2 consist almost totally of unspecific leakage current. This is in contrast to frog myelinated nerve fibres in which voltage-dependent potassium currents of large amplitude are regularly present (see review of Stämpfli & Hille 1976).

The ionic hypothesis (Hodgkin & Huxley 1952) explains repolarization of the action potential by inactivation of sodium channels and by activation of potassium channels. In mammalian myelinated nerve fibres the kinetics of the sodium current suffice to explain the upstroke of the action potential. Provided that the sodium channels are closed, repolarization takes place almost instantaneously because of the

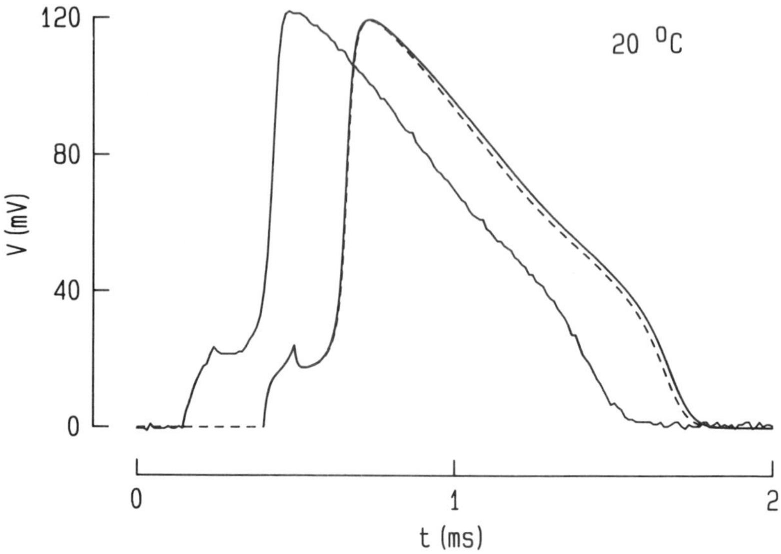

Fig. 3.—Action potential elicited by a 0.1 ms depolarizing current stimulus, temperature 20°C. Superimposed and shifted by 0.2 ms to the right were two computed action potentials. They were calculated with (dotted line) and without (smooth line) allowing for the small K permeability present in this particular fibre.

large resting leakage conductance. Fig. 3 presents a measured action potential and an action potential computed on the basis of the voltage clamp data of this particular fibre. The duration, amplitude, and shape of the recorded and the computed action potential are very similar. The amount of action potential shortening induced by the small potassium permeability present in this fibre is almost negligible (dotted line in Fig. 3; Schwarz & Eikhof 1987).

The resting conductance in mammalian myelinated nerve fibres is large, and is due to the large unspecific leakage conductance and to the large resting potassium conductance (Brismar & Schwarz 1985). The magnitude of the latter can be determined by increasing the driving force for potassium ions. This is illustrated in the left part of Fig. 4. After exchanging the Ringer for isotonic KCl solution a steady-state inward current of 4 nA occurred, indicating the existence of potassium channels which are in the open state at the normal resting potential. These channels could be blocked by tetraethylammoniumchlorid, or they could be closed upon a hyperpolarization (Schwarz & Röper 1988).

7.6.2.2 Paranodal axolemma

To characterize the paranodal potassium channels the paranode was demyelinated with 0.2% pronase. Superfusion of the node under investigation for 15 min resulted in loosening of the myelin until potassium currents of large amplitude occurred. These currents were activated and reached a steady state during a depolarizing potential step (right part of Fig. 4). Upon repolarization large tail currents occurred. Fig. 4 shows that the tail currents decreased with a multiexponential time course. Least squares fits yielded best results when at least three exponentials were used. In

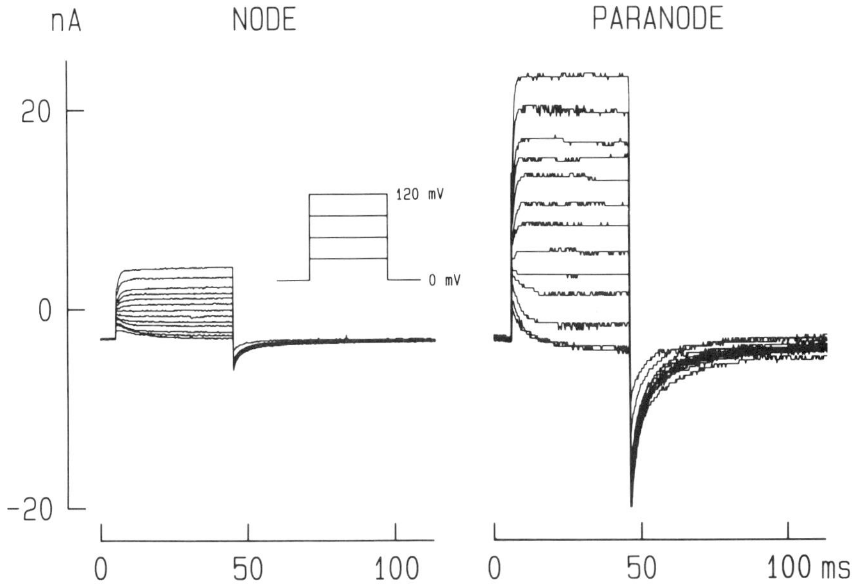

Fig. 4.—Membrane currents recorded in isotonic KCl solution before (left) and after (right) paranodal demyelination with 0.2% pronase. 300 nM tetrodotoxin were added to the solution to block Na channels.

addition to this kinetic separation, three types of potassium channels (K_{2-4}) could also be distinguished pharmacologically; for example, application of 1 mM 4-aminopyridine selectively blocked the fast tail current components. Furthermore, Fig. 4 shows that despite the increase in the exposed axolemma by paranodal demyelinization the steady-state inward current did not increase. The same was true in all other experiments in which demyelination was performed. From this one can conclude that the potassium channels which are open at the normal resting potential are confined to the nodal area and that they are not present in the axolemma covered by myelin. Furthermore, paranodal demyelination was never accompanied by an increase in the sodium current, indicating that sodium channels are concentrated in the nodal membrane.

7.6.3 CONCLUSION

Fig. 5 illustrates the distribution of ionic channels in the mammalian axolemma. Voltage-dependent sodium channels are located in high concentration only in the nodal area which in mammalian myelinated nerve fibres is about 20 μm^2. They are closed at the resting potential and opened by a depolarization, e.g. by local circuit current. They initiate the upstroke of the action potential, which has a duration of 0.25 ms at 37°C (Schwarz 1986). Quick repolarization is provided by the leakage conductance and the open K_1 channels. These open potassium channels may also be responsible for the high resting potential of about −80 mV (Brismar & Schwarz 1985).

Sodium, leakage, and K_1 channels which are responsible for the resting and action potential are confined to the nodal membrane. In contrast, the potassium channels

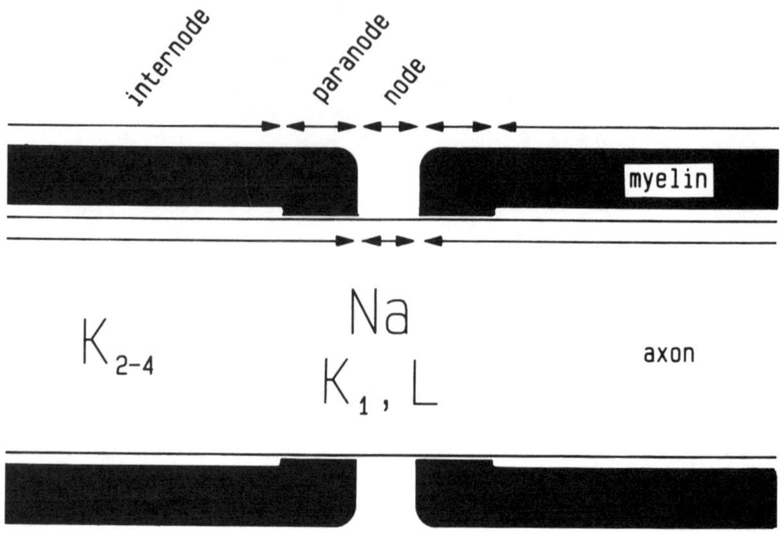

Fig. 5.—Schematic illustration of the segregation of ionic channels in the mammalian node–paranode region.

which have the properties of the classical axonal delayed rectifiers (Hille 1984) are located in the internode. At present, three populations of potassium channels were distinguished (K_{2-4}) by kinetic and pharmacological criteria which were equal to those described in the frog node (Dubois 1981). The functional significance of these paranodal and internodal potassium channels which are normally buried under the myelin is as yet unclear. They do not contribute to the resting potential and do not repolarize the action potential. Perhaps they could serve as a 'chemical' voltage clamp preventing the node to fire repetitively after an action potential. Furthermore, they may contribute in modulating the various states of hyperexcitability in pathological changes of excitability occurring in peripheral nerve fibre diseases. This point has to be established in experiments using isolated mammalian nerve fibres with structural changes either induced by chronic diseases or by chronic exposure to toxins.

REFERENCES

Brismar, T. (1979). Potential clamp experiments on myelinated nerve fibres from alloxan diabetic rats. *Acta Physiol. Scand.* **105**, 384–386.

Brismar, T. (1980). Potential clamp analysis of membrane currents in rat myelinated nerve fibres. *J. Physiol.* **298,** 171–184.

Brismar, T. & Schwarz, J. R. (1985). Potassium permeability in rat myelinated nerve fibres. *Acta Physiol. Scand.* **124,** 141–148.

Chiu, S. Y. & Ritchie, J. M. (1981). Evidence for the presence of potassium channels in the internodal region of acutely demyelinated mammalian single nerve fibres. *J. Physiol.* **313,** 415–437.

Chiu, S. Y., Ritchie, J. M., Rogart, R. B., & Stagg, D. (1979). A quantitative description of membrane currents in rabbit myelinated nerve. *J. Physiol.* **292,** 149–166.

Dubois, J. M. (1981). Evidence for the existence of three types of potassium channels in the frog ranvier node membrane. *J. Physiol.* **318,** 297–316.

Frankenhaeuser, B. & Huxley, A. F. (1964). The action potential in the myelinated nerve fibre of *Xenopus laevis* as computed on the basis of voltage clamp data. *J. Physiol.* **171,** 302–315.

Hille, B. (1984). *Ionic channels of excitable membranes.* Sinauer Associates, Inc., Sunderland, Massachusetts.

Hodgkin, A. L. &. Huxley, A. F. (1952). A quantitative description of membrane current and its application to conduction and excitation in nerve. *J. Physiol.* **117,** 500–544.

Huxley, A. F. & Stämpfli, R. (1949). Evidence for saltatory conduction in peripheral myelinated nerve fibres. *J. Physiol.* (Lond.) **108,** 315–339.

Neucmke, B. & Stämpfli, R. (1982). Sodium currents and sodium dependent fluctuations in rat myelinated nerve fibres. *J. Physiol.* **329,** 163–184.

Neumcke, B., Schwarz, J. R., & Stämpfli, R. (1987). A comparison of sodium currents in rat and frog myelinated nerve, normal and modified sodium inactivation. *J. Physiol.* **382,** 175–191.

Noda, M., Shimizu, S., Tanabe, T., Takai, T., Kayano, T., Ikeda, T., Takahashi, H., Nakayama, H., Kanaoka, Y., Minamina, N., Kangawa, K., Matsuo, H., Raftery, M. A., Hirose, T., Iniyama, S., Hayashida, H., Miyata, T., & Numa, S. (1984). Primary structure of *Electrophorus electricus* sodium channel deduced from cDNA sequence. *Nature* **312,** 121–127.

Noda, M., Ikeda, T., Suzuki, H., Takeshima, H., Takahashi, H., Kuno, M., & Numa, S. (1986). Expression of functional sodium channels from coned cDNA. *Nature* **322,** 826–828.

Nonner, W. (1969). A new voltage clamp method for Ranvier nodes. *Pflügers Arch.* **309,** 176–192.

Schwarz, J. R. (1986). The effect of temperature on Na currents in rat myelinated nerve fibres. *Pflügers Arch.* **406,** 397–404.

Schwarz, J. R. & Eikhof, G. (1987). Na currents and action potentials in rat myelinated nerve fibres at 20 and 37°C. *Pflügers Arch.* **409,** 569–577.

Schwarz, J. R. & Röper, J. (1988). Properties of nodal and paranodal K channels in rat myelinated nerve fibres. *Pflügers Arch.* (in press).

Stämpfli, R. & Hille, B. (1976). Electrophysiology of the peripheral nerve. In: Llinàs, R. & Precht, W., *Handbook of frog neurobiology*, 3–32. Springer, Berlin, Heidelberg, New York.

Tasaki, I. (1953). *Nervous transmission.* Springfield, Illinois, Charles C. Thomas.

7.7 Amino azaheterocycles: friend of foe?

J. W. Gorrod & S. P. Lam†

(1) Amino azaheterocycles occur widely as natural compounds and medicinal agents.
(2) These compounds may be metabolized at the exo-amino group to produce potential genotoxic hydroxylamines or at the ring nitrogen to form innocuous N-oxides.
(3) N-Hydroxylation appears to involve a high-spin cytochrome P-448 isozyme, whereas N-oxide formation is mediated by a phenobarbital inducible P-450 isozyme.
(4) Electronic, lipophilic, tautomeric, and stereochemical properties of these compounds have been considered as factors influencing the site of N-oxidation of amino azaheterocycles and hence their toxicity.

7.7.1 OCCURRENCE OF AMINO AZAHETEROCYCLES

The frequent occurrence of nitrogen in different forms and various structures in organic molecules has consequently attracted extensive metabolic studies on this chemical function (Gorrod 1978a, Gorrod & Damani 1985). The less often encountered but equally important group of compounds are the amino azaheterocycles, particularly those possessing an exo-amino group *ortho* to a ring nitrogen. The widespread existence of these compounds as natural products and as synthetic pharmacologically active medicinal agents has, nevertheless demonstrated their importance (Fig. 1). These compounds include the natural occurring vitamin thiamine and the nucleic acid bases adenine, guanine, and cytosine. A large number of drugs also possess this structure and cover a wide spectrum of pharmacological activities: the anti-anaemic, folic acid; the antimalarials, pyrimethamine and cycloguanil; the broad spectrum antibacterial, cefotaxime; the antileprotic, thiazolesulphone; the new anti-hypertensive, SM-2470; the diuretics, triamterene and amiloride; the respiratory stimulant, amiphenazole; and the muscle relaxant, zoxazolamine, are a few examples.

The repeated occurrence of the structure consisting of an amino group which is directly attached to a carbon next to a ring nitrogen in a heteroaromatic system is of metabolic significance, as biotransformation of this part of the molecule may have pharmacologically desirable or undesirable toxic effects. The frequency of amino azaheterocycles occurring as medicinal compounds is greatly increased if those which are formed after metabolic conversion of the parent drugs are included. Cussans *et al.* (1986) reported that the anti-hypertensive agent, doxazosin, was metabolically converted to the 2-amino product. A similar situation where a piperazine ring was

† Chelsea Department of Pharmacy, King's College London, Chelsea Campus, University of London, Manresa Road, London SW3 6LX, UK

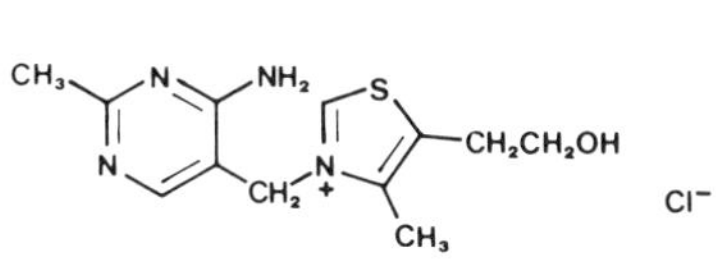

Thiamine
Vitamin

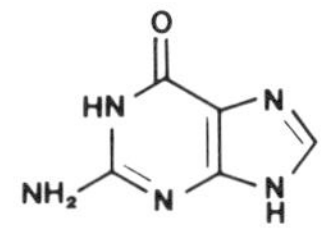

Guanine
Nucleic acid base

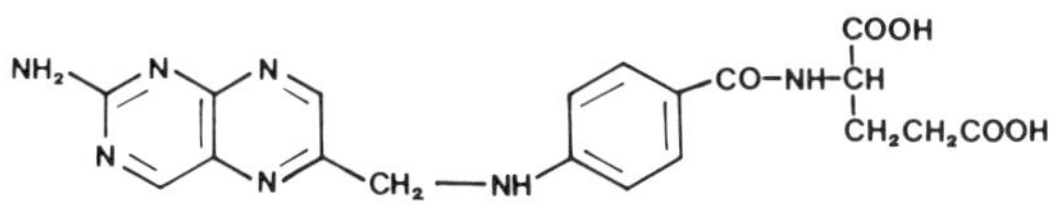

Folic Acid
Anti-anaemic

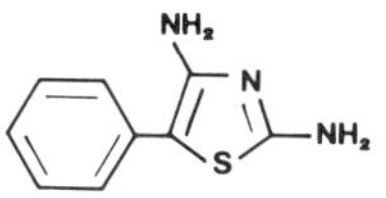

Amiphenazole
Respiratory Stimulant

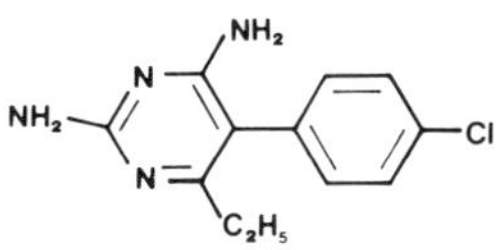

Pyrimethamine
Antimalarial

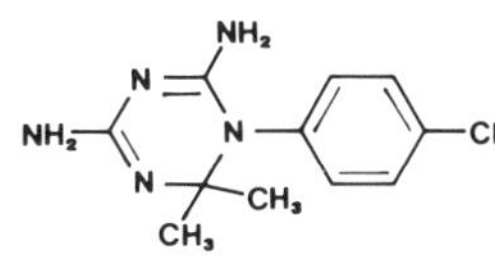

Cycloguanil
Antimalarial

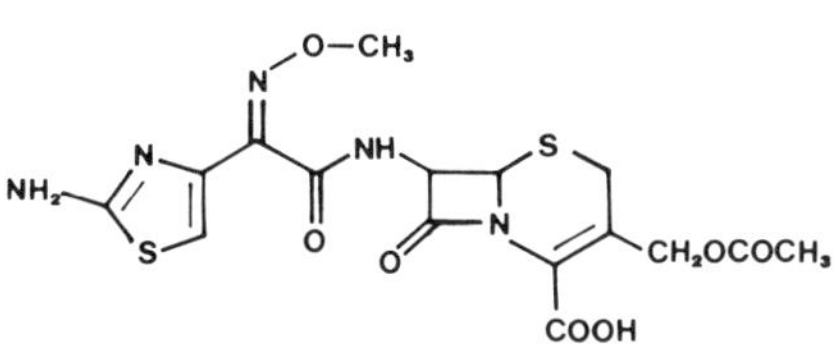

Cefotaxime
Antibacterial

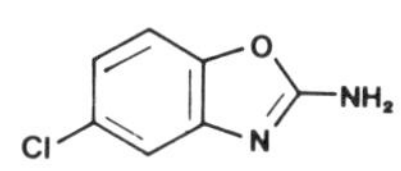

Zoxazolamine
Muscle Relaxant

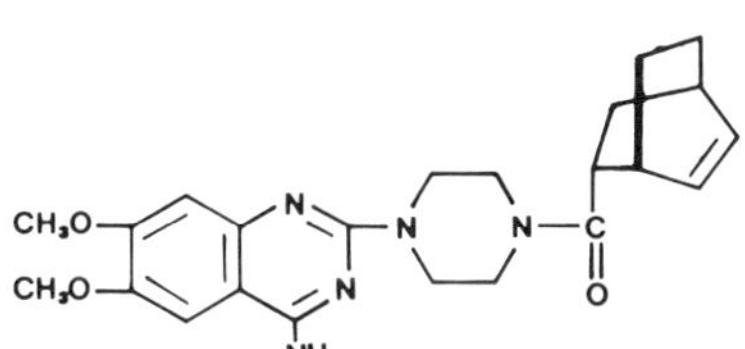

SM-2470
Anti-hypertensive

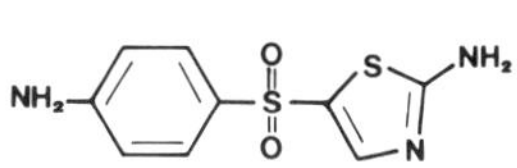

Thiazolesulphone
Antileprotic

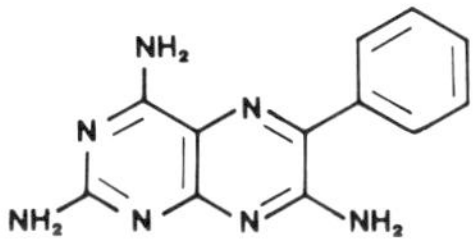

Triamterene
Diuretic

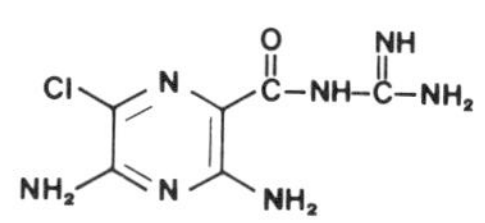

Amiloride
Diuretic

Fig. 1.—Some medicinal amino azaheterocyclic compounds

metabolized to release the amino azaheterocyclic moiety of the drug VK 774 was reported by Prox *et al.* (1973). Piromidic acid was metabolized at the pyrrolidine ring to form the amino metabolite (Sekine *et al.* 1976). Another process by which amino azaheterocycles may be formed is by metabolic cyclization as occurs during the metabolism of proguanil (Crowther & Levi 1953) (Fig. 2).

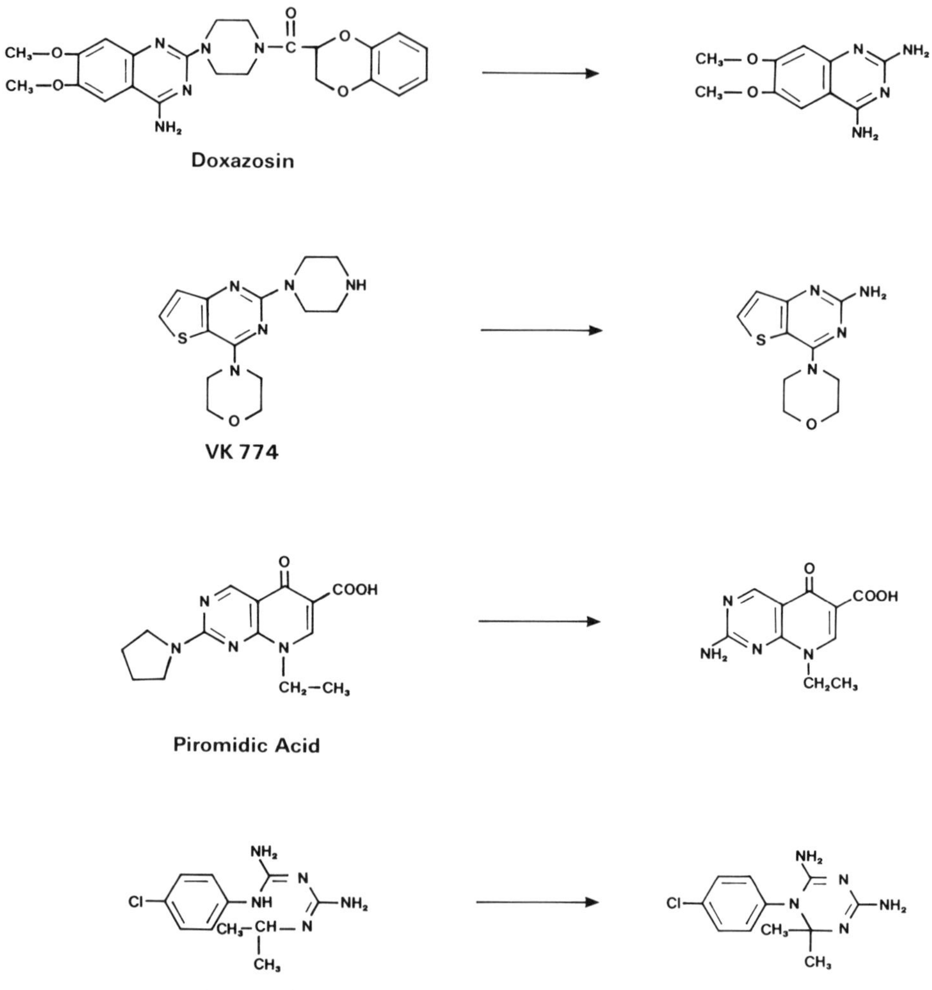

Fig. 2.—Examples of amino azaheterocycles formed from medicinal compounds following metabolic transformation

Amino azaheterocycles are also detected in charred meat and broiled fish, and in pyrolysates of protein and amino acids (Sugimura & Nagao 1979, Sugimura & Sato 1983). It was shown that many of this group of compounds have mutagenic activity very much higher than, or comparable to, many typical carcinogens when examined in the presence of a metabolic oxidizing system (Table 1). These discoveries led to an increasing concern of a potential hazard derived from food. Ishida *et al.*

Table 1—Mutagenic activities of mutagens isolated from pyrolysis products in comparison with typical carcinogens

Test compounds	Mutagenic activity (revertants/μg) TA98
Pyrolysis products	
MeIQ	661 000
IQ	433 000
Trp-P-2	104 200
Glu-P-1	49 000
Trp-P-1	39 000
Glu-P-2	1 900
AαC	300
MeAαC	200
Lys-P-1	86
Phe-P-1	41
Typical carcinogens	
AF-2	6 500
Aflatoxin B_1	6 000
4-Nitroquinoline 1-oxide	970
Benao[*a*]pyrene	320
Diethylnitrosamine	0.02

Note: Mutagenicity was tested with optimal amount of 9000 × *g* supernatant fraction of liver from PCB-treated rats (Kato 1986)

(1987) reported that in the presence of liver S-9 obtained from rhesus monkey, the compound with strongest mutagenic activity was MeIQ (2-amino-3,4-diethylimidazo-[4,5-f]quinoline). This and another mutagenic compound IQ (2-amino-3-methyl-imidazo[4,5-f]quinoline) were first isolated from broiled sardines (Kasai *et al.* 1980a,b). Felton *et al.* (1984) isolated at least ten mutagenic amino azaheterocycles from fried ground beef in which the major mutagen was identified as MeIQx (2-amino-3,8-dimethylimidazo[4,5-f]quinoxaline). 7,8-DiMeIQx (2-amino-3,7,8-trimethylimidazo[4,5-f]quinoxaline) formation was demonstrated by Negishi *et al.* (1984) during the pyrolysis of a mixture of creatinine, glycine, and glucose. This compound was shown to be fifteen times more potent in mutagenic activity than MeIQx in the same system using a liver preparation from rhesus monkey for metabolic activation. Amino acid pyrolysates contain another group of mutagenic compounds, Trp-P-1 (3-amino-1,4-dimethyl-5H-pyrido[4,3-b]indole) and Trp-P-2 (3-amino-1-methyl-5H-pyrido[4,3-b]indole) and are produced during tryptophan pyrolysis (Sugimura *et al.* 1977), while Glu-P-1 (2-amino-6-methyldipyrido-[1,2-a:3′,2′-d]-imidazole) and Glu-P-2 (2-aminodipyrido[1,2-a:3′,2′-d]imidazole) are products of glutamic acid pyrolysis (Yamamoto *et al.* 1978). These amino azaheterocycles, when given to rats and mice, have been shown to be carcinogenic as well as mutagenic in the bacterial test system (Sugimura 1985). Recently, Felton *et al.* (1986) isolated from fried ground beef a new mutagen which was identified as PhIP (2-amino-1-methyl-6-phenylimidazo-[4,5-b]pyridine). PhIP possibly represents a new class of mutagenic amino azaheterocycles belonging to the amino-imidazoazaarenes. Although PhIP is not as mutagenic as other compounds isolated, it is the most abundant mutagenic compound in fried ground beef (Fig. 3).

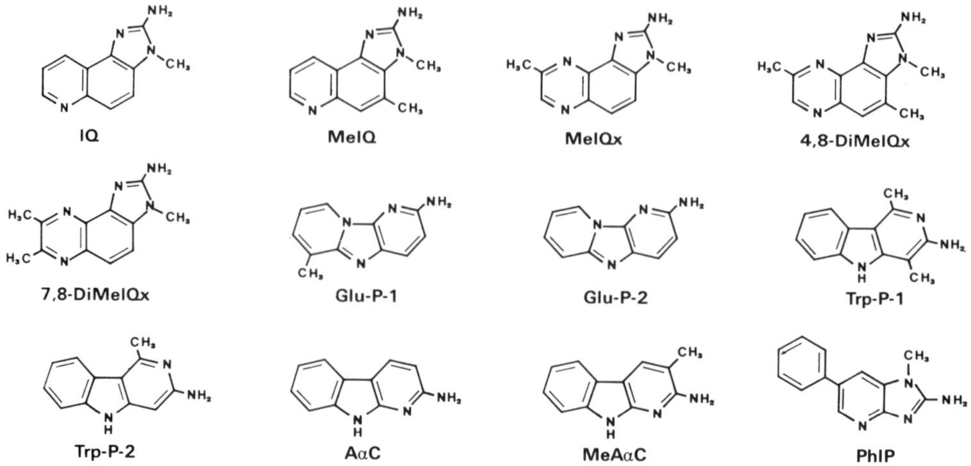

Fig. 3.—Chemical structures of mutagenic amino azaheterocycles

7.7.2 AMINO AZAHETEROCYCLES METABOLIZED TO GENOTOXIC HYDROXYLAMINES

It is important to realize that these compounds are not themselves mutagens, but require metabolic activation by a microsomal system to produce a mutagenic effect (Nemoto *et al.* 1979). Investigations of the enzymology of this process revealed that a cytochrome P-450 isozyme was involved, and that all these amino azaheterocycles were N-oxidized at the exo-amino group to produce mutagenic hydroxylamines (Yamazoe *et al.* 1980, Hashimoto *et al.* 1980, Kato *et al.* 1983, Nagao *et al.* 1983) (Fig. 4). Studies using various specific enzyme inhibitors, inducers, and purified enzymes strongly suggested that the P-448 isoenzymes of cytochrome P-450 were largely responsible for metabolically N-hydroxylating these compounds (Kawajiri *et al.* 1983). Kamataki *et al.* (1983), using purified low and high spin forms of the P-448 species, demonstrated that the high-spin form was capable of N-hydroxylating the amino azaheterocycles, whereas the low-spin form, which was responsible for

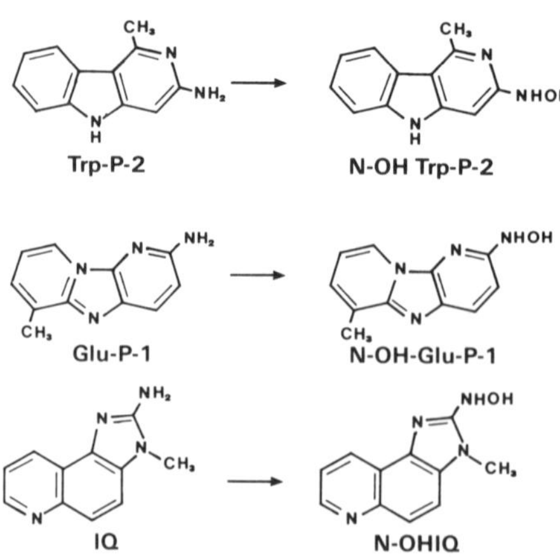

Fig. 4.—Amino azaheterocycles converted to genotoxic hydroxylamines

metabolically activating benzo[a]pyrenes and other aromatic hydrocarbons (Ryan *et al.* 1979), showed low activity in the N-hydroxylation of these amino azaheterocycles. Another study by Yamazoe *et al.* (1984) further substantiated the involvement of the high-spin form of P-448 in the N-hydroxylation process. Metabolic activation of mutagenic amino azaheterocycles has been reviewed by Kato (1986).

7.7.3 AMINO AZAHETEROCYCLES METABOLIZED TO INNOCUOUS N-OXIDES

Other amino azaheterocyclic compounds have apparently no mutagenic and/or carcinogenic activity, and are widely used in medicinal compounds (Fig. 1). Amongst this group are the 2,4-diaminopyrimidines which include the anticancer agent metoprine (2,4-diamino-5-(3,4-dichlorophenyl)-6-methylpyrimidine), and antimalarial pyrimethamine (2,4-diamino-5-(p-chlorophenyl)-6-ethylpyrimidine), and the anti-bacterial trimethoprim (2,4-diamino-5-(3,4,5-trimethoxybenzyl)pyrimidine). These are all inhibitors of dihydrofolate reductase (Hubbel *et al.* 1978, Meshi & Sato 1972, Sykes & Schwalbe 1987). These drugs are highly lipid-soluble, a property which appears to be essential for their activity. Early *in vivo* metabolic studies on these compounds reported that N-oxidation occurred at the ring nitrogens to form N-1 or N-3 oxides (Fig. 5) (Sigel 1973, Sigel & Brent 1973, Brooks *et al.* 1973, Hubbel

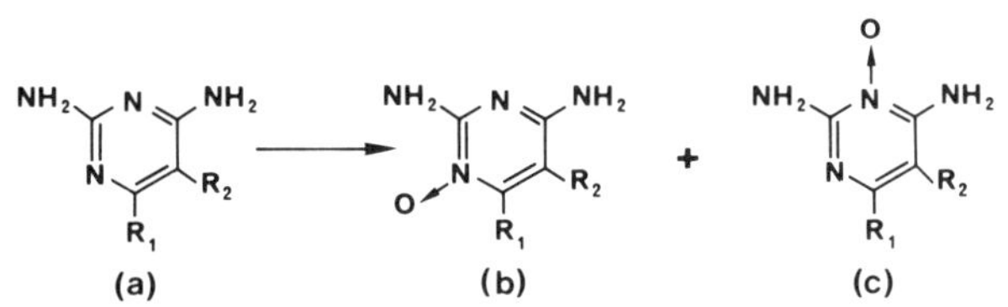

		R_1	R_2
1.	Trimethoprim (a)	H	3,4,5-trimethoxybenzyl
2.	Metoprine (a)	CH_3	3,4-dichlorophenyl
3.	Pyrimethamine (a)	C_2H_5	4-chlorophenyl

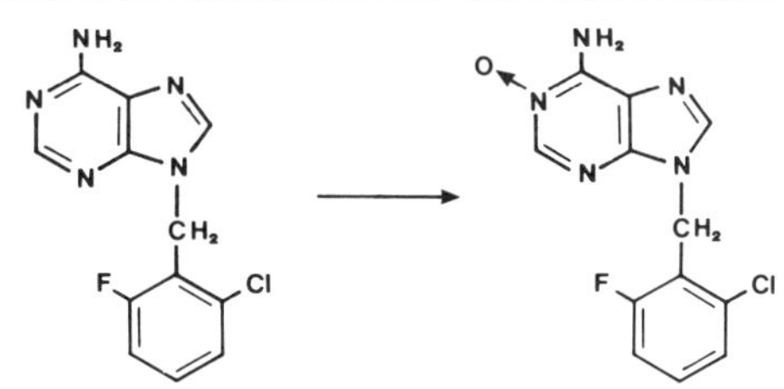

Arprinocid

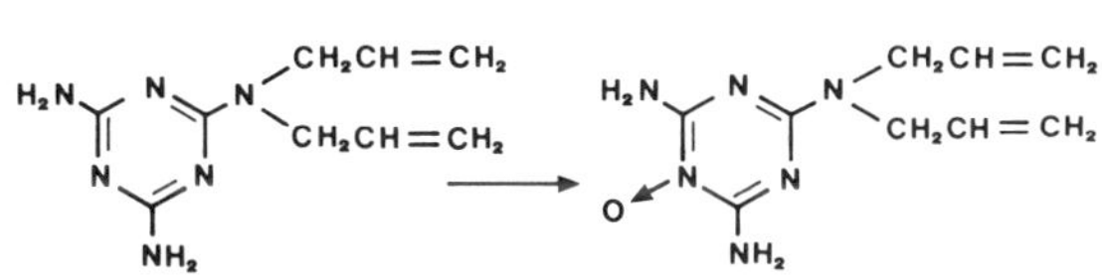

Diallylmelamine

Fig. 5.—Amino azaheterocycles converted to innocuous amine oxides

et al. 1978, Hubbel *et al.* 1980). Another example is N,N-diallylmelamine which causes vasodilation in rats and dogs with only a marginal response in man. The effect is delayed and is due to the metabolic production of the N-oxide (Fig. 5) (Zins 1965, Zins *et al.* 1968). The anticoccidial agent arprinocid (6-amino-9-(2-chloro-6-fluoro-benzyl)purine) was found to yield the N-oxide as minor metabolite. It was later confirmed that the N-oxide was the active cocciostatic agent (Fig. 5) (Wolf *et al.* 1978, Wang & Simashkevich 1980). Another example of an amino azaheterocyclic drug in which the N-oxide is an active compound is minoxidil (2,4-diamino-6-piperidinopyrimidine-N-3-oxide) (Fig. 6). This is an effective hypotensive compound in rats, dogs, monkeys, and humans (Thomas & Harpoolian 1975). This is an example of a synthetic N-oxide being used as a drug.

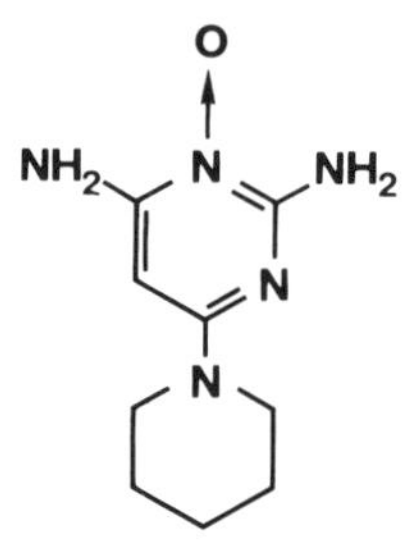

Fig. 6.—Structure of the hypotensive medicinal agent minoxidil

These examples confirm the general observation that N-oxidation at a nitrogen in a ring results in a product which is non-genotoxic to the host system, whereas N-oxidation at an exo-amino group results in the formation of a hydroxylamine with extremely potent toxic effects.

7.7.4 FACTORS AFFECTING N-OXIDATION OF AMINO AZAHETEROCYCLES

It can be seen that a situation exists where very similar molecules are being metabolized by similar processes and yet different types of products, with different toxicological properties, are formed (Fig. 7). Gorrod (1985) proposed that amine–imine

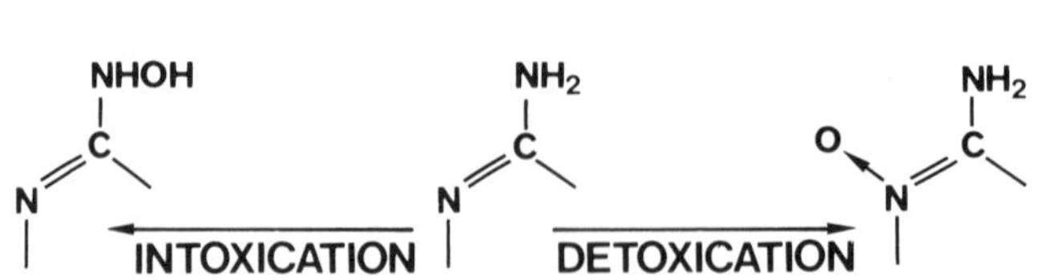

Fig. 7.—Metabolic pathways of amino azaheterocycles to hydroxylamine or amine-oxide

tautomerism could be a determinant of the site of N-oxidation of amino azaheterocycles. It was suggested that the substrate binds at a different orientation with different isozymes to produce various products; binding of the substrate with the enzyme at the exo-amino group would lead to N-oxidation at the basic ring nitrogen, whereas binding at the ring nitrogen might induce the exo-amino group to tautomerize to the more basic imino form which could then be oxidized to produce the hydroxylamine. Our laboratory has been interested in elucidating the physico-chemical as well as structural factors which determine the site of N-oxidation of amino azaheterocycles. Watkins & Gorrod (1987) investigated the *in vitro* N-oxidation of 5-substituted 2,4-diaminopyrimidines. Using hepatic microsomes from various species it was found that N-oxidation of trimethoprim occurred at the ring nitrogens and that both 1- and 3-trimethoprim-N-oxides were formed. In the case of the 6-substituted 2,4-diaminopyrimidines (El-Ghomari & Gorrod 1987), only the 3-N-oxides of some substrates were detected. We have also looked at the microsomal N-oxidation of 9-substituted 6-aminopurines (Lam *et al.* 1987). These investigations revealed that only a ring nitrogen next to an exo-amino group was N-oxidized, suggesting the involvement of the exo-nitrogen. In the study of 6-substituted 2,4-diaminopyrimidines, the 3-N-oxides of 6-piperidino-, 6-diethylamino-, 6-morpholino-, 6-methyl-, and 6-chloro-substituted 2,4-diaminopyrimidines were formed. However, no N-oxidative metabolite of the 6-hydroxy-, 6-amino-, and unsubstituted 2,4-diaminopyrimidines or melamine was detected. El-Ghomari & Gorrod (1988) thus examined the pKa of these compounds, and the data obtained indicated that pKa alone could not have accounted for the difference in the N-oxidation results. The pKa values for 6-methyl-, 6-diethylamino-, 6-piperidino-, and 6-morpholino-substituted 2,4-diaminopyrimidines which form 3-N-oxides are 7.62, 7.41, 7.05, and 6.63 respectively. These values are not dissimilar from those of the 6-amino (pKa = 6.93) and unsubstituted (pKa = 7.33) 2,4-diaminopyrimidines which do not form N-oxides. Furthermore, the pKa of 6-chloro-2,4-diaminopyrimidine, which forms a 3-N-oxide, is 3.55 and is not much different from the non N-oxidizable 6-hydroxy derivative (pKa = 3.81). These observations suggest that although the basicity of the nitrogen atom is important in N-oxidation generally (Gorrod 1978b), it does not seem to be the sole determining factor when considering the amino azaheterocycles.

In fact, these metabolic results have possible implications for the involvement of amine–imine tautomerism in these compounds; the lack of hydrogen on the tertiary amino group substituted on position 6 of diethylamino-, piperidino-, and morpholino-substituted compounds suppresses the formation of any imino tautomeric form associated with the 1-N position. This phenomenon always seems to be associated with an ability to form a 3-N-oxide. In other analogues i.e. where $6 = NH_2$ or OH, it appears that tautomerism at the 1-N-position (Fig. 8) produces a redistribution of electrons and so suppresses 3-N-oxidation. In this respect, it is particularly relevant to note that 2-N,N-diallylmelamine forms the 5-N-oxide in rats, dogs, and man (Zins 1965, Zins *et al.* 1968) whereas melamine does not. However, the role of tautomerism needs careful assessment as it has also been reported that the 2-N-allylmelamine, a substrate having a proton on the secondary amino group and therefore capable of tautomerism, formed a 5-N-oxide in the rat (Zins *et al.* 1968).

The lipophilicity of these 6-substituted 2,4-diaminopyrimidines has also been measured. The partition coefficients of these compounds obtained indicated that the compounds which form the 3-N-oxides are lipophilic, whereas the ones which do not yield the N-oxides are hydrophilic when measured in a water/octanol system. Lipophilicity appears also to be an essential characteristic in relation to N-oxide formation in the metabolism of 9-substituted aminopurines (Lam *et al.* 1987). The hydrophilic adenine and 9-methyladenine are not N-oxidized, whereas the lipophilic

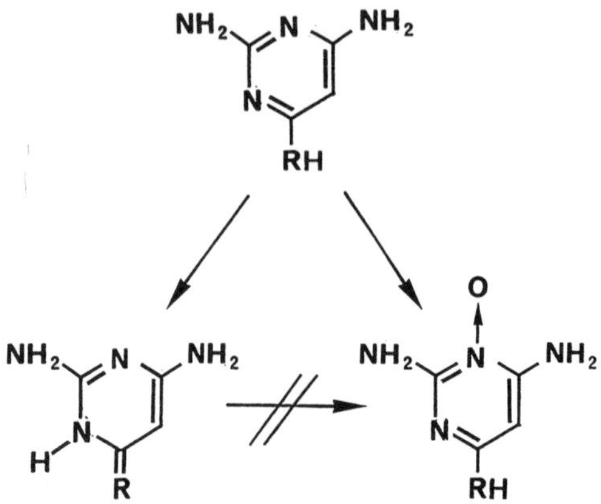

Fig. 8.—Role of tautomerism in the 3-N oxidation of 6-substituted 2,4-diaminopyrimidines

9-benzyl-, and 9-benzhydryladenines form the 1-N-oxides. However, the highly lipophilic 9-trityladenine does not form the 1-N-oxide, indicating that other factors are involved.

We have investigated the possible correlation of the stereochemical properties of 9-substituted adenines and their 1-N-oxidation using computer graphic modelling and ^{1}H NMR techniques. The results obtained suggest that 9-benzyl- and 9-benzhydryladenines, which are N-oxidized, have similar favourable conformations which are not found in the other non N-oxidizable analogues (Lam, Barlow & Gorrod 1989).

The possible relation of N-electron density and its oxidizability of pyridine and pyrimidine was discussed by Gorrod (1987). Webb (1986) further calculated the 'lone pair availability' as the ratio of lone pair probability on N to the lone pair energy on N for 2-aminopyridine and 2-aminopyrimidine. It was found that in 2-aminopyridine, the 'lone pair availability' index values were 0.961 and 0.714 for the ring nitrogen and the exo-amino nitrogen respectively, suggesting that the ring nitrogen should oxidize before the exo-amino group. Similarly for 2-aminopyrimidine, values of 0.697 and 0.786 were obtained for the ring and exo-amino nitrogens respectively, implying a reverse situation to that found for 2-aminopyridine. These two sets of values are in good agreement with the general observations that the ring nitrogen of pyridine compounds are more susceptible to N-oxidation than pyrimidine compounds (Katritsky & Lagowski 1971, Cowan *et al.* 1978, Gorrod & Damani 1979a,b, Wareing 1983). It is of course too early to postulate or extrapolate these results to structurally more complicated amino azaheterocycles. Nevertheless, this method may provide useful information as to the factors influencing the site of N-oxidation of these compounds.

Studies on the enzymology of these processes in our laboratory indicated that a phenobarbital-inducible form of cytochrome P-450 was involved in the formation of these N-oxides (Gorrod 1987, El-Ghomari & Gorrod 1987, Lam *et al.* 1987, Watkins & Gorrod 1987). This cytochrome species is different from the high-spin form of P-448 which is believed to be responsible for the metabolic N-hydroxylation of amino azaheterocycles derived from amino acid pyrolysates and responsible for their mutagenic activation (Kamataki *et al.* 1983, Yamazoe *et al.* 1984).

We do not yet have sufficient evidence to conclude which are the controlling factors which determine the site of N-oxidation of amino azaheterocycles. Experiments designed to investigate these factors are in progress, as it would be of tremendous value in drug design if we can predict the factors that determine whether a potential drug candidate is metabolized by the P-450 or P-448 isoenzymes to an innocuous N-oxide or a genotoxic hydroxylamine. Until such time, we have to accept that 'Amino azaheterocycles: can be either a friend or foe'.

ACKNOWLEDGEMENTS

The authors acknowledge the permission to use unpublished data from K. El-Ghomari. S.P.L. wishes to thank the Croucher Foundation for a Scholarship and the ORS scheme for an award.

REFERENCES

Brooks, M. A., de Silva, J. A. F., & D'Arconte L. (1973). Determination of trimethoprim and its N-oxide metabolites in urine of man, dog and rat by differential pulse polarography. *J. Pharm. Sci.* **62,** 1776–1779.

Cowan, D. A., Damani, L. A., & Gorrod, J. W. (1978). Metabolic N-oxidation of 3-substituted pyridines: identification of products by mass spectrometry, *Biomedical Mass Spectrometry* **5,** 551–556.

Crowther, A. F., & Levi, A. A. (1953). Proguanil—the isolation of a metabolite with high antimalarial activity, *Brit. J. Pharmacol.* **8,** 93–97.

Cussans, N. J., Kaye, B., Faulkner, J. K., & Stopher, D. A. (1986). The metabolism and kinetics of doxazosin in man, rat, mouse and dog. In: *Development of drugs and modern medicines* (eds Gorrod, J. W., Gibson, G. G., & Mitchard, M.), Ellis Horwood Ltd, Chichester, U.K. p. 527–537.

El-Ghomari, K. & Gorrod, J. W. (1987). Metabolic N-oxygenation of 2,4-diamino-6-substituted pyrimidines, *Europ. J. Drug Metab. Pharmacokin.* **12,** 253–258.

El-Ghomari, K. & Gorrod, J. W. (1988). Unpublished Data.

Felton, J. S., Knize, M. G., Shen, N. H., Lewis, P. R., Andersen, B. D., Happe, J., & Hatch, F. T. (1986). The isolation and identification of a new mutagen from fried ground beef: 2-amino-1-methyl-6-phenylimidazo[4,5-b]pyridine (PhIP), *Carcinogenesis* **7,** 1081–1086.

Felton, J. S., Knize, M. G., Wood, C., Wuebbles, B. J., Healy, S. K., Stuermer, D. H., Bjeldanes, L. F., Kimble, B. J., & Hatch, F. T. (1984). Isolation and characterization of new mutagens from fried ground beef, *Carcinogenesis* **5,** 95–102.

Gorrod, J. W. (1978a). *Biological oxidation of nitrogen*, Elsevier, Amsterdam.

Gorrod, J. W. (1978b). The current status of pKa concept in the differentiation of enzymic N-oxidation. In: *Biological oxidation of nitrogen* (ed. Gorrod, J. W.). Elsevier, Amsterdam, p. 201–210.

Gorrod, J. W. (1985). Amine–imine tautomerism as a determinant of the site of biological N-oxidation. In: *Biological oxidation of nitrogen in organic molecules* (eds Gorrod, J. W. & Damani, L. A.). Ellis Horwood Ltd, Chichester, UK. p. 219–230.

Gorrod, J. W. (1987). The *in vitro* metablism of amino azaheterocycles. In: *Drug metabolism from molecules to man* (eds Benford, D. J., Bridges J. W., & Gibson, G. G.). Taylor & Francis, London, p. 456–461.

Gorrod, J. W. & Damani, L. A. (1979a). Some factors involved in the N-oxidation of 3-substituted pyridines by microsomal preparations *in vitro*. *Xenobiotica* **9,** 209–218.

Gorrod, J. W. & Damani, L. A. (1979b). The effect of various potential inhibitors, activators and inducers on the N-oxidation of 3-substituted pyridines *in vitro*. *Xenobiotica* **9,** 219–226.

Gorrod, J. W. & Damani, L. A. (1985). *Biological oxidation of nitrogen in organic molecules*, Ellis Horwood Ltd, Chichester, UK.

Hashimoto, Y., Shudo, K., & Okamoto, T. (1980). Activation of a mutagen, 3-amino-1-methyl-5H-pyrido[4,3-b]indole. Identification of 3-hydroxyamino-1-methyl-5H-pyrido[4,3-b]indole and its reaction with DNA, *Biochem. Biophys. Res. Commun.* **96,** 355–362.

Hubbel, J. P., Henning, M. L., Grace, M. E., Nichol, C. A., & Sigel, C. W. (1978). N-Oxide metabolites of the 2,4-diaminopyrimidine inhibitors of dihydrofolate reductase, trimethoprim, pyrimethamine and metoprine. In: *Biological oxidation of nitrogen* (ed Gorrod, J. W.), Elsevier, Amsterdam, p. 177–182.

Hubbel, J. P., Kao, C. J., Sigel, C. W., & Nichol, C. A. (1980). Sex dependent disposition of metoprine by mice. In: *Current chemotherapy and infectious disease* (eds Nelson, J. D. & Grassi, C.), American Society for Microbiology, Washington, p. 1620–1621.

Ishida, Y., Negishi, C., Umemoto, A., Fujita, Y., Sato, S., Sugimura, T., Thorgeirsson, S. S., & Adamson, R. H. (1987). Activation of mutagenic and carcinogenic heterocyclic amines by S-9 from the liver of a Rhesus monkey, *Toxic. in Vitro* **1,** 45–48.

Kamataki, T., Maeda, K., Yamazoe, Y., Matsuda, N., Ishii, K., & Kato, R. (1983). A high spin form of cytochrome P-450 highly purified from polychlorinated biphenyl-treated rats, *Mol. Pharmacol.* **24,** 146–155.

Kasai, H., Yamaizumi, Z., Wakabayashi, K., Nagao, M., Sugimura, T., Yokoyama, S., Miyazawa, T., Springam, N. E., Weisburger, J. H., & Nishimura, S. (1980a). Potent novel mutagens produced by broiling fish under normal conditions, *Proc. Jpn. Acad. Ser. B* **46,** 278–283.

Kasai, H., Yamaizumi, Z., Wakabayashi, K., Nagao, M., Sugimura, T., Yokoyama, S., Miyazawa, T., & Nishmura, S. (1980b). Structure and chemical synthesis of Me-IQ, a potent mutagen isolated from broiled fish, *Chem. Lett.* p. 1391–1394.

Kato, R. (186). Metabolic activation of mutagenic heterocyclic aromatic amines from protein pyrolysates, *CRC Crit. Rev. Toxicol.* **16,** 307–347.

Kato, R., Kamataki, T., & Yamazoe, Y. (1983). N-Hydroxylation of carcinogenic and mutagenic aromatic amines, *Environ. Health Perspct.* **49,** 21–25.

Katritsky, A. R. & Lagowski, J. M. (1971). *Chemistry of the heterocyclic N-oxides*. Academic Press, London, UK.

Kawajiri, K., Yonehawa, H., Gotoh, O., Wantanabe, J., Igarashi, S., & Tagashira, Y. (1983). Contributions of two inducible forms of cytochrome P-450 in rat liver microsomes of the metabolic activation of various chemical carcinogens, *Cancer Res.* **43,** 819–823.

Lam, S. P., Devinsky, F., & Gorrod, J. W. (1987). Biological N-oxidation of adenine and 9-alkyl derivatives, *Europ. J. Drug Metab. Pharmacokin.* **12,** 239–243.

Lam, S. P., Barlow, D. J., & Gorrod, J. W. (1989). Conformational analysis of 9-substituted adenines in relation to their microsomal 1-N-oxidation. *J. Pharm. Pharmacol.* (in press).

Meshi, T. & Sato, Y. (1972). Studies on sulfamethoxaole/trimethoprim. Absorption, distribution, excretion and metabolism of trimethoprim in rat, *Chem. Pharm. Bull. (Japan)* **20,** 2079–2090.

Nagao, N., Fujita, Y., Wakabayashi, K., & Sugimura, T. (1983). Ultimate forms of mutagenic and carcinogenic heterocyclic amines produced by pyrolysis, *Biochem. Biophys. Res. Commun.* **114,** 626–631.

Negishi, C., Wakabayashi, K., Tsuda, M., Sato, S., Sugimura, T., Saito, H., Maeda, M., & Jagerstad, M. (184). Formation of 2-amino-3,7,8-trimethylimidazo[4,5-f]-quinoxaline, a new mutagen, by heating a mixture of creatinine, glucose and glycine, *Mutat. Res.* **140,** 55–59.

Nemoto, N., Kusumi, S., Takayama, S., Nagao, M., & Sugimura, T. (1979). Metabolic activation of 3-amino-5H-pyrido[4,3-b]indole, a highly mutagenic principle in tryptophan pyrolysate, by rat liver enzymes, *Chem. Biol. Interact.* **27,** 191–198.

Prox. A., Zimmer, A., & Machleidt, H. (1973). Rapid structure elucidation of drug metabolites by use of stable isotopes, *Xenobiotica* **3,** 103–112.

Ryan, D. E., Thomas, P. E., Karzenlowski, D., & Levin, W. (1979). Separation and characterization of highly purified forms of liver microsomal cytochrome P-450 from rats treated with polychlorinated biphenyls, phenobarbital, and 3-methylcholanthrene, *J. Biol. Chem.* **254,** 1365–1374.

Sekine, Y., Miyamoto, M., Hashimoto, M., & Nakamura, K. (1976). Metabolism in rats and man of piromidic acid, a new antibacterial agent, *Xenobiotica* **6,** 185–198.

Sigel, C. W. (1973). Metabolism of trimethoprim in man and measurement of a new metabolite: a new fluorescence assay, *J. Infec. Dis. Suppl.* **128,** 580–583.

Sigel, C. W., & Brent, D. A. (1973). Identification of trimethoprim 3-N-oxide as a new urinary metabolite of trimethoprim in man. *J. Pharm. Sci.* **62,** 694–695.

Sugimura, T. (1985). Carcinogenicity of mutagenic heterocyclic amines formed during the cooking process, *Mutat. Res.* **150,**33–41.

Sugimura, T., Kawachi, T., Nagao, M., Yahagi, T., Seino, Y., Okamoto, T., Shudo, K., Kosuge, T., Tsuji, K., Wakabayashi, K., Itaka, Y., & Itai, A. (1977). Mutagenic principle(s) in tryptophan and phenylalanine pyrolysis products, *Proc. Jpn. Acad.* **53,** 58–61.

Sugimura, T., & Nagao, M. (1979). Mutagenic factors in cooked foods, *CRC Crit. Rev. Toxicol.* **8,** 189–209.

Sugimura, T., & Sato, S. (1983). Mutagens–carcinogens in foods, *Cancer Res.* **43,** 2415s–2421s.

Sykes, G., & Schwalbe, C. H. (1987). Preferred conformations of pyrimethamine and triamterene with impications for binding to dihydrofolate reductase, *J. Pharm. Pharmacol.* **39s,** 114p.

Thomas, R. C., & Hartpoolian, H. (1975). Metabolism of minoxidil, a new hypotensive agent II: Biotransformation following oral administration to rats dogs and monkeys, *J. Pharm. Sci.* **64,** 1366–1371.

Wang, C. C., & Simashkevich, P. M. (1980). A comparative study of the biological activities of arprinocid and arprinocid-1-N-oxide, *Mol. Biochem. Parasitol.* **1,** 335–345.

Wareing, M. P. A. (1983). Metabolic studies on isomeric monosubstituted pyridines, PhD thesis, University of London.

Watkins, P. J., & Gorrod, J. W. (1987). Studies on the *in vitro* biological N-oxidation of trimethoprim, *Europ. J. Drug Metab. Pharmacokin.* **12,** 245–251.

Webb, G. A. (1986). Dept. of Chemistry, University of Surrey (personal communication).

Wolf, F. J., Steffens, J. J., Alvaro, R. F., & Jacob, T. A. (1978). Microsomal conversion of MK-302, arprinocid [6-amino-9-(2-chloro-6-fluorobenzyl)purine to 6-amino-9-(2-chloro-6-fluorobenzyl)purine-1-N-oxide by liver microsomes from the chicken and the dog and to the 2-chloro-6-fluorobenzyl alcohol by liver microsomes from rat and mouse, *Fed. Proc.* **37,** 814.

Yamamoto, T., Tsuji, K., Kosuge, T., Okamoto, T., Shudo, K., Takeda, K., Iitaka, Y., Yamaguchi, K., Seino, Y., Yahagi, T., Nagao, M., & Sugimura, T. (1978). Isolation and structure determination of mutagenic substances in L-glutamic acid pyrolysate, *Proc. Jpn. Acad.* **54,** 248–250.

Yamazoe, Y., Ishii, K., Kamataki, T., Kato, R., & Sugimura, T. (1980). Isolation and characterization of active metabolites of tryptophan-pyrolysate mutagen, Trp-P-2, formed by rat liver microsomes, *Chem. Biol. Interns.* **30,** 125–138.

Yamazoe, Y., Shimada M., Maeda, K., Kamataki, T., & Kato, R. (1984). Specificity of four forms of cytochrome P-450 in the metabolic activation of several aromatic amines and benzo[a]pyrene, *Xenobiotica* **14,** 549–552.

Zins, G. R. (1965). The *in vivo* production of a potent, long acting hypotensive metabolite from diallylmelamine, *J. Pharmacol. Exptl. Therap.* **150,** 109–117.

Zins, G. R., Emmert, D. W., & Walker, R. A. (1968). Hypotensive metabolite producton and sequential metabolism of N,N-diallylmelamine in rats, dogs and man, *J. Pharmacol. Exptl. Therap.* **159,** 194–205.

7.8 DNA interaction with carbonyl-labelled methyl or ethylnitrosoureas

D. Kanduc & E. Quagliariello†

(1) The carbonyl group of (m)ethylnitrosoureas was found to interact with DNA both *in vitro* and *in vivo*.
(2) (^{14}C-carbonyl)-radioactivity remained associated to DNA after a number of ethanolic precipitations as well as after RNase and protease treatments, but was extremely labile to DNA enzymic and acid digestion.
(3) Detectable amount of (^{14}C-carbonyl)-radioactivity was still found in DNA of various rat tissue 18 days after i.p. administration of carbonyl-labelled methylnitrosourea.

7.8.1 INTRODUCTION

The main current hypothesis in chemical carcinogenesis by N-nitroso compounds and alkylating reagents is that the neoplastic transformation could result from DNA alkylation with consequent changes in the genetic structure of the cell (Singer & Grunberger 1983, O'Neill *et al.* 1984). Some specific alkylation products have received much attention during recent years, and, successively, 7-alkylguanosines (Magee & Farber 1962, Beranek *et al.* 1983, Kadlubar *et al.* 1984), O^6-alkylguanosine (Loveless 1969, Goth & Rajewsky 1974), 1,7-dialkylguanosine (Kanduc 1982, 1985), and O^4- and O^2-alkylthymines (Swemberg *et al.* 1984, Preston *et al.* 1986) have been implicated as main or contributing factors in tumorigenesis. Despite the intensive and extensive studies on nucleic acid alkylation, it can be concluded that at present the possible link between carcinogenesis and alkylating agents remains obscure. It is possible that nucleic acid alkylation is not related to carcinogenesis, as well as that some type of interaction not yet considered, or other alkyl products, are the important ones in tumorigenesis (Lijinsky 1976).

Recent data obtained in this laboratory have shown a RNA-ethylnitrosourea reaction which could not be accounted for by an alkylation reaction (Kanduc *et al.* 1987a), and it was shown that both ethyl and carbonyl functions of ethylnitrosourea interact *in vivo* with rat liver tRNA (Kanduc *et al.* 1987b). Here we present data to demonstrate *in vivo* and *in vitro* DNA interaction with the carbonyl function of N-methyl- and N-ethyl-N-nitrosourea.

† Dipartimento di Biochimica e Biologia Molecolare, Facoltà di Scienze, Università di Bari, Via Amendola 165/, 70126—Bari, Italy
Abbreviations: MNU, N-methyl-N-nitrosurea; ENU, N-ethyl-N-nitrosourea.

7.8.2 MATERIALS AND METHODS

(^{14}C-carbonyl)-methyl and ethylnitrosoureas were prepared by reacting (^{14}C)urea (6 or 7 mCi/mmol, New England Nuclear, Boston, MA), with methylamine or ethylamine hydrochloride (Vogel 1964). Enzymes were from Boehringer, Mannheim. In *in vitro* reaction, calf thymus DNA was reacted with (^{14}C-carbonyl)methyl- or ethylnitrosourea at 37°C for 1 h in 10 mM Bis Tris, pH 6.5 and recovered by ethanol precipitations and dissolved in 10 mM NaCl. In *in vivo* reaction, Wistar male albino rats were injected i.p. with the labelled reagents and killed at different times. DNA was isolated (Abanobi *et al.* 1980), treated with RNases, proteinase K and pronase and digested (Beranek *et al.* 1980, Den Engelse *et al.* 1986). The enzymatic or acid hydrolysate were analyzed by h.p.l.c. using a Partisil-10 SCX column (Whatman) and a gradient which brought the buffer ammonium-formate, pH 4.0 from 0.018 to 0.18 M in 35 min. Two ml/min fractions were collected and assayed for radioactivity by liquid scintillation counting.

7.8.3. RESULTS

When calf thymus DNA was treated *in vitro* with methyl- or ethylnitrosourea labelled in the carbonyl group, detectable (^{14}C)-radioactivity was bound to the nucleic acid as shown in Table 1. The extent of reaction measured as μmol of carbonyl group

Table 1—*In vitro* DNA labelling by carbonyl-labelled methyl and ethylnitrosoureas

	Overall extent of reaction (μmol of carbonyl group/mol DNA P)
MNU	465 ± 37
ENU	150 ± 18

Calf thymus DNA (6 mM DNA-P) in 10 mM Bis Tris, pH 6.5 (3 ml) treated with labelled MNU (50 mM) or ENU (78 mM), at 37°C for 1 h, isolated by ethanolic precipitation and analysed for ^{14}C-CPM. Data represent average of 4 determinations from 2 experiments ±S.D.

per mol DNA-P shows that the different reactivity characterizing the two nitrosoureas in relation to alkylating potential, as the methyl is more reactive than the ethyl compound (Swenson & Lawley 1978), is also present in the carbonyl-DNA reaction. Specifically, the reactivity ratio of methylnitrosourea versus ethylnitrosourea, expressed as ratio of the overall extent of reaction (μmol of carbonyl group per mol DNA P) to the molar concentration of the carcinogen, was 5.4.

Extents of *in vivo* DNA interaction in different rat organs at various times after injection of the two carcinogens isotopically labelled in the carbonyl group, are recorded in Table 2. To exclude unequivocally a possible labelling due to protein contamination, DNA purification procedure always included a double protease treatment as described under *Materials and methods*. Moreover, when a control was run by administrating a high amount of (^{14}C)-urea to rats (2.5 mCi, 95 mg/kg b.w.) no significant radioactivity binding to DNA was observed 1.5 h after (^{14}C)urea administration.

Table 2—DNA labelling in various rat organs after single intraperitoneal injection of (^{14}C-carbonyl)-alkylnitrosureas

Compound	Dose	Time (h)	Brain	Liver	Spleen	Lung	Kidney
(^{14}C)urea (2)	95	1.5	n.d.	3 ± 2	n.d.	n.d.	n.d.
ENU (2)	170	1.5	176 ± 31	49 ± 17	109 ± 33	89 ± 40	15 ± 9
ENU (3)	205	3	—	158 ± 15	—	—	—
MNU (2)	85	1.5	444 ± 67	220 ± 43	212 ± 61	106 ± 29	106 ± 45
MNU (2)	85	72	228 ± 38	46 ± 19	163 ± 33	37 ± 5	20 ± 11
MNU (3)	85	432	104 ± 21	19 ± 13	77 ± 44	19 ± 11	27 ± 8

Extent of modification reported as μmol of carbonyl group per mol DNA-P. Dose expressed as mg of carcinogen per kg body weight. Data represent the mean average of at least 6 determinations from experiments shown in parentheses $\pm$S.D., —, not determined; n.d. not detectable.

Overall, the extents of DNA modification by (^{14}C-carbonyl)-alkynitrosoureas paralleled the values obtained *in vitro* regarding both reaction extents and reactivity ratio of the carbonyl function of the two compounds. At 1.5 h after injection of MNU and ENU, in hepatic DNA the reactivity ratio of the methyl versus the ethyl compound was 7.9 (expressed as the ratio of reaction extent to dose, i.e mmol carcinogen/kg). Moreover, another important datum was the high index of persistence of this lesion: in fact, ^{14}C-radioactivity was still found in DNA even 18 days after (^{14}C-carbonyl) MNU administration.

Table 3 shows that ^{14}C-radioactivity was stable in a number of treatments and remained tightly bound to DNA. In fact RNase digestion, protease treatments and neutral thermal treatment at 100°C did not alter the extent of interaction of the carbonyl group to DNA. On the other hand, a marked loss of DNA-bound radioactivity was found after enzymic digestion, and, to a lesser extent, after mild acid hydrolysis.

H.p.l.c. analyses of enzymic and acid digests of (^{14}C-carbonyl)-DNA (not shown) showed only one early eluting radioactive peak, and no counts were found corresponding to deoxynucleosides or bases. Residual radioactivity after enzymic or

Table 3—Lability to enzymic and acid hydrolyses of (^{14}C-carbonyl)-radioactivity bound to DNA following *in vivo* and *in vitro* exposure to carbonyl-labelled (m)ethylnitrosoureas

Treatment	DNA from: Mode: Time (h): Compound: Dose:	Rat liver *in vivo* 1.5 ENU 250 mg/kg	Calf thymus *in vitro* 1 ENU 78 mM	Rat liver *in vivo* 1.5 MNU 85 mg/kg	Calf thymus *in vitro* 1 MNU 50 mM	Rat brain *in vivo* 432 MNU 85 mg/kg
After extraction and ethanol precipitation		151		209		97
RNases		148		197		101
Proteinase K		162		231		79
Pronase		158		220		104
Neutral thermal treatment		151		201		106
8 ethanolic precipitations			150		465	
Enzymic hydrolysis		28	12	17	18	13
Mild acid hydrolysis		61	85	97	188	27

DNA isolated at time stated and analysed for ^{14}C-cpm after various treatments listed. Data expressed as μmol of carbonyl group per mole DNA-P and represent the average of at least 4 determinations.

acid digestion may probably be ascribed to undigested material rather than to specific adducts which presumably are labile to the hydrolyses procedures and, are consequently, undetectable. Concentration under vacuum of the early-eluted radioactive fractions resulted in a further loss of radioactivity, thus increasing the difficulty of any attempt to characterize the carbonyl-induced lesion more completely.

7.8.4 DISCUSSION

The two important observations here reported are (i) occurrence and persistence of a DNA interaction with the carbonyl function of (M)ENU, and (ii) lability of such interaction to the hydrolytic procedures usually employed in DNA analysis.

The binding of the carbonyl group to DNA is proved by the fact that (^{14}C)-radioactivity remained tightly associated to the nucleic acid on ethanol precipitations as well as after the long and numerous DNA purification procedures. The absence of radioactivity in the bases and deoxynucleosides allows for exclusion of metabolic incorporation due to entry of the ^{14}C-label in the one-carbon pool. Likewise, double protein digestion excludes possible protein contamination.

The second important point is the extreme lability of ^{14}C-carbonyl radioactivity to mild hydrolytic procedures usually employed in DNA analysis, with the practical consequence the objective difficulty of exactly quantifying and chemically identifying the lesion(s) produced. The second consequence is theoretical. In fact, existing literature on chemical carcinogenesis by N-nitroso compounds and alkylating agents has focused mainly on the possible carcinogenic role of alkylation, thus neglecting the possibility of other kinds of DNA interaction. But, as already underlined by other authors (Miller & Miller 1974), it could be that, though attention has been predominantly placed on covalent interactions, other kinds of reactions (tight non-covalent binding, chemical interaction with no carcinogen retention, etc.) could alter the function of a macromolecule in such a way as to modify the status of a cell and possibly of its progeny.

Thus, the experimental data reported here are of particular interest in the light of the possibility of a direct or indirect effect by this type of DNA damage on the normal cell metabolism, especially when considering both the quantitatively significant extent of the reaction and its high index of persistence *in vivo*.

ACKNOWLEDGEMENTS

This work was supported by a grant from CNR Special project 'Oncology'. We thank Mr M. Cinquepalmi for secretarial assistance.

REFERENCES

Abanobi, S. E., Columbano, A., Mulivor, R. A., Rajalakshmi, S., & Sarma, D. S. R. (1980) *In vivo* replication of hepatic deoxyribonucleic acid of rats treated with dimethylnitrosoamine: presence of dimethylnitrosamine induced O^6-methylguanine, N^7-methylguanine and N^3-methyladenine in the replicated hybrid deoxyribonucleic acid. *Biochemistry* **19**, 1382–1387.

Beranek, D. T., Weis, C. C., & Swenson, D. H. (1980) A comprehensive quantitative analysis of methylated and ethylated DNA using high pressure liquid chromatography. *Carcinogenesis* **1,** 595–606.

Beranek, D. T., Weis, C. C., Evans, F. E., Chetsanga, C. J., & Kadlubar, F. F. (1983) Identification of N^5-methyl-N^5-formyl 2,5,6-triamino-4-hydroxypyrymidine as a major adduct in rat-liver DNA after treatment with the carcinogens N,N-dimethylnitrosamine or 1,2-dimethylhydrazine. *Biochem. Biophys. Res. Commun.* **110,** 625–631.

Den Engelse, L., Menkveld, G. J., De Brij, R. J., & Tates, A. D. (1986) Formation and stability of alkylated pirimidines and purines (including imidazole ring opened 7-alkylguanine) and alkyl phosphotiesters in liver DNA of adult rats treated with ethylnitrosourea or dimethylnitrosamine. *Carcinogenesis* **7,** 393–403.

Goth, R. & Rajewsky, M. F. (1974) Persistence of O6-ethylguanine in rat brain DNA: correlation with nervous system specific carcinogenesis by ethylnitrosourea. *Proc. Natl. Acad. Sci. USA* **71,** 639–643.

Kadlubar, F. F., Beranek, D. T., Weis, C. C., Evans, F. E., Cox, R., & Irving, C. C. (1984) Characterization of the purine ring opened 7 methylguanine and its persistence in rat bladder epithelial DNA after treatment with the carcinogen N-methylnitrosourea. *Carcinogenesis* **5,** 587–592.

Kanduc, D. (1982) tRNA chemical methylation. *In vitro* and *in vivo* formation of 1,7-dimethylguanosine at high concentrations of methylating agents. *Biochim. Biophys. Acta* **698,** 336–343.

Kanduc, D. (1985) 1,7-diethylguanosine formation in tRNA chemical ethylation by ethionine and ethylnitrosourea. *Biochim. Biophys. Acta* **840,** 218–227.

Kanduc, D., Casalino, E., & Liuzzi, M. G. (1987a) *In vitro* DNA-ethylnitrosourea reaction under anhydrous and aqueous conditions. *Bull. Mol. Biol. Med.* **12,** 1–10.

Kanduc, D., Liuzzi, M. G., & Casalino, E. (1987b) *In vivo* tRNA interaction with ethyl- and carbonyl-labelled ethylnitrosourea. *Bull. Mol. Biol. Med.* **12,** 11–18.

Lijinsky, W. (1976) Interaction with nucleic acids of carcinogenic and mutagenic N-nitroso compounds. *Prog. Nucleic Acid Res. Mol. Biol.* **17,** 247–269.

Loveless, A. (1969) Possible relevance of O6-alkylation of deoxyguanoscine to the mutagenicity and carcinogenicity of nitrosamines and nitrosomides. *Nature* **223,** 206–207.

Magee, P. N. & Farber, E. (1962) Toxic liver injury and carcinogenesis methylation of liver nucleic acids by dymethylnitrosamine *in vivo. Biochem. J.* **83,** 114–124.

Miller, E. C. & Miller, J. A. (1974) Biochemical mechanisms of chemical carcinogenesis. In: H. Busch (ed.), *The molecular biology of cancer*, pp. 377–402, Academic Press, New York and London.

O'Neill, I. K., Von Borstel, R. C., Miller, C. T., Long, J., & Bartsch, H. (eds) (1984) *N-Nitroso compounds: occurrence, biological effects and relevance to human cancer*, IARC, Lyon.

Preston, B. D., Singer, B., & Loeb, L. A. (1986) Mutagen potential of O^4-methylthymine *in vivo* determined by an enzymatic approach to site-specific mutagenesis. *Proc. Natl. Acad. Sci. USA* **83,** 8501–8505.

Singer, B. & Grunberger, D. (1983) *Molecular biology of mutagens and carcinogens*, Plenum Press, New York.

Swenson, D. H. & Lawley, P. D. (1978) Alkylation of deoxyribonucleic acid by carcinogens dimethyl sulphate, ethyl methanesulphonate, N-ethylnitrosourea and M-methyl-M-nitrosourea. *Biochem. J.* **171,**575–587.

Swemberg, J. A., Dyroff, M. C., Bedell, M. A., Popp, J. A., Huh, N., Nirstein, U., & Rajewsky, M. F. (1984) O^4-ethyldeoxythymidine, but not O^6-ethyldeoxyguanosine, accumulates in hepatocyte DNA of rats exposed continuously to diethylnitrosamine. *Proc. Natl. Acad. Sci. USA* **81,** 1692–1696.
Vogel, A. I. (1964) *Practical organic chemistry*, p. 969, Longmans, London

7.9 Effects of anthracycline antibiotics on the reconstituted tricarboxylate carrier

I. Stipani, V. Zara, V. Bonvino, C. Manfreda, & G. Prezioso†

The partially purified tricarboxylate carrier system eluted by hydroxyapatite column has been used to study the effect of the anthracycline antibiotics adriamycin (doxorubicin) and Br-daunomycin.

(1) The reconstituted citrate/citrate exchange activity is inhibited by both anthracycline antibiotics. Br-daunomycin, however, is much more effective than adriamycin.

(2) The inhibition of the reconstituted citrate transport activity by Br-daunomycin and adriamycin is concentration- and time-dependent.

(3) Cardiolipin protects the reconstituted citrate transport activity against the inhibition by Br-daunomycin.

(4) The reconstituted citrate/citrate exchange activity of the hydroxyapatite eluate depends upon the ratio of cardiolipin/Br-daunomycin added to the mitochondrial extract.

7.9.1 INTRODUCTION

The inner mitochondrial membrane contains a specific carrier system that catalyses an electroneutral exchange of citrate, malate, and phosphoenolpyruvate (Palmieri *et al.* 1972).

We have partially purified the tricarboxylate carrier protein from rat liver mitochondria by chromatography on hydroxyapatite (Stipani & Palmieri 1983, Palmieri *et al.* 1986).

The purified tricarboxylate carrier fraction incorporated into liposomes exhibits transport properties which are distinctive features of the citrate transport system as characterized in intact mitochondria (Stipani & Palmieri 1983, Palmieri *et al.* 1986).

Furthermore, as it has been found for the phosphate carrier (Kadenbach *et al.* 1982), the tricarboxylate carrier has an essential requirement for cardiolipin (Stipani & Palmieri 1983, Stipani *et al.* 1984).

It is known that the anthracycline antibiotic adriamycin (doxorubicin) segregates membrane cardiolipin by forming a cardiolipin–adriamycin complex with a molar ratio of 1:2 (Goormaghtigh *et al.* 1980).

It has been reported that adriamycin and Br-daunomycin strongly inhibit the reconstituted phosphate transport activity in cardiolipin-containing liposomes (Cheneval *et al.* 1983).

† Department of Pharmaco-Biology, Laboratory of Biochemistry, University of Bari, Italy and CNR Unit for the Study of Mitochondria and Bioenergetics, University of Bari, 70126 Bari, Italy.

In this paper we have investigated the effect of the anthracycline antibiotics adriamycin and Br-daunomycin on the partially purified tricarboxylate carrier. Br-daunomycin, and less efficiently adriamycin, inhibit the reconstituted citrate/citrate exchange activity. Cardiolipin protects against anthracycline antibiotics.

7.9.2 MATERIALS AND METHODS

Adriamycin and Br-daunomycin were a gift of Farmitalia-Carlo Erba (Milano). Rat liver mitochondria were solubilized with 3% Triton X-100 in the presence of 2 mg/ml of cardiolipin and the tricarboxylate carrier was purified by hydroxyapatite chromatography as described by Stipani & Palmieri (1983), Palmieri *et al.* (1986). The mitochondrial extract or hydroxyapatite eluate was incubated in the presence and in the absence of the anthracycline antibiotics before its reconstitution into liposomes. The citrate/citrate exchange activity was measured by adding 0.6 mM ^{14}C-citrate to the proteoliposomes. After 10 min the reaction was stopped with 10 mM 1,2,3-benzenetricarboxylate.

7.9.3 RESULTS AND DISCUSSION

In the experiment illustrated in Fig. 1, the hydroxyapatite eluate obtained from solubilized rat liver mitochondria was incubated with increasing concentration of adriamycin and Br-daunomycin for 60 min at 0°C. After this incubation the eluate was incorporated into liposomes, and the reconstituted citrate/citrate exchange activity was measured. The data show that citrate transport is inhibited by both

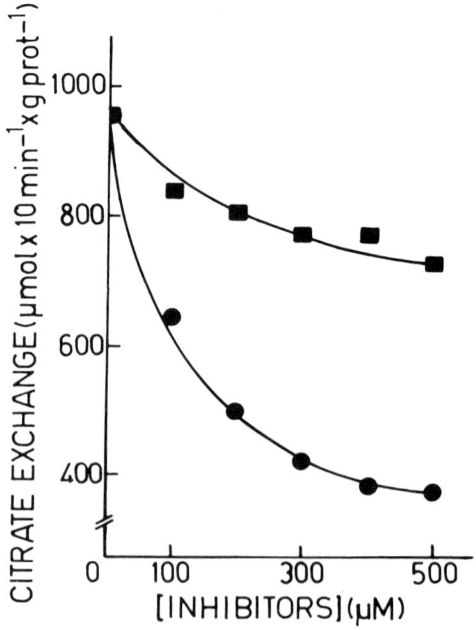

Fig. 1.—Effect of increasing concentrations of Br-daunomycin and adriamycin on the reconstituted tricarboxylate transport activity. Br-daunomycin (●) or adriamycin (■) was incubated for 60 min at 0°C with the hydroxyapatite eluate before reconstitution into liposomes.

antibiotics. Br-daunomycin, however, is much more effective than adriamycin. At 500 μM Br-daunomycin inhibits the citrate/citrate exchange activity 63%, whereas adriamycin only 17%. This contrasts to what found with the mitochondrial phosphate carrier (Cheneval *et al.* 1983). In this case, the two antibiotics have about the same inhibitory effect on the reconstituted phosphate transport activity. Furthermore, tricarboxylate carrier is less sensitive to the two inhibitors than the phosphate carrier.

Almost identical inhibition curves to those shown in Fig. 1 were obtained when the proteoliposomes, instead of the hydroxyapatite eluate, were incubated with the inhibitors for 40 min at 30°C.

The time course of the inhibition of the reconstituted citrate transport activity caused by 500 μM adriamycin and 500 μM Br-daunomycin is shown in Fig. 2. With

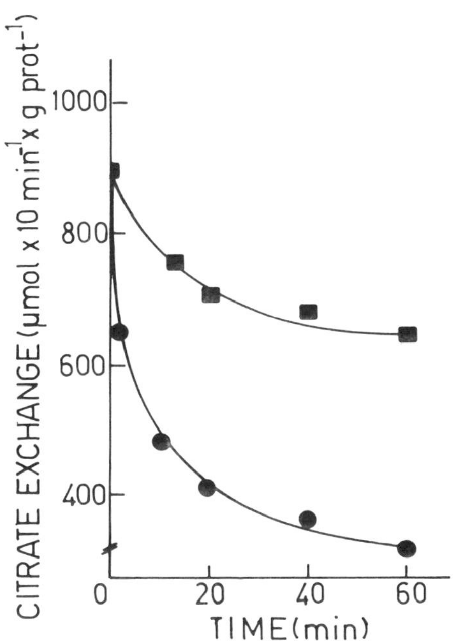

Fig. 2.—Time course of the inhibition of the reconstituted tricarboxylate activity by Br-daunomycin and adriamycin. The hydroxyapatite eluate was incubated with 500 μM Br-daunomycin (●) or adriamycin (■) at 0°C for the times indicated before reconstitution into cardiolipin-containing liposomes.

both antibiotics the inhibition is time-dependent and reaches its maximum after 60 min incubation of the hydroxyapatite eluate with adriamycin or Br-daunomycin. In Fig. 3 the protection by cardiolipin of the tricarboxylate carrier against inhibition by Br-daunomycin is shown. In the control, that is, in the absence of inhibitor, the cardiolipin markedly increases the activity of the citrate/citrate exchange. Maximum activity is obtained in the presence of 10–15 mg/ml cardiolipin. The activation of the solubilized and partially purified tricarboxylate carrier by cardiolipin agrees with our previous observations (Stipani *et al.* 1984). The data of Fig. 3 clearly indicate that the inhibition of the citrate/citrate exchange caused by Br-daunomycin decreases with increasing concentrations of cardiolipin. This is shown more clearly in the inset of Fig. 3. The percentage of inhibition by Br-daunomycin decreases from 85% without cardiolipin to 20% with 15–20 mg/ml cardiolipin.

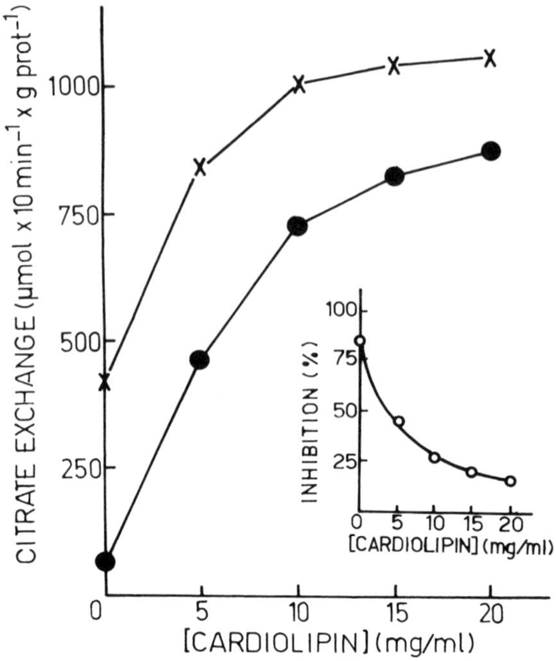

Fig. 3.—Protection by cardiolipin of the reconstituted citrate transport activity against inhibition of Br-daunomycin. The hydroxyapatite eluate was incubated with the indicated amounts of cardiolipin for 30 min at 0°C and then incubated for a further 60 min at 0°C with (●) or without (×) 500 μM Br-daunomycin before reconstitution into liposomes. The inset shows the inhibition of Br-daunomycin at the indicated concentrations of cardiolipin.

As mentioned in the *Introduction*, Br-daunomycin segregates cardiolipin, and it has been found that 2 molecules of adriamycin bind 1 molecule of cardiolipin (Goormaghtigh *et al.* 1980). It should be expected, therefore, that cardiolipin and the anthracycline antibiotic are ineffective when they are added at a ratio of 1:2. At ratios higher or lower than 1:2, activities higher and lower than the control (without cardiolipin) should be obtained. To check this hypothesis we have incubated the mitochondrial extract with both cardiolipin and Br-daunomycin at molar ratios ranging from 4:1 to 1:8. After 60 min incubation at 0°C the mitochondrial extract was subjected to hydroxyapatite chromatography, and the reconstituted citrate transport activity was measured in the eluate. Fig. 4 shows that when the ratio cardiolipin:Br-daunomycin is 1:2 the activity of the reconstituted citrate/citrate exchange is 350 nmol $\times$ 10 min^{-1} $\times$ mg protein^{-1}, i.e. about the same value obtained in the control without cardiolipin (see Fig. 3). The activity, on the other hand, is increased when more cardiolipin is added than Br-daunomycin. Vice versa, the activity is decreased when the ratio between cardiolipin and Br-daunomycin is lowered.

These results can be explained by assuming that the anthracycline antibiotics complexe cardiolipin, which is necessary for the activity of the carrier (Stipani & Palmieri 1983, Stipani *et al.* 1984). It remains, however, to be clarified why the inhibition of the reconstituted citrate/citrate exchange activity by the anthracycline antibiotics is not complete at high concentrations of inhibitors. It is also not clear why adriamycin is much less effective than Br-daunomycin in inhibiting the tricarboxylate carrier.

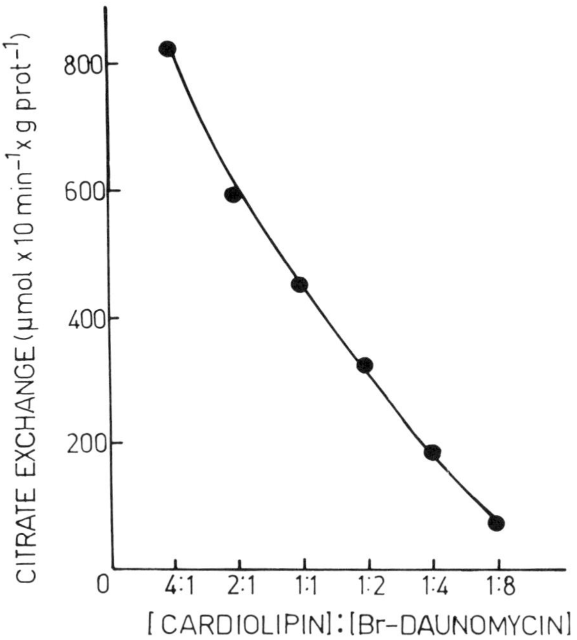

Fig. 4.—Effect on citrate transport of the addition of both cardiolipin and Br-daunomycin at various molar ratios. The mitochondrial extract was treated with the indicated molar ratios of cardiolipin to Br-daunomycin. The hydroxyapatite eluate was incorporated into liposomes, and the citrate/citrate exchange activity was measured. Cardiolipin was added at 2 mg/ml, whereas the concentration of the inhibitor was varied to give the indicated molar ratios.

REFERENCES

Cheneval, D., Muller, M., & Carafoli, E. (1983). The mitochondrial phosphate carrier reconstituted in liposomes is inhibited by doxorubicin. *FEBS Lett.* **159,** 123–126.

Goormaghtigh, E., Chatelain, P., Caspers, J., & Ruysschaert, J. M. (1980). Evidence of a specific complex between adriamycin and negatively-charged phospholipids. *Biochim. Biophys. Acta* **597,** 1–14.

Kadenbach, B., Mende, P., Kolbe, H. V. J., Stipani, I., & Palmieri, F. (1982). The mitochondrial phosphate carrier has an essential requirement for cardiolipin. *FEBS Lett.* **139,** 109–112.

Palmieri, F., Stipani, I., Quagliareillo, E., & Klingenberg, M. (1972). Kinetic study of the tricarboxylate carrier in rat liver mitochondria. *Eur. J. Biochem.* **26,** 587–594.

Palmieri, F., Stipani, I., Prezioso, G., & Kramer, R. (1986). Partial purification and reconstitution of the tricarboxylate carrier from rat liver mitochondria. *Methods in Enzymol.* **125,** 692–696.

Stipani, I. & Palmieri, F. (1983). Purification of the active mitochondrial tricarboxylate carrier by hydroxylapatite chromatography. *FEBS Lett.* **161,** 269–274.

Stipani, I., Prezioso, G., Zara, V., Iacobazzi, V., & Genchi, G. (1984). Activation by cardiolipin of the Triton X-100-inhibited tricarboxylate carrier purified from rat liver mitochondria. *Bull. Mol. Biol. Med.* **9,** 193–201.

Part 8
Defence and repair mechanisms

8.1 DNA repair and human malignancy

P. Karran†

Human cells are able to remove damage to their DNA. This damage may result from exposure to agents such as ultraviolet radiation and exogenous chemicals including the environmentally important alkylnitrosamines. Unrepaired damage may be mutagenic, and, as a consequence, DNA repair reactions in multicellular organisms are beneficial and act to prevent cellular transformation and tumour induction.

The cytotoxicity of the alkylating compounds has led to their use as anti-tumour chemotherapeutic agents in man. The cytotoxic properties of these agents depend on their ability to react with cellular DNA. Unfortunately, the efficiency with which DNA repair reactions can recognize and remove alkylation adducts reduces the effectiveness of many alkylating drugs. A disturbing feature of alkylating agent based chemotherapy has been the appearance of secondary malignancies. This implies the persistence of potentially mutagenic (as distinct from cytotoxic) alkylation damage in the DNA of non-target cells.

8.1.1 DNA REPAIR AND PROTECTION AGAINST TRANSFORMATION

Pathways which protect DNA against the consequences of damage are widely distributed in living systems (see Friedberg 1985 for review). Analogous enzymes which act on damaged DNA can be found in species as diverse as simple prokaryotes and man, indicating selective pressures for their conservation. The kinds of damage inflicted on DNA range from intrinsic hydrolytic reactions, which occur as a consequence of the maintenance of DNA at normal growth temperatures in an aqueous environment, to the products of attack by complex exogenous 'environmental' chemical agents. These diverse molecular alterations in DNA show the common feature that their persistence can result in heritable change in the genome (mutations) with the consequent possibility of aberrant gene expression and growth control. Almost all chemical and physical agents which are carcinogenic in man and animals have been shown by direct experimental investigation to be mutagens, and most of them interact directly with DNA. Fortunately, cells are well protected against such DNA damage by a battery of repair enzymes. We now understand the mechanisms by which many of these enzymes act, and also the consequences of their impaired function.

† Imperial Cancer Research Fund, Clare Hall Laboratories, Blanche Lane, South Mimms, Potters Bar, Herts, EN6 3LD, UK

8.1.2 HUMAN CANCER AND IMPAIRED DNA REPAIR

Probably the most dramatic examples of a defect in DNA repair in humans is afforded by xeroderma pigmentosum (XP) (Friedberg 1985). This genetic disease, which is inherited in an autosomal recessive mode, is characterized by an extreme sensitivity of the homozygotes to sunlight exposure accompanied by a dramatic increase in the incidence of melanoma at sites exposed to ultraviolet radiation (UV). The sensitivity to UV is also observed at the cellular level, and cell lines derived from XP homozygotes are hypersensitive to the cytotoxic and mutagenic effects of UV *in vitro*. Although the disease is complex (XP patients fall into 10 genetic complementation groups), it is characterized at the molecular level by an inability to repair certain UV-induced photoproducts in DNA. These photoproducts which are formed by the reaction of adjacent pyrimidines in the DNA strands (cyclobutane pyrimidine dimer and pyrimidine (6,4) pyrimidones) are normally recognized and removed by a process of excision repair (Fig. 1). Although the precise details of the steps in the repair pathway are still unclear, Fig. 1 gives the general outline. The overall effect is the removal of the potentially harmful photoproduct along with a limited region of adjacent DNA and resynthesis of the correct DNA sequences. In most cases, cells from XP patients are unable to perform one of the early steps in this process which is related to incision of the damaged DNA strand. Of additional interest is the observation that this particular DNA repair pathway is not restricted to the repair of pyrimidine photoproducts. Some large organic chemical carcinogens such as activated benz(α)pyrene react covalently with DNA bases. Many of the resulting adducts, which share the property of inducing considerable distortion of the DNA helix, are also recognized by the UV-photoproduct excision system. Thus, a failure of this damage-monitoring system results in hypersensitivity to a number of structurally unrelated transforming chemicals.

A second important example of defective DNA repair in human disease is Bloom's syndrome. In this case, the homozygous state is characterized by the early onset of various malignancies including Wilms tumour (German 1983). At the cellular level, Bloom's syndrome cells exhibit an intrinsic chromosomal instability and are sensitive *in vitro* to a variety of DNA-damaging agents. It has recently been established that the molecular defect in Bloom's syndrome involves a DNA ligase (Willis & Lindahl 1987). Since the formation of breaks in one of the strands is a essential step in many reactions involving DNA, including excision repair (Fig. 1), the observed reduction in activity of this enzyme may result in varied and profound effects on DNA replication, recombination, and repair.

Not all DNA repair reactions of human cells exhibit the broad specificity of the excision repair system. An example of a more stringent mechanism which is restricted to repair of a single alteration in DNA in a very straightforward fashion, is provided by O^6-alkylguanine-DNA alkyltransferase. The alkylated base O^6-alkylguanine is a product of the reaction of guanine with a number of alkylating agents such as N-methyl-N-nitrosourea (MNU) and the activated form of dimethyl- and diethyl-nitrosamine (DMN and DEN). The nitrosamines represent an important class of environmental chemicals, and agents of this type are potent carcinogens and mutagens. The mutagenic (and by inference carcinogenic) properties of such agents have been ascribed to the production of O^6-alkylguanine in DNA (although other alkylated species may also contribute), and human cells express an alkyltransferase which recognizes and repairs this damaged base in DNA. During repair of this base, the alkyl group is transferred from the guanine base to a particular cysteine residue within the transferase molecule. In this case, DNA repair is completed without any requirement for the excision and resynthesis of segments of DNA; guanine is regenerated in the intact DNA strand, and an alkylated protein is produced. This alkylated protein is non-functional and is neither able to effect the transfer of, nor to accept, additional alkyl groups. Active enzyme is not subseqently regenerated by dealkylation of the protein. In other words, the cell is protected by its pool of preformed alkyltransferase molecules, each of which acts only once, and when this pool is exhausted, new proteins have to be synthesized to restore protection. During this regenerative phase, the cell is presumably at increased risk of trasformation by alkylating agents.

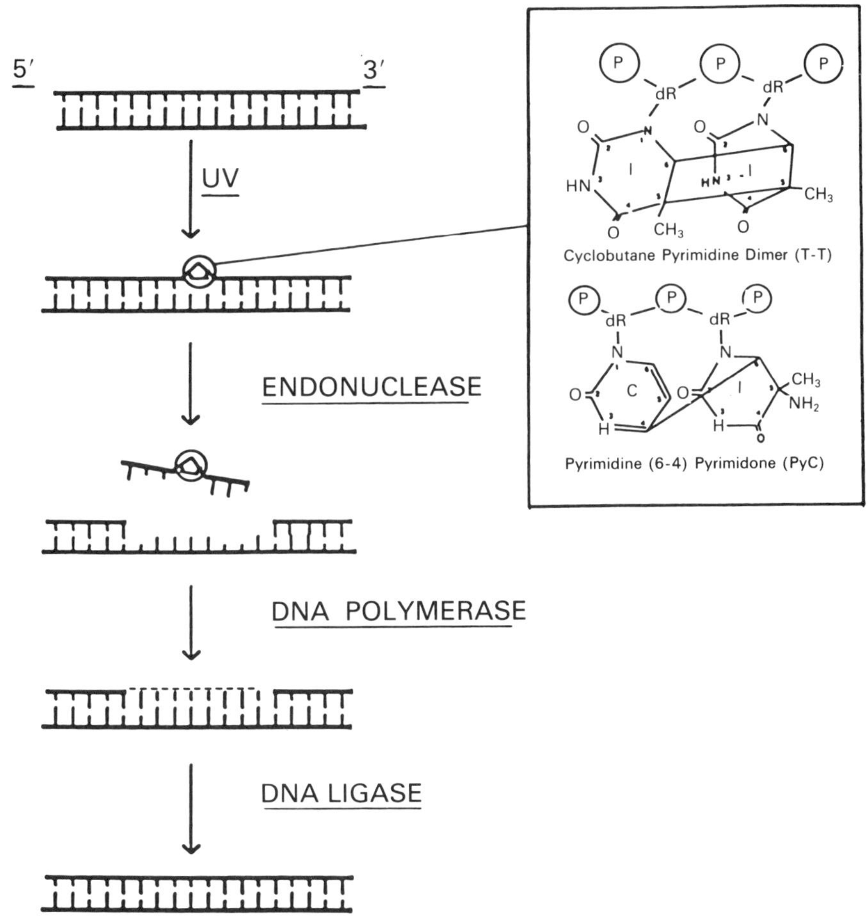

Fig. 1.—Steps in the removal of UV-induced damage in DNA. Two common photoproducts, the cyclobutane-pyrimidine dimer and the pyrimidine (6-4) pyrimidone product, are shown boxed. The cellular repair enzymes recognize the distortion introduced in the double helix by the presence of these products. An incision is made adjacent to the damaged region, and a segment of DNA is excised. The missing section is resynthesized by DNA polymerase utilizing the complementary strand coding sequences. Repair is completed by ligation of this newly-synthesized 'patch' to the existing DNA strand by DNA ligase.

The importance of this single enzyme in protecting against mutation and transformation by alkylating agents is indicated by the existence of human (and other mammalian) cell lines which lack alkyltransferase activity (Mex$^-$ or Mer$^-$) (Sklar & Strauss 1981, Day *et al.* 1980). Such cell lines are highly sensitive to the genotoxic effects of alkylating chemicals (but not unrelated compounds). These effects may be reversed by the stable integration and expression of alkyltransferase coding sequences from an exogenous source (Samson *et al.* 1986, Brennand & Margison 1986, Ishizaki *et al.* 1986, Kataoka *et al.* 1986). Interestingly, the levels of alkyltransferase in man exhibit not only considerble variation between body tissues but also wide interindividual differences for each tissue (Myrnes *et al.* 1983). This raises interesting implications for the pharmacology of alkylating agents and the tissue distribution of human cancers.

8.1.3 DNA REPAIR AND CHEMOTHERAPEUTIC DRUGS

During the last 20 years or so, a considerable number of cytotoxic drugs have been introduced into the treatment of human neoplastic disease. Such chemotherapeutic agents can be crudely classified as acting either as anti-metabolites or interacting with DNA directly to prevent replication. The former compounds (e.g. methotrexate) generally interfere with some important metabolic process linked to cell multiplication, such as the provision of precursor nucleoside triphosphates, whereas the latter group cause covalent alkylation of DNA constituents. Many structural similarities exist between the 'environmental' cytotoxic compounds which the cell is armed naturally to withstand and the clinically employed alkylating agents. This similarity, allied to the relatively broad substrate specificity of some of the DNA repair enzymes, undoubtedly leads to reduction in therapeutic effectiveness as target tumour cells are able to excise large numbers of otherwise lethal DNA adducts. A specific example of this can be seen with the chloroethylnitrosourea analogues BCNU and CCNU, both of which break down spontaneously to produce an alkylating species. A substantial proportion of the cytotoxic effect of these drugs resides in their ability to generate cross-links between the two strands of the DNA double helix. An obligatory first step in the formation of such cytotoxic cross-links is chloroethylation of the O^6-position of guanine in DNA. The product of this reaction can be recognized and removed by the O^6-alkylguanine alkyltransferase, thus preventing the formation of the cytotoxic adduct (Robins *et al.* 1983). Evidence of this protective effect has come from three complementary approaches. Firstly, the dealkylation of O^6-chloroethylguanine by purified alkyltransferase has been demonstrated *in vitro* (Robins *et al.* 1983). Secondly, Kohn and co-workers have demonstrated that Mex$^-$ human cell lines are more sensitive than Mex$^+$ cell lines to the cytotoxicity of the clinically used nitrosoureas (Erickson *et al.* 1980). However, Mex$^+$ cells may be rendered sensitive to killing by these chloroethylating agents following inactivation of the cellular alkyltransferase by growth in the presence of free O^6-methylguanine, a non-toxic specfic inhibitor of the alkyltransferase (Karran & Williams 1985, Day *et al.* 1987). Finally, the expression of an exogenous alkyltransferase gene in Mex$^-$ cells restores their resistance to chloroethylating agents (Samson *et al.* 1986, Brennand & Margison 1986, Kataoka *et al.* 1986).

8.1.4 DNA REPAIR AND SECONDARY MALIGNANCIES

A disturbing consequence of the successful clinical application of alkylating agents in chemotherapy has been the appearance of secondary neoplasms (IARC 1982). Ironically, it is presumably the prolongation of survival which allows sufficient time for these secondary tumours to develop. Thus, the successful treatment of Hodgkin's disease and non-Hodgkin's lymphoma with combined chemotherapy which includes the alkylating agents nitrogen mustard and procarbazine carries with it a greatly increased risk of leukaemia compared to radiation treatment. Interestingly, procarbazine (which is highly carcinogenic in animal systems) is metabolized to a methylating species and would be expected to produce the same spectrum of DNA damage as the potent mutagens MNU and DMN (Zedeck 1984). Many other alkylating agents which have been widely used in clinical practice (e.g. cyclophosphamide) have been shown to induce DNA damage and mutations in test systems.

8.1.5 CONCLUSIONS

The role of DNA repair in reducing the effectiveness of chemotherapeutic agents and its involvement in the avoidance of cellular transformation presents a number of significant challenges. The DNA repair enzymes expressed by humans cells confer a survival advantage upon those cells; they repair potentially *cytotoxic* lesions in DNA. As we find out more about the precise mechanisms of DNA repair enzymes and the way in which they interact with their substrates, it may be possible to design cytotoxic compounds producing lesions in DNA which block DNA synthesis but do not resemble the substrates normally recognized by DNA repair enzymes. Alternatively, synergistic enhancement of cytotoxicity may be brought about by the simultaneous administration of cytotoxic drug and a non-toxic inhibitor of a particular DNA repair enzyme. An example of this is the potentiation of chloroethylating agent cytotoxicity by O^6-methylguanine. By such means, the cellular defences could be outwitted.

The induction of secondary malignancies presents a challenge of a different nature. We assume that such malignancy results from persistence, in non-target tissue, of promutagenic DNA damage introduced by the drug. While the potential for mutation induction or cell killing may sometimes reside in a single type of DNA lesion, this is not always the case. Certain lesions may exert more profound effects on cytotoxicity than on mutagenicity. One challenge for the future may be to define carefully the genotoxicity of particular DNA adducts in order to allow design of compounds whose ultimate reaction products with DNA have overwhelmingly cytotoxic potential with little or no promutagenic potential.

REFERENCES

Brennand, J. & Margison, G. P. (1986) Reduction of the toxicity and mutagenicity of alkylating agents in mammalian cells harbouring the *Escherichia coli* alkyltransferase gene. *Proc. Natl. Acad. Sci. USA* **83,** 6282–6296.

Day, R. S., Ziolkowski, C. H. J., Scudiero, D. A., Meyer, S. A., Lubiniecki, A. S., Girardi, A. J., Galloway, S. M., & Bynum, G. D. (1980) Defective repair of alkylated DNA by human tumour and SV40 transformed human cells strains. *Nature* **288,** 724–727.

Day, R. S., Babich, M. A., Yarosh, D. B., & Scudiero, D. A. (1987) The role of O^6-methylguanine in cell killing, sister chromatid exchange induction and mutagenesis. A review. *J. Cell Sci.* (**Suppl. 6**), 333–353.

Erickson, L. C., Laurent, G., Sharkey, N. A., & Kohn, K. W. (1980) DNA cross-linking and monoadduct repair in nitrosourea-treated human tumour cells. *Nature* **288,** 727–729.

Friedberg, E. C. (1985) *DNA repair*. W.H. Freeman and Company, New York, USA.

German, J. (1983) Bloom's syndrome X. The cancer-proneness points to chromosome mutation as a crucial event in human neoplasia. In: *Chromosome mutation and neoplasma*. J. German (ed) Alan R. Liss Inc., New York, USA, pp. 347–357.

IARC (1982) Chemicals, industrial processes and industries associated with cancer in humans. *IARC Monographs Vol. 1–29, Supplement 4*. International Agency for Research on Cancer, Lyon, France.

Ishizaki, K., Tsujimura T., Yawata, H., Fujio, C., Nakabeppu, U., Sekiguchi, M., & Ikenaga, M. (1986) Transfer of the *Escherichia coli* O^6-methylguanine methyltransferase gene into repair deficient human cells and restoration of cellular resistance to N-methyl-N′-nitro-N-nitrosoguanidine. *Mutat. Res.* **166,** 135–141.

Karran, P. & Williams, S. (1985) The cytotoxic and mutagenic effects of alkylating agents on human cells are caused by different DNA lesions. *Carcinogenesis* **6,** 789–792.

Kataoka, H., Hall, J., & Karran, P. (1986) Complementation of sensitivity to alkylating agents in *Escherichia coli* and Chinese hamster ovary cells by expression of a cloned bacterial DNA repair gene. *EMBO J.* **5,** 3195–3200.

Myrnes, B., Giercksky, K. E., & Krokan, H. (1983) Inter-individual variation in the activity of O^6-methylguanine-DNA methyltransferase and uracil-DNA glycosylase in human organs. *Carcinogenesis* **4,** 1565–1568.

Robins, P., Harris, A. L., Goldsmith, I., & Lindahl, T. (1983) Cross-linking of DNA induced by chloroethylnitrosourea is prevented by O^6-methylguanine-DNA methyltransferase. *Nucl. Acids Res.* **11,** 7743–7758.

Samson, L., Derfler, B., & Waldstein, E. (1986) Suppression of human DNA alkylation-repair defects by *Escherichia coli* DNA repair genes. *Proc. Natl. Acad. Sci. USA* **83,** 5607–5610.

Sklar, R. & Strauss, B. (1981) Removal of O^6-methylguanine from DNA of normal and xeroderma pigmentosum derived lymphoblastoid lines. *Nature* **289,** 417–420.

Willis, A. E. & Lindahl, T. (1987) DNA ligase I deficiency in Bloom's syndrome. *Nature* **325,** 355–357.

Zedek, M. S. (1984) Hydrazine derivatives, Azo and Azoxy compounds and methylazoxymethanol and cycasin. In: *Chemical carcinogens* (2nd ed.) *A.C.S. Monograph* **182,** American Chemical Society, Washington D.C., USA, pp. 915–944.

8.2 Protection against drug toxicity by modification of drug metabolism or reactivation of cellular defence mechanisms *in vivo*

Gerard J. Mulder, J. Fred Nagelkerke, & John H. N. Meerman†

(1) Many drugs interact irreversibly with receptors in their target organ for toxicity, e.g. through chemically reactive metabolites or depletion of essential endogenous compounds.
(2) Bioactivation of toxicants can be inhibited by selective inhibitors of biotransformation, while the reactive intermediates formed can be trapped by various types of nucleophiles.
(3) Depleted endogenous compounds (like uridine or glutathione) can be repleted by administration of precursors.
(4) Some thiols prevent (by unknown mechanisms) toxicity to develop even when they are administered up to 12 hours after the toxicant.
(5) More insight in mechanisms of drug toxicity is required in order to prevent full expression of drug toxicity *in vivo* by preventive drug therapy.

8.2.1 INTRODUCTION

Overt drug toxicity in animals or man is the final outcome of a number of subsequent steps that start with the initial interaction between the drug (or any of its metabolites) with the receptor coupled to that particular effect. The receptor binding may be reversible, but also interactions leading to irreversible changes may occur, especially when a drug is converted into a reactive intermediate. In this paper the discussion will be limited primarily to those toxic interactions of drugs that ultimately lead to irreversible changes at the cellular level in the liver. Because reactive intermediates, owing to their chemical reactivity, may bind covalently to any appropriate chemical group on (macro-)molecules in the cell where they are formed, the definition of 'receptor' becomes something of a problem. For instance, paracetamol is converted to the reactive N-acetyl-*p*-iminobenzoquinone (NAIQ), which initially binds to the thiol group of reduced glutathione (GSH) so long as GSH is available (Hinson 1980). When GSH becomes depleted, NAIQ binds to thiol groups of proteins, amongst which are those essential for the maintenance of cell homoeostasis. It has been suggested that depletion of GSH may already lead to cell toxicity (Reed & Fariss

† Division of Toxicology, Center for Bio-Pharmaceutical Sciences University of Leiden, P.O. Box 9503, 2300 RA Leiden, The Netherlands

1984). If that in itself were a mechanism of toxicity, what would one then call the receptor for toxicity? If, however, toxicity is due to covalent binding of the paracetamol moiety to a thiol group of an essential enzyme, clearly that enzyme could be called the receptor. A similar problem arises with D-galactosamine which seems to be toxic through depletion of the uridine pool (Macdonald *et al.* 1984).

The localization of the receptor involved in the toxic effect (that is, the mechanism of the initial toxic interaction) is essential to prevent toxicity. If depletion of GSH is directly responsible for toxicity, then repletion of GSH is essential and sufficient to prevent toxicity. However, if the receptor is a single enzyme that is inhibited, can one circumvent that blockage, for instance by reactivation, as for some acetylcholinesterase inhibitors, or by supply of an enzyme product as for some inhibitors of nucleotide synthesis?

Fig. 1 summarizes the tentative sequence of events that can be postulated to occur between the initial attack of a toxic compound and the final overt toxicity: an avalanche of derangements is very likely. We shall discuss, almost exclusively, the *in vivo* situation.

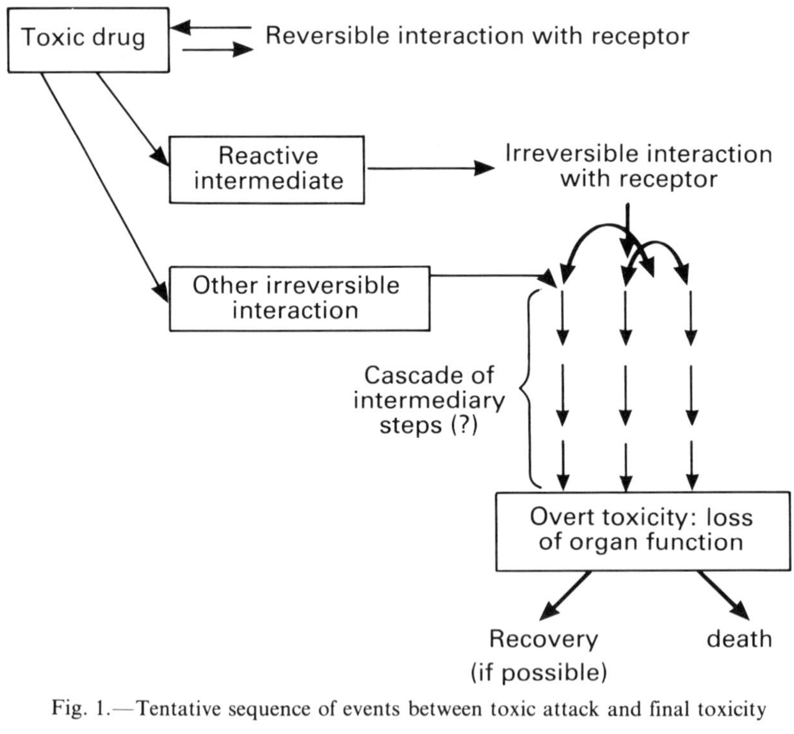

Fig. 1.—Tentative sequence of events between toxic attack and final toxicity

Let us assume that only one component is responsible for the initial toxic interaction. When this is a reactive intermediate it may be trapped before it can react with the receptor, by endogenous protective compounds such as GSH or methionine, or by similar, exogenous compounds (see below). Moreover, the formation of a reactive intermediate may be prevented.

Recent studies of isolated cell preparations have led to a better understanding of the processes involved in drug toxicity resulting in cell death. Very different processes may be set in motion by toxicants as different as cyanide (Belinsky *et al.* 1986), carbon tetrachloride (Macdonald *et al.* 1986), or cystamine (Nicotera *et al.* 1986). However, as yet the *in vivo* situation is not so clear: do these processes play a role *in vivo* as well, or are they to a certain extent artifacts of the isolated cells *in vitro*? For instance, cystamine is toxic to isolated hepatocytes (Nicotera *et al.* 1986), while *in vivo* it may prevent hepatotoxicity of a number of toxins (see below).

8.2.2 INHIBITION OF BIOACTIVATION

An obvious approach to alleviation of drug toxicity is to prevent the formation of a toxic metabolite, if the pathway of activation is known. For instance methoxsalen, a suicide inhibitor of cytochrome P450, completely prevents CCl_4 toxicity, because it prevents CCl_4 bioactivation (Labbe *et al.* 1987). For such model studies in animals various inhibitors are available for cytochrome P450, monoamino oxidase, and some conjugating enzyme such as sulfotransferase (Meerman 1986). In man, possibilities for interference with drug metabolism are more limited. Except for some H_2-blockers like cimetidine (Mitchell *et al.* 1984), no (relatively) safe and effective inhibitors that might be used clinically are available. Salicylamide, which may inhibit sulfate and glucuronide conjugation in animal studies (Mulder & Scholtens 1977) has only an extremely short duration of action, and therefore is not effective *in vivo*.

Obviously, experiments in which drug activation is prevented require drug administration before, or at the same time as, the toxic compound. This complicates the interpretation of the site of action of such drugs, because they may interfere not only with activation, but also at the level of the receptor, and the subsequent events.

8.2.3 AVAILABILITY OF THE TOXIC AGENT: EFFECTS ON CELLULAR UPTAKE IN RELATION TO ORGAN SPECIFIC TOXICITY

When a drug is quite lipid-soluble it will reach most cells in the body by diffusion. However, when it does not so easily cross lipid membranes it may be taken up selectively in certain cells by carrier transport. The latter can in principle be inhibited by uptake-inhibitors. Thus 1-methyl-4-phenyl-1,2,3,6-tetrahydropyrdine (MPTP), is selectively toxic *in vivo* to the nigrostriatal dopaminergic system. It is converted to its toxic metabolite (MPP) by monoamino oxidase B, so that inhibitors of this enzyme (such as pargyline) will also protect against MPTP toxicity (Markey *et al.* 1986). MPP is taken up by a dopamine carrier system in dopaminergic neurones, where it is selectively toxic. This uptake can be prevented by mazindol, an inhibitor of the dopamine carrier system which prevents this toxicity. Toxicity of MPTP in isolated rat hepatocytes could also be inhibited by pargyline (DiMonte *et al.* 1986). Although the experiment was not reported, one would expect that in hepatocytes an inhibitor of dopamine uptake would have no effect.

Many drugs damage hepatocytes in the liver *in situ*, presumably because the liver accumulates many xenobiotics. Clearly it would not be easy to influence such massive uptake without major interference with organ function.

The lung has an uptake system for amines. Uptake of pulmonary toxicants which use that carrier might be prevented by appropriate compounds.

8.2.4 TRAPPING OF REACTIVE INTERMEDIATES AND PREVENTION OF DEPLETION OF ENDOGENOUS PROTECTIVE AGENTS

The reactive intermediates generated by drug metabolism are electrophilic agents (Anders 1985). One of the main protections of the cell against them is the —SH group of GSH, while the —SCH_3 of methionine may also afford protection against certain reactive intermediates (Reed 1985). The efficiency of trapping by various nucleophiles depends on the chemical properties of the reactive intermediate. Thus while GSH and cysteine are very effective with the paracetamol reactive intermediate NAIQ, they are much less so for the nitrenium ion of N-hydroxy-2-acetylaminofluorene (NOHAAF) sulfate (Table 1). Methionine and guanine, on the other hand, are more

Table 1—Differences in trapping efficiency of reactive intermediates by various agents

Agent	(mM)	Percentage inhibition of covalent binding to BSA† of	
		N-acetyl-*p*-iminobenzoquinone‡	2-acetylaminofluorene-N-sulfate
Glutathione	0.25	98	13
L-Cysteine	0.25	95	30
L-Methionine	20	4	87
Guanine	2	0	60
Adenine	2	0	15

† Binding to bovine serum albumine at pH 7.4 during generation of both substrates by rat liver cytosol.
‡ Generated from the N-O-sulfate of N-hydroxyphenacetin. Data taken from Mulder *et al.* (1978).

efficient towards the NOHAAF reactive intermediate and not at all towards NAIQ. By overloading of the cell with reactive intermediates, the availability of the endogenous protective compounds may decrease so that the endogenous protection fails. This clearly occurs after paracetamol overdosing, and the common therapy, intravenous administration of N-acetylcysteine to prevent GSH depletion, has proved to be very effective if it is applied in time (Corcoran & Wong 1986, Hazelton *et al.* 1986).

An alternative is to administer a thiol that itself can trap the reactive metabolite such as 2-mercaptopropionylglycine (Labadarios *et al.* 1977, Harman & Self 1986). Like N-acetylcysteine this compound has to be administered soon after paracetamol, because otherwise the initial toxic interaction of NAIQ has already taken place. Propylthiouracil (PTU) may also trap the reactive intermediate of paracetamol and thus reduce hepatotoxicity. However, PTU was fed for 12 days preceding the paracetamol administration (Linscheer *et al.* 1980). Thus, the mechanism of the protective effect of PTU (which has several more effects on the animal) is not unambiguously proved to be trapping of the reactive intermediate (Raheja *et al.* 1983). Various other thiols have been tested. In view of the fact that they seem to have several effects, such as on cellular calcium accumulation, cytochrome P450 activity or on hormones such as prolactin (Miners *et al.* 1984, MacDonald *et al.* 1985, Scott *et al.* 1987), the resulting effect may be of a mixed nature.

Recent work by Van den Goorbergh *et al.* (1987) showed that some thioethers were very efficient trapping agents for the nitrenium ion derived from NOHAAF-

Table 2—Trapping of the reactive metabolite of N-hydroxy-2-acetylaminofluorene (NOHAAF) sulfate by various thioethers *in vitro* and *in vivo*

Thioethers	% inhibition of			
	^{14}C-NOHAAF sulfate binding *in vitro*		^{14}C-NOHAAF induced	
	to BSA	to RNA	DNA-binding *in vivo*	transaminases *in vivo*
Thiazolidine	33	38	21	45
2-(Methylthio)-benzimidazole	43	80	44	83
Methyl-4-(methylthio)-benzoate	24	72	54	71

In vitro, the covalent binding of [9-^{14}C]-NOHAAF-sulfate to either RNA or bsa was measured in the presence or absence of 5 mM of the thioethers. *In vivo*, 360 μmol/kg [^{14}C]-NOH2AAF was given i.p., with or without 0.7 mmol/kg of the thioethers. DNA binding was measured in rat liver, and the activity of the transaminases was determined in blood after 24 hours. For details: see Van den Goorbergh *et al.* (1987).

sulfate, both *in vitro* and, in the rat, *in vivo*. Binding to macromolecules such as albumin, RNA, or DNA was prevented by these agents, as well as hepatotoxicity of NOHAAF *in vivo* (Table 2).

8.2.5 PREVENTION OF HEPATOTOXICITY BY -THIOL-CONTAINING COMPOUNDS

Sipes and co-workers have extensively investigated D-galactosamine hepatotoxicity, which does not seem to involve reactive intermediates. Its toxicity is due to depletion of the uridine pool as the initial step. Toxicity can, therefore, be prevented when the uridine pool is replenished immediately. Cysteamine effectively prevented D-galactosamine at a time when toxicity could not be further prevented by administration of uridine (MacDonald *et al.* 1984, 1985b, 1987). This was not correlated with an alteration of free protein thiol groups or cellular calcium, while the leakage of lactate dehydrogenase was also little affected by cystamine (MacDonald *et al.* 1985, 1987). At present the mechanism of this protective effect is unknown, which is not surprising, because the sequence of events involved in D-galactosamine toxicity is not known either. Several other compounds also show protection against D-galactosamine toxicity (MacDonald *et al.* 1985a), such as calcium chelators (EDTA, EGTA), aminoethanethiol derivatives (cysteamine, penicillamine), and precursors (N-acetylcysteine, 2-aminoethylisothiourea, cysteamine). Further, taurine alleviated toxicity of D-galactosamine *in vivo*, presumably by decreasing free intracellular calcium.

Cysteamine is also effective against CCl_4 toxicity when it is administered up to 12 hours after CCl_4 (MacDonald *et al.* 1986). Interestingly, the release of transaminases from the liver or the rise in liver calcium are not prevented by cysteamine; but histologically evaluated necrosis is decreased *in vivo*. When cystamine is administered before CCl_4 it is much more effective, presumably because it prevents 'early effects' such as activation of CCl_4 by cytochrome P450. Moreover, treatment with cystamine after CCl_4 administration also resulted in an increased mitotic index, indicating a more rapid regeneration process.

Recovery of isolated hepatocytes was also stimulated by dithiothreitol after paracetamol or NAIQ treatment (Harman & Self 1986, Albano *et al.* 1985). Whether such effects could also occur *in vivo* is unknown.

8.2.6 OTHER PROTECTIVE DRUGS

Various drugs have been tested more or less extensively *in vivo* for their protective properties against a number of hepatotoxins. Their mechanism of action is usually not understood, and they may be effective against only a limited number of drugs. A few will be mentioned here. A synthetic muramyl dipeptide [N-acetylmuramyl-L-alaninyl-D-iso-glutamine (MDP)] protects against CCl_4 and a number of cytostatics such as nitrogen mustard, cytosine arabinoside, and cyclophosphamide (Farghali *et al.* 1984). It was suggested that MDP and similar immunomodulatory drugs somehow 'stabilize' the cells against toxic insults.

A prostaglandin derivative, 16,16-dimethylprostaglandin E_2, markedly decreased the hepatotoxicity of bromobenzene in mice, without affecting biotransformation or covalent binding of bromobenzene reactive metabolites (Funck-Brentano *et al.* 1984). This prostaglandin derivative strongly increases DNA synthesis, and may stimulate regeneration of hepatocytes after the toxic insult (McNeill *et al.* 1985).

Nifedipine and chlorpromazine were highly effective against liver toxicity caused by various toxins. A reduction in liver cell calcium was assumed to be the mechanism of the protective action of these calcium channel blockers (Landon *et al.* 1986). However, the agents were administered before the hepatotoxin, so that other effects cannot be excluded.

A pronounced reduction in paracetamol toxicity was observed when acetylsalicylic acid was administered, although rather high doses were required (De Vries *et al.* 1984). An explanation is not evident, although a decreased calcium availability and increased glucose availability have been suggested (De Vries 1983).

8.2.7 CONCLUSIONS

The above review suggests that in the near future the therapeutic possiblities of preventing drug toxicity will expand into the period of 12–24 hours after administration of the toxicant. Protective mechanisms to be used in the liver may also be available in other organs. However, extrapolation is severely limited by our lack of knowledge about the protective mechanisms of, for example, cystamine *in vivo*. Yet even if this knowledge becomes available, the period after which protection still can be provided will always be limited by the extent of cell death: if too many cells have already died before therapy begins, the residual organ capacity may be insufficient for survival.

REFERENCES

Albano, E., Rundgren, M., Harvison, P. J., Nelson, S. D., & Moldéus, P. (1985) Mechanisms of N-acetyl-*p*-benzoquinone imine cytotoxicity. *Molec. Pharmacol.* **28,** 306–311.

Anders, M. W. (ed) (1985) *Bioactivation of foreign compounds.* Academic Press Inc. Orlando, Florida.

Belinsky, S. A., Badr, M. Z., Kauffman, F. C., & Thurman, R. G. (1986) Mechanism of hepatotoxicity in periportal regions of the liver lobule due to allyl alcohol: studies on thiols and energy status. *J. Pharmacol. exp. Ther.* **238,** 1132–1137.

Corcoran, G. B. & Wong, B. K. (1986) Role of glutathione in prevention of acetaminophen-induced hepatotoxicity by N-acetyl-L-cysteine *in vivo*: studies with N-acetyl-D-cysteine in mice. *J. Pharmacol. exp. Ther.* **238,** 54–61.

De Vries, J. (1983) Induction and prevention of biochemical disturbances in hepatic necrosis. *TIPS* **4,** 393–394.

De Vries, J., De Jong, J., Lock, F. M., Van Bree, L., Mullink, H. & Veldhuizen, R. W. (1984) Protection against paracetamol-induced hepatotoxicity by acetylsalicyclic acid in rats. *Toxicology* **30,** 297–304.

DiMonte, D., Jewell, S. A., Ekström, G., Sandy, M. S., & Smith, M. T. (1986) MPTP and MPP cause rapid ATP depletion in isolated hepatocy s. *Biochem. Biophys. Res. Commun.* **137,** 310–315.

Farghali, H., Machková, Z., Kameniková, L., Jankü, I., Masek, K. (1984) The protection from hepatotoxicity of some compounds by the synthetic immunomodulator muramyl dipeptide (MDP) in rat hepatocytes and *in vivo. Meth. Find exptl. Clin. Pharmacol.* **6,** 449–454.

Funck-Bretano, C., Tinel, M., Degott, C., Letteron, P., Babany, G., & Pessayre, D. (1984) Protective effect of 16,16-dimethyl prostaglandin E_2 on the hepatotoxicity of bromobenzene in mice. *Biochem. Pharmacol.* **35,** 89–96.

Harman, A. W. & Self, G. (1986) Comparison of the protective effects of N-acetylcystein, 2-mercaptopropionylglycine and dithiothreitol against acetaminophen toxicity in mouse hepatocytes. *Toxicology* **41,** 83–91.

Hazelton, G. A., Hjelle, J. J., & Klaassen, C. D. (1986) Effects of cysteine pro-drugs on acetaminophen-induced hepatotoxicity. *J. Pharmacol. exp. Ther.* **237,** 341–349.

Hinson, J. A. (1980) Biochemical toxicology of acetaminophen. In: *Revs in Biochem. Toxicol.* (eds by Hodgson, E., Bend, J. R., & Philpot, R.), **2,** pp. 103–129. Elsevier/North Holland, Amsterdam.

Labadarios, D., Davis, M., Portmann, B., & Williams, R. (1977) Paracetamol-induced hepatic necrosis in the mouse—Relationship between covalent binding, hepatic glutathione depletion and the protective effect of α-mercaptopropionylglycine. *Biochem. Pharmacol.* **26,** 31–34.

Labbe, G., Desctoire, V., Letteron, P., Degott, C., Tinel, M., Larrey, D., Carrion-Pavlov, Geneve, J., Maouyal, G., & Pessayre, D. (1987) The drug methoxsalen, a suicide substrate for cytochrome P450, decreases the metabolic activation, and prevents the hepatotoxicity of carbon tetrachloride in mice *Biochem. Pharmacol.* **36,** 907–914.

Landon, E. J., Naukam, R. J., & Rama Sastry, B. V. (1986) Effects of calcium channel blocking agents on calcium and centrilobular necrosis in the liver of rats treated with hepatotoxic agents. *Biochem. Pharmacol.* **35,** 697–705.

Linscheer, W. G., Raheja, K. L., Cho, C., & Smith, K. L. (1980) Mechanism of the protective effect of propylthiouracil against acetaminophen (Tylenol) toxicity in the rat. *Gastroenterology* **78,** 100–107.

MacDonald, J. R., Gandolfi, A. J., & Sipes, I. G. (1984) Cysteamine modulation of galactosamine-induced hepatotoxicity. *Toxicol. Appl. Pharmacol.* **73,** 551–558.

MacDonald, J. R., Gandolfi, A. J., & Sipes, I. G. (1985a) Structural requirements for cytoprotective agents in galactosamine-induced hepatic necrosis. *Toxicol Appl. Pharmacol.* **81,** 17–24.

MacDonald, J. R., Gandolfi, A. J., & Sipes, I. G. (1985b) Hepatic cysteamine and non-protein sulfhydryl levels following cystamine or cysteamine treatment of galactosamine-poisoned rats. *Drug Chem. Toxicol.* **8,** 483–494.

MacDonald, J. R., Gandolfi, A. J., & Sipes, I. G. (1986) Amelioration of carbon tetrachloride-induced hepatic necrosis by post-toxicant treatment with cystamine. *Toxicology* **39,** 135–148.

MacDonald, J. R., Thayer, K. J., White, C. (1987) Inhibition of galactosamine cytotoxicity in an *in vivo/in vitro* hepatocellular toxicity model. *Toxicol. Appl. Pharmacol.* **89**, 269–277.

Markey, S. D., Castagnoli, N., Trevor, A., Kopin, I. J. (1986) *MPTP: a neurotoxin producing Parkinsonian syndrome*. Academic Press, New York.

McNeil, G. E., Chen, T. S., & Leevy, C. M. (1985) Reversal of ethanol and indomethacin-induced suppression of hepatic DNA synthesis by 16,16-dimethyl prostaglandin E_2. *Hepatology* **5,** 43–46.

Meerman, J. H. N. (1986) Experimental modification of biotransformation of xenobiotics: consequences for hepatotoxicity. In: *Hepatotoxicity of drugs* (ed. Fillastre, J. P.), pp. 269–286. Edit. INSERM, University of Rouen, France.

Miners, J. O., Drew, R., & Birkett, D. J. (1984) Mechanism of action of paracetamol protective agents in mice *in vivo*. *Biochem. Pharmacol.* **33,** 2995–3000.

Mitchell, M. C., Schenker, S., & Speeg, K. V. (1984) Selective inhibition of acetaminophen oxidation and toxicity by cimetidine and other histamine H_2-receptor antagonists *in vivo* and *in vitro* in the rat and man. *J. Clin. Invest.* **73,** 383–391.

Mulder, G. J. & Scholtens, E. (1977) Phenolsulphotransferase and UDP glucuronyl-transferase from rat liver *in vivo* and *in vitro*. 2,6-dichloro-4-nitrophenol as selective inhibitor of sulfation. *Biochem. J.* **165,**553–559.

Mulder, G. J., Hinson, J. A., & Gillette, J. R. (1978) Conversion of the N-O-glucuronide and N-O-sulfate conjugates of N-hydroxyphenacetin to reactive intermediates. *Biochem. Pharmacol.* **27,** 1641–1649.

Nicotera, P., Hartzell, P., Baldi, C., Svensson, S. A., Bellomo, G., & Orrenius, S. (1986) Cystamine induces toxicity in hepatocytes through the elevation of cytosolic Ca^{2+} and the stimulation of a non-lysosomal proteolytic. *J. Biol. Chem.* **261,** 14628–14635.

Raheja, K. L., Linscheer, W. G., & Cho, C. (1983) Prevention of acetaminophen hepatotoxicity by propylthiouracil in the glutathione depleted rat. *Comp. Biochem. Physiol.* **76C,** 9–14.

Reed, D. J. (1985) Cellular defence mechanisms against reactive metabolites. In: *Bioactivation of foreign compounds* (ed. Anders, M. W.), pp. 71–108. Academic Press Inc., Orlando, Florida.

Reed, D. J. & Fariss, M. W. (1984) Glutathione depletion and susceptibility. *Pharmacol. Revs.* **36,** 25S–33S.

Scott, J. S., Lakin, C. A., & Oliver, J. R. (1987) The effect of cysteamine, cystamine and the structurally related compounds taurine, N-acetylcysteine and D-penicillamine on plasma prolactin levels in normal, and estrogen primed hyperprolactinemic rats. *Endocrinology* **121,** 812–820.

Van den Goorbergh, J. A. M., De Wit, H., Tijdens, R. B., Mulder, G. J., & Meerman, J. H. N. (1987) Prevention by thioethers of the hepatotoxicity and covalent binding to macromolecules of N-hydroxy-2-acetylaminofluorene and its sulfate ester in rat liver *in vivo* and *in vitro*. *Carcinogenesis* **8,** 275–279.

8.3 On the way to a recombinant vaccine for pertussis

Aldo Tagliabue M. Teresa De Magistris, Miriam Romano, & Rino Rappuoli†

A population of healthy adults who had suffered from whooping cough in childhood, was screened for humoral and cellular immunity against *Bordetella pertussis*. Out of these subjects, an immune donor defined by positive anamnesis, high serum levels of IgG against pertussis toxin and strong lymphocyte proliferation in response to inactivated *B. pertussis*, was selected to generate T-cell clones. Fourteen clones were obtained, and their specificity against *B. pertussis* and five Tn5-induced mutants or against *B. bronchiseptica* and *B. parapertussis* was tested. On the basis of the different pattern of reactivity of the T-cell clones in response to the bacteria tested the *Bordetella* antigens responsible for anamnestic responses can be predicted.

8.3.1 INTRODUCTION

The need for a safer, efficacious vaccine against whooping cough is widely recognized. While field trials are in progress with the new acellular vaccines from *Bordetella pertussis* in Japan and Sweden, where the disease has reappeared after the withdrawal of the cellular vaccine, recombinant proteins which may be used as third generation anti-whooping cough vaccines are becoming more easily available (Nicosia *et al.* 1987). On the other hand, the immune mechanisms which induce protection against *B. pertussis* infection are still poorly understood.

In an attempt to develop tools which might be useful to define the antigens which are most important in inducing immunity against *B. pertussis*, an analysis at the T-cell clonal level was performed in a donor who had suffered from whooping cough in childhood. In fact it is likely that the understanding of the mechanisms and/or the specificity of the T-cell dependent immunological memory may represent a model to predict the minimal antigenic structures capable of inducing protection against pertussis.

Thus, the availability of new *in vitro* techniques to investigate immunity against pertussis in humans can be viewed as an interesting alternative to the unsatisfactory animal models for *B. pertussis* infection. Here, preliminary results obtained with 14 human T-lymphocyte clones specific for *B. pertussis* are reported.

† Sclavo Research Center, Via Fiorentina 1, 53100 Siena, Italy.

8.3.2 IDENTIFICATION OF AN IMMUNE DONOR TO GENERATE T-CELL CLONES

In the past, the presence of antibodies against *B. pertussis* antigens in serum and the ability of peripheral blood mononuclear cells (PBMC) to express cell-mediated immunity against the whole microorganisms were investigated mainly in vaccinees and/or infected patients (Burstyn *et al.* 1983, Granström *et al.* 1985, Andersen *et al.* 1977). We performed a series of studies employing 30 adults of both sexes (25–50 years old) with negative or positive anamnesis of whooping cough in their childhood. Sera from these donors were tested in sandwich ELISA where goat antibodies against highly purified pertussis toxin were used as space layer between the solid phase and the antigen. After the addition of anti-human IgG conjugated to alkaline phosphatase it was found that the majority of donors with negative anamnesis (10/12 donors) have absorbance values at 405 nm below 0.150, whereas in the donors with positive anamnesis, two major populations could be observed: one below 0.150 (7/18 donors) and one between 0.150 and 0.600 (11/18 donors). Then, PBMC (10^5/0.2 ml per wel) from donors negative for ELISA and pertussis anamnesis or positive for both parameters were tested for proliferation in response to increasing numbers (from 0.05 to 40×10^5 bacteria per well) or inactivated *B. pertussis* cells by ^{3}H-Thymidine incorporation in a 5-day assay. As shown in Fig. 1, a good correlation was found (correlation coefficient $r = 0.697$, $P < 0.01$) between the level of antibodies against

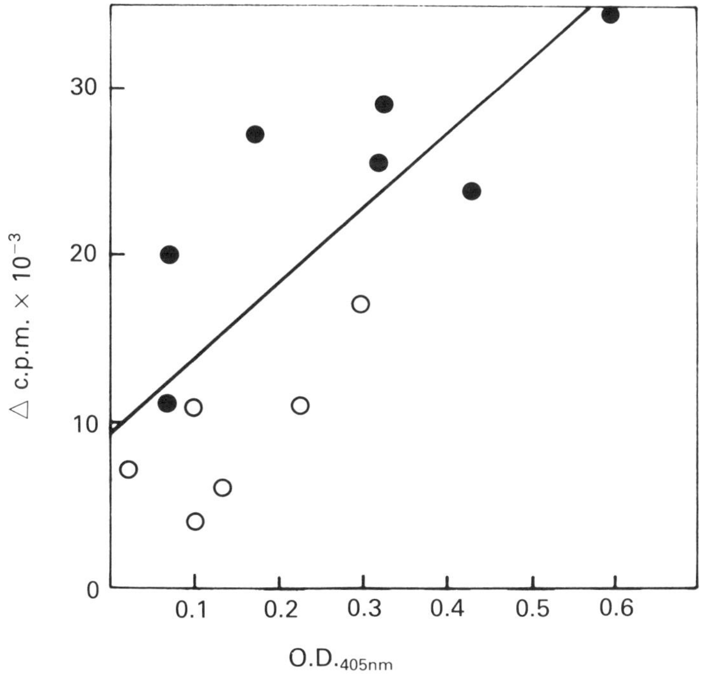

Fig. 1.—Humoral and cellular immunity of normal adults with positive (●) and negative (○) anamnesis of whooping cough in childhood. On the *x* axis, absorbance values determined by ELISA against pertussis toxin and on the *y* axis, proliferative response expressed in ^{3}H-thymidine incorporation of peripheral blood mononuclear cells in response to inactivated *B. pertussis*. Correlation coefficient was $r = 0.697$ ($p < 0.01$).

pertussis toxin and the optimal proliferative response to *B. pertussis*. Based on these results, a donor positive in anamnesis, with high antibody level against pertussis toxin (OD = 0.310) and significant proliferative response (30 000 cpm), was chosen for generation of T-cell clones against *B. pertussis*.

8.3.3 GENERATION OF T-CELL CLONES SPECIFIC FOR *B. PERTUSSIS*

As shown in Fig. 2, PBMC from the supposed immune donor were restimulated *in vitro* for 7 days with killed bacteria (Lanzavecchia 1985). Recombinant IL-2 (rIL-2) was then added to expand immune T lymphocytes, which were then cloned by limiting dilution and tested for specificity against *B. pertussis*. In this case, parallel cultures of autologous B lymphocytes were established *in vitro* by immortalization with Epstein–Barr virus (EBV) in the presence of cyclosporin A (CyA). Fourteen clones (out of 46) specific for *B. pertussis* antigens were obtained by determining their proliferative response to inactivated bacteria (Fig. 2, bottom left).

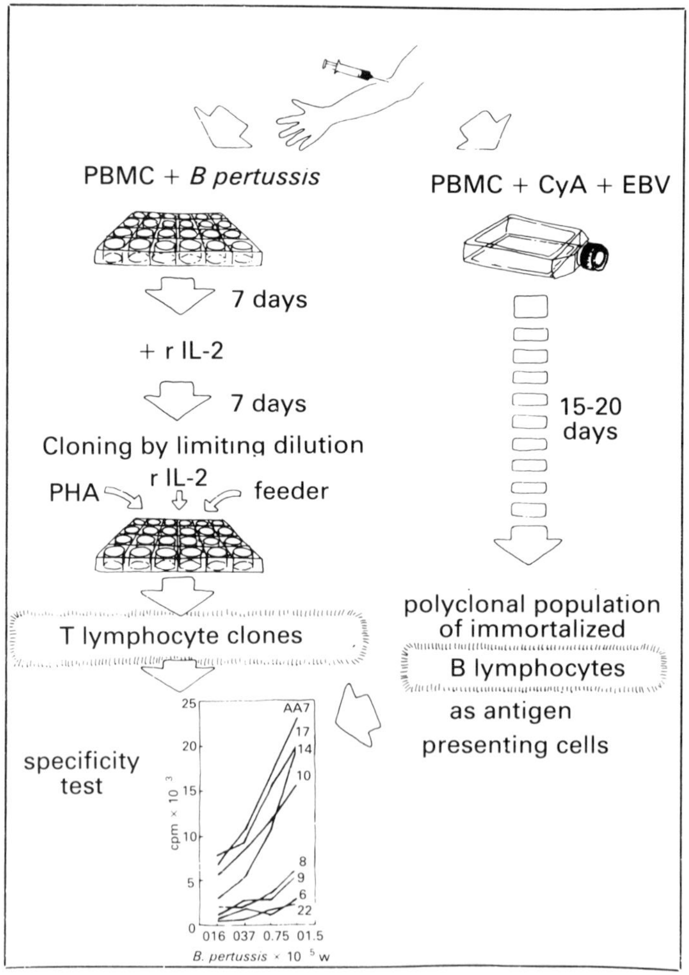

Fig. 2.—Schematic representation of the generation of T-cell clones in response to *B. pertussis*.

8.3.4 ANALYSIS OF THE SPECIFICITY OF T-CELL CLONES

To gain further information about the specificity of the T-cell clones, two other species of *Bordetella* and four Tn5-induced mutants defective in the production of *B. pertussis* virulence factors (Weiss *et al.* 1983) were employed after inactivation as antigen in the proliferative assay (Table 1). It was found that T-cell clones recognize different antigens on *B. pertussis*. In fact, as shown in Fig. 3, the pattern of reactivity in response to the other *Bordetella* species and/or to the mutants differs widely. However, some clones can be clustered. The specificity of the T-cell clones was further confirmed by the lack of responsiveness to *Salmonella typhi* (Fig. 3).

Table 1—Bacteris used as antigens in T-cell clone proliferation assay

Bordetella pertussis *Bordetella parapertussis* *Bordetella bronchiseptica*
Tn5 mutants: BP 353 deficient for filamentous hemagglutinin BP 356 deficient for subunit 3 of the pertussis toxin BP 348 deficient for adenylate cyclase BP 347 deficient for hemolysin
Salmonella typhi

	CLONES	*B. pertussis*	*B. parapertussis*	*B. bronchiseptica*	BP 353 (FHA^-)	BP 356 (S_3^-)	BP 348 (AC^-, HLY^-)	BP 347 (vir^-)	*S. typhi*
	6	■	■	□	□	■	■	□	□
	18	■	■	■	□	■	■	■	□
	22	■	■	■	■	■	■	□	□
Group I	23, 32	■	□	□	■	■	■	□	□
Group II	7, 8, 31, 34	■	■	□	■	■	■	□	□
Group III	9, 17, 26, 28, 30	■	■	■	■	■	■	■	□
Number of responding clones:		14/14	12/14	7/14	12/14	14/14	14/14	6/14	0/14

Fig. 3.—Summary of the results obtained with 14 human T-cell clones against *B. pertussis* in response to different bacteria. A positive response (■) was considered as incorporation of more than 1000 cpm over the control by 2×10^4 lymphocytes in the presence of 3×10^6 bacteria, whereas less than that was considered a negative response (□).

Even though these results must be considered still preliminary, it may be suggested that whooping cough is able to induce T-cell memory which is expressed against a variety of *B. pertussis* antigens. The possibility of stimulating T-cell clones with bacteria which are identical to *B. pertussis* but lack some virulence antigens, seems to be of interest in defining which antigenic determinants are important in inducing protection against the disease. This is based on the hypothesis that the immunological memory represents the specific antibacterial defences which determined the overcoming of the disease. One may predict the antigens recognized by some T-cell clones. For instance, it is quite likely that clones 23 and 32 might recognize pertussis toxin. This hypothesis must be confirmed by direct experiments where the soluble antigen is employed. Differing from group I, group III is formed by a cluster of clones that recognize all the *Bordetella* species and mutants. These clones may be used as probes to define important antigens on *Bordetella* which may not be associated with virulence but may still play an important role in protection. In conclusion, the T-cell clonal approach seems to be a useful technique to define the specificity of immunity against whooping cough. Of particular interest is the fact that this approach may also serve to define the immunogenic epitopes within the antigens which induce protection. And this may lead to short, synthetic, or recombinant peptides to be used as potential vaccines.

REFERENCES

Andersen, V., Hertz, J. B., Sorensen, S. F., Baekgaard P., Christensen, P. E., Ramhoj, W., Hansen, G. A., Wardlaw, A. C., & Sato, Y. (1977). *In vitro* stimulation of human lymphocytes by *Bordetella pertussis. Acta Path. Microbiol. Scand. Sect. C* **85,** 65–72.

Burstyn, D. G., Baraff, L. J., Peppler, M. S., Leake, R. D., Geme, J. St. Jr., & Manclark, C. R. (1983). Serological response to filamentous hemagglutinin and lymphocytosis-promoting toxin of *Bordetella pertussis. Infect. Immun.* **41,** 1150–1156.

Granström, M. Granström, G., Gillenius, P., & Askelöf, P. (1985). Neutralizing antibodies to pertussis toxin in whooping cough. *J. Infect. Dis.* **151,** 646–649.

Lanzavecchia, A. (185). Antigen-specific interaction between T and B cells. *Nature* **314,** 537–539.

Nicosia, A., Bartoloni, A., Perugini, M., & Rappuoli, R. (1987). Expression and immunological properties of the five subunits of pertussis toxin. *Infect. Immun.* **55,** 963–967.

Weiss, A. A., Hewlett, E. L., Myers, G. A., & Falkow, S. (1983). Tn5-induced mutations affecting virulence factors of *Bordetella pertussis. Infect. Immun.* **42,** 33–41.

8.4 Adenylate cyclase toxin of *Bordetella pertussis*

Octavian Bârzu, Daniel Ladant, & Agnes Ullmann†

(1) *Bordetella pertussis* adenylate cyclase was purified from culture supernatants or urea-extracts of whole organisms by affinity chromatography using a genetically engineered calmodulin, immobilized on agarose beads.
(2) The enzyme exists as 'high' and 'low' molecular weight form, each interacting with free or agarose-immobilized calmodulin.
(3) The 'low' molecular weight component of *Bordetella pertussis* adenylate cyclase consists of three structurally related peptides of 50, 45 and 43K. Trypsin converts the 50 and 45K components to the 43K specie with no loss of activity.
(4) Limited proteolysis with trypsin in the presence of calmodulin and use of a photoactivable derivative of calmodulin, showed that the 43K peptide consists of two separate domains of 25 and 18K respectively, each interacting with calmodulin.
(5) *Bordetella pertussis* and rat brain adenylate cyclase showed immunological cross-reactivity which might suggest that the bacterial enzyme arose by gene transfer from the host eukaryote to the bacterium.

8.4.1 INTRODUCTION

Bordetella pertussis, a Gram-negative bacterium, is the causative agent of whooping cough. Several compounds are secreted by this organism (pertussis toxin, filamentous hemagglutinin, dermonecrotic toxin, hemolysin, adenylate cyclase) and are incriminated in the virulence of *Bordetella pertussis* (Weiss & Hewlett 1986).

Pertussis toxin, known under different names (lymphocytosis promoting factor, islet-activating protein, histamine sensitivity factor), is the most extensively studied product (Ui *et al.* 1984). It is a hexamer composed of five different peptides; the largest subunit catalyses the transfer of ADP-ribose moiety of NAD^+ to the subunit of one or more guanine nucleotide-binding (G or N) proteins (Katada & Ui 1982).

Adenylate cyclase of *Bordetella pertussis* occupies a particular place among several factors incriminated as playing a role in the virulence of this organism. It is activated by an eukaryotic regulatory protein, calmodulin (Wolff *et al.* 1980), and enters animal cells, thus causing an elevation of the intracellular cAMP content (Confer & Eaton 1982).

† Unité de Biochimie des Régulations Cellulaires, Institut Pasteur, 75742 Paris, France

8.4.2 PURIFICATION OF *BORDETELLA PERTUSSIS* ADENYLATE CYCLASE

The first attempt to purify the enzyme from culture supernatants was reported by Hewlett & Wolff (1976). It soon became evident that enzyme was sensitive to calmodulin stimulation both in the presence and the absence of calcium ions (Wolff *et al.* 1980, Greenlee *et al.* 1982), and that the specific activity was much higher than that originally suggested (Shattuck *et al.* 1985). On the other hand, adenylate cyclase showed molecular heterogeneity, both in molecular weight and its capacity to enter animal cells (Kessin & Francke 1986, Hanski & Farfel 1985).

Ladant *et al.* (1986) purified extracellular enzyme nearly to homogeneity from a highly virulent strain of *Bordetella pertussis* by taking the advantage of the fact that calmodulin complexed enzyme, unlike free adenylate cyclase, was able to bind to DEAE–Sephacel at neutral pH. The complex was recovered in high yield and purity from the anion-exchanger by salt elution. Another property of *Bordetella pertussis* adenylate cyclase, namely its strong interaction with bovine brain calmodulin immobilized on agarose beads, allowed its purification from culture supernatants or bacterial extracts by elution with 8 M urea (Ladant *et al.* 1986). An engineered calmodulin (VU-8 calmodulin) which differs in its ability to activate *Bordetella pertussis* adenylate cyclase, has been used recently as a basis for a new purification protocol for the adenylate cyclase (Haiech *et al.* 1988). VU-8 calmodulin, in which three glutamic acid residues (residues 82–84) have been substituted with three lysine residues) showed a thousand-fold lower apparent affinity for *Bordetella pertussis* adenylate cyclase compared to vertebrate calmodulin. Immobilized VU-8 camodulin was tested as a calcium-dependent, affinity-based absorption chromatography step in the purification of the cyclase from culture media or bacterial extract. The specific activity of such an enzyme preparation was 2400 μmol/min/mg of protein. This procedure allowed the isolation of 50–70 μg of pure protein from 4 litres of culture supernatants or from 1.5 g of bacteria (Haiech *et al.* 1988).

8.4.3 MOLECULAR HETEROGENEITY OF *BORDETELLA PERTUSSIS* ADENYLATE CYCLASE

Gel permeation chromatography using both culture supernatants and urea extracts of *Bordetella pertussis* indicated the existence of 'low' and 'high' molecular weight forms of adenylate cyclase (Hanski & Farfel 1985, Kessin & Francke 1986). The smaller species correspond to a molecular weight between 50 and 79K, whereas the higher molecular weight species have variable sizes ranging between 120and 700K. Kessin & Francke (1986) showed that there was increased conversion of the high molecular weight enzme to the low molecular weight form upon 2% Triton X-100 or acetone–ethanol treatment. In fact, the high molecular weight form of adenylate cyclase separated from the low molecular weight component by gel permeation chromatography, purified by affinity chromatography, and further analysed by SDS-polyacrylamide gel electrophoresis and western blot, was shown to contain a large proportion of 50K, 45K, and 43K polypeptides (Bârzu *et al.*, unpublished). This seems to indicate that hydrophobic interactions are partly responsible for holding the enzyme in its high molecular weight form. It is worthwhile mentioning also that the 'invasive' form of adenylate cyclase (approximately 190K) does not correspond to the major peaks of adenylate cyclase activity (Hanski & Farfel 1985, Friedman *et al.* 1987). This and other evidence suggest that intracellular penetration of adenylate cyclase might require the presence of another factor. This is not an unprecedented case, since *Bacillus anthracis* adenylate cyclase, identified as the oedema factor, enters animal cells by means of another protein called protective antigen (Leppla 1982).

Each of the three polypeptides belonging to the low molecular weight species of adenylate cyclase (50K, 45K, and 43K, respectively) possesses enzyme activity. They can be separated by SDS-polyacrylamide gel electrophoresis, excised from the gel, then extratced and renatured to active, calmodulin-dependent forms (Ladant 1988). Moreover, the 50K and 45K polypeptides can be converted to the 43K form by limited proteolysis with trypsin, which suggests that the three peptides are structurally related and arose from a different processing of a common precursor during secretion.

8.4.4 MOLECULAR PROPERTIES OF *BORDETELLA PERTUSSIS* ADENYLATE CYCLASE

Adenylate cyclase of *Bordetella pertussis* is very sensitive to trypsin digestion (Wolff *et al.* 1984, Ladant *et al.* 1986). Calmodulin greatly increases resistance of the enzme to proteolytic inactivation (Ladant *et al.* 1986, Ladant 1987). After conversion of 50K and 45K peptides to the 43K form with no loss of activity, these were further digested to 25K and 18K fragments. The two-dimensional tryptic map of these last peptides called T25 and T18 was significantly different, indicating that they represent indeed two different, complementary, fragments of adenylate cyclase. Analysis of the trypsin-cleaved adenylate cyclase ^{125}I-calmodulin complex by gel permeation chromatography revealed a unique peak of adenylate cyclase activity comigrating with the main peak of radioactivity. Its apparent molecular weight of 70K was identical to that of the undigested complex. In other words, after proteolysis, T25, T18, and calmodulin remained associated by non-covalent interactions in an active, native-like structure. The 43K, T25, and T18 peptides were further cleaved with N-chlorosuccinimide (known to cleave specifically peptide bonds involving tryptophan residues), then analysed by SDS-polyacrylamide gel electrophoresis. The number and the size of resulting fragments allowed localization of T25 at the N-terminal side of 43K polypeptide. Furthermore, knowing the primary structure of the *Bordetella pertussis* adenylate cyclase as deduced from the nucleotide sequence of the cloned gene (Glaser *et al.* 1988), we can assign the 43K polypeptide as representing the first 400 residues of a large precursor comprising 1706 amino acids.

Photolysis of a mixture of adenylate cyclase and ^{125}I-labelled azido-calmodulin (before or after trypsin digestion of the complex), allowed identification of several crosslinked products of 70K, 63K, 45K, and 38K respectively. Since the apparent molecular weight of calmodulin or azido-calmodulin on SDS-polyacrylamide gel electrophoresis is 20K, the crosslinked products probably correspond to covalent attachment of one azido-calmodulin molecule to the 50K, 43K, T25, and T18 peptides, respectively. These results strongly suggested that both T25 and T18 domains of adenylate cyclase interact with calmodulin most probably through their C- and N-terminal sequences, respectively.

Kinetic experiments showed that the photoactivable analog of ATP, Bz_2ATP (3′-O-(benzoyl)benzoyl adenosine 5′-triphosphate) acts as a competitive inhibitor of bacterial enzyme, having a 60-fold higher affinity for the active site than its natural substrate (K_m for ATP is 0.6 mM, K_i for Bz_2ATP is 0.01 mM). Photolysis of a mixture of Bz_2ATP and adenylate cyclase irreversibly inactivated the enzyme. Adenylate cyclase was covalently labelled when ^{32}P labelled Bz_2ATP was used in photolysis experiments. Therefore, proteolytic 'dissection' combined with crosslinking experiments using photoactivable derivatives of calmodulin and ATP allowed localization of two important interacting sites of *Bordetella pertussis* adenylate cyclase.

8.4.5 IMMUNOLOGICAL PROPERTIES OF *BORDETELLA PERTUSSIS* ADENYLATE CYCLASE

Antibodies against *Bordetella pertussis* adenylate cyclase raised in rabbits or guinea-pigs recognized all three polypeptides of 50K, 45K, and 43K in immunoblots. Other *Bordetella pertussis* proteins such as pertussis toxin or filamentous hemagglutinin, were not recognized by the immune sera. Interestingly, the sera obtained from animals immunized against purified rat brain adenylate cyclase (Monneron *et al.* 1987) gave the same recognition pattern of *Bordetella pertussis* adenylate cyclase. Control experiments made with pre-immune sera or with *E. coli* adenylate cyclase gave negative results. Conversely, when antibodies raised against *Bordetella pertussis* adenylase cyclase were tested for cross-reaction with the rat brain adenylate cyclase catalytic subunit, they gave positive reactions comparable to those obtained with the anti-rat brain adenylate cyclase antibodies. On the basis of the evolutionary distance between bacteria and mammals, a convergent evolution of the two addeylate cyclases seems unlikely. The immunological relatedness could indicate that the two enzymes originate from a common ancestor to bacteria and mammals. However, since calmodulin is not known to occur in bacteria, we would rather suggest that the bacterial enzyme arose by gene transfer from the host eukaryote to the bacterium (Monneron *et al.* 1988).

8.4.6 CLONING AND EXPRESSION IN *E. COLI* OF *BORDETELLA PERTUSSIS* ADENYLATE CYCLASE

Several adenylate cyclase genes have been cloned in *E. coli* or *S. cerevisiae* by screening complementing cyclase defective clones on selective media. Attempts to clone the *Bordetella pertussis* adenylate cyclase gene using the same screening procedures failed, and no functional clones have been obtained until recently. Glaser *et al.* (1988) chose a *E. coli* adenylate cyclase defective strain harbouring a plasmid, pVUC-1 that expressed high levels of a synthetic calmodulin. This strain was used as a recipient for a library of total *Bordetella pertussis* DNA, constructed in a compatible replicon. Several clones complementing the *E. coli* defects were found. The *Bordetella pertussis* adenylate cyclase gene was sequenced and shown to encode a 1706 amino acids protein (Glaser *et al.* 1988). Several truncated proteins possessing adenylate cyclase activity were expressed in *E. coli* and purified by affinity chromatography as previously described. All proteins are calmodulin-dependent and react with antibodies directed against the 50K, 45K, and 43K polypeptides from *Bordetella pertussis*.

8.4.7 FUTURE PROSPECTS

Purification of *Bordetella pertussis* adenylate cyclase, cloning and expression of the gene in *E. coli*, open new ways ins understanding the molecular evolution of this enzyme, and its involvement in the virulence of *Bordetella pertussis*. The high molecular weight of the adenylate cyclase precursor as compared to the catalytically active species might suggest another function of the large remaining fragment. It is possible that adenylate cyclase, like other protein toxins, exhibits beside the catalytic activity a function that enables the toxin to interact with host cells.

ACKNOWLEDGEMENTS

This work was supported by grants from the Centre National de la Recherche Scientifique (UA 1129).

REFERENCES

Confer, D. L. & Eaton, J. W. (1982) Phagocyte impotence caused by an invasive bacterial adenylate cyclase. *Science* **217,** 948–950.

Friedman, E., Farfel, Z., & Hanski, E. (1987) The invasive adenylate cyclase of *Bordetella pertussis*. Properties and penetration kinetics. *Biochem. J.* **243,** 145–151.

Glaser, P., Ladant, D., Sezer, O., Pichot, F., Ullmann, A., & Danchin, A. (1988) The calmodulin sensitive adenylate cyclase of *Bordetella pertussis*: cloning and expression in *E. coli*. *Mol. Microbiol.* 2, 19–30.

Greenlee, D. V., Andreasen, T. J., & Storm, D. R. (1982) Calcium independent stimulation of *Bordetella pertussis* adenylate cyclase by calmodulin. *Biochemistry* **21,** 2759–2764.

Haiech, J., Predeleanu, R., Watterson, D. M., Ladant, D., Bellalou, J., Ullmann, A., & Bârzu, O. (1987) Affinity-based chromatography using genetically engineered proteins: purification of *Bordetella pertussis* adenylate cyclase. *J. Biol. Chem.* **263**, 4259–4262.

(submitted).

Hanski, E. & Farfel, Z. (1985) *Bordetella pertussis* invasive adenylate cyclase. *J. Biol. Chem.* **260,** 5526–5532.

Hewlett, E. & Wolff, J. (1976) Soluble adenylate cyclase from the culture medium of *Bordetella pertussis*: purification and characterization. *J. Bacteriol.* **127,** 890–898.

Katada, T. & Ui, M. (1982) ADP-ribosylation of the specific membrane protein of C_6 cells by islet-activating protein associated with modification of adenylate cyclase activity. *J. Biol. Chem.* **257,** 7210–7216.

Kessin, R. H. & Francke, J. (1986) Secreted adenylate cyclase of *Bordetella pertussis*: calmodulin requirements and partial purification of two forms. *J. Bacteriol.* **166,** 290–296.

Ladant, D., Brezin, C., Alonso, J.-M., Crenon, I., & Guiso, N. (1986) *Bordetella pertussis* adenylate cyclase: purification, characterization and immunoassay. *J. Biol. Chem.* **261,** 16264–16269.

Ladant, D. (1988) Interaction of *Bordetella pertussis* adenylate cyclase with calmodulin: identification of two separate calmodulin binding domains. *J. Biol. Chem.* **263**, 2612–2618.

Leppla, S. H. (1982) Anthrax toxin oedema factor: a bacterial adenylate cyclase that increases cyclic AMP concentrations in eukaryotic cells. *Proc. Natl. Acad. Sci. USA* **79,** 3162–3166.

Monneron, A., d'Alayer, J., & Coussen, F. (1987a) Purification of the catalytic subunit of adenylate cyclase in vertebrates: state of the art in 1987. *Biochimie* **69,** 263–270.

Monneron, A., Ladant, D., d'Alayer, J., Bellalou, J., Bârzu, O., & Ullmann, A. (1988) Immunological relatedness between *Bordetella pertussis* and rat brain adenylyl cyclases. *Biochemistry* (in press).

Shattuck, R. L., Oldenberg, D. J., & Storm, D. R. (1985) Purification and characterization of a calmodulin-senstive adenylate cyclase from *Bordetella pertussis*. *Biochemistry* **24,** 6356–6362.

Ui, M., Katada, T., Murayama, T., Kurose, H., Yajima, M., Tamura, M., Nakamura, T., & Nogimori, K. (1984) Islet-activating protein, pertussis toxin: a specific uncoupler of receptor-mediated inhibition of adenylate cyclase. *Adv. Cyclic Nucleotide and Protein Phosphorylation Research* **17,** 145–151.

Weiss, A. A. & Hewlett, E. L. (1986) Virulence factors of *Bordetella pertussis*. *Ann. Rev. Microbiol.* **40,** 661–686.

Wolff, J., Hope Cook, G., Goldhammer, A. R., & Berkowitz, S. A. (1980) Calmodulin activates prokaryotic adenylate cyclase. *Proc. Natl. Acad. Sci. USA* **77,** 3841–3844.

Wolff, J., Hope Cook, G., Goldhammer, A. R., Londos, C., & Hewlett, E. L. (1984) *Bordetella pertussis*: multiple attacks on host cell cyclic AMP regulation. *Adv. Cyclic Nucleotide and Protein Phosphorylation Research* **17,** 161–172.

8.5 Mechanisms of liver injury and protection

E. Altomare, G. Vendemiale, N. Antonacci, G. Palasciano, & O Albano†

In recent years many studies have been accumulated concerning the mechanisms of hepatotoxicity of a number of toxic agents, including hydrogen peroxides, free radicals, and foreign compounds.

Among the defence mechanisms, the tripeptide glutathione (gamma-glutamyl-cysteinyl-glycine, GSH) is known to play a key role in limiting chemically induced injury to cells and tissues. GSH performs, indeed, a variety of physiological and metabolic functions such as thiol transfer reactions, thiol-disulfide reactions, detoxification of free radicals, organic peroxides, and toxic metabolites.

Decreases in GSH levels have been associated with the enhancement of toxicity of many compounds, and in a number of animal studies ethanol consumption has been reported to cause hepatic GSH depletion and altered biliary GSH concentration.

In two different studies we have recently observed decreased GSH levels in liver biopsies from patients with alcoholic and non-alcoholic liver diseases, in respect to a well-selected group of subjects without any liver injury. The depression of GSH concentration seems to be a consistent characteristic of patients with chronic liver diseases which occurs even in the absence of evident liver damage.

It would be of interest to evaluate the efficacy of administration of glutathione and glutathione precursors during chronic liver injury and to assess whether GSH restoration could modify the progression of hepatic damage.

8.5.1 INTRODUCTION

It is well known that a wide variety of chemical and biological agents can induce hepatic injury. Clinical and experimental observations have led to general agreement that there are two main categories of hepatotoxicants. The first group consists of intrinsically toxic agents whose toxicity appears to be a fundamental property to which most exposed individuals are susceptible. The other group includes agents that produce hepatic injury only in unusually susceptible humans; their toxic effects, in other words, result from the special vulnerability of the affected subjects, rather than from their intrinsic toxicity.

Hepatic injury due to medical agents is, of course, of most interest for clinicians. There are a large number of drugs capable of causing cellular damage, depending on the dose of the chemical and the status of certain cellular protections systems. Among mechanisms of hepatotoxicity, the peroxidation of polyunsaturated fatty acids, as components of biological membranes, is considered to be the starting point of many toxic processes (Comporti 1985).

† Institute of Clinica Medica I, University of Bari, Bari, Italy

Lipid peroxidation is known to proceed in three different steps: (a) initiation by which the lipid radicals are generated, (b) the propagation reactions in which the number of free radicals is conserved, and (c) the termination reaction.

Lipid radical formation may be accomplished in two different ways, either by reactive oxygen species ($OH^{\cdot}$, O_2^{-}) or by chemicals (Ekstrom & Ingelman-Sundberg 1986). In addition, Di Luzio (1966) suggested that lipid peroxidation might also play a role in the liver damage produced by alcohol, and more recently Shaw *et al.* (1981) have confirmed the ethanol-induced lipid peroxidation in association with gutathione (GSH) depression. As is known, GSH is a tripeptide, gamma-glutamil-cysteinyl-glycine, which appears to have a key role in protective mechanisms. It participates in detoxification reactions of electrophilic substances, such as carcinogen epoxide metabolites and certain drugs by conjugation between nucleophilic thiol of GSH and an electrophilic site on another molecule. Hydrogen peroxide and lipid peroxides are also detoxified by reduced glutathione generating oxidized glutathione (GSSG), in addition, the ratio of reduced to oxidized glutathione is critical in regulating protein and enzyme functions and protein synthesis, and the maintenance of the redox state (Kaplowitz 1981).

Decreases in GSH levels have been associated with the enhancement of toxicity of many compounds, including carbontetrachloride, acetaminophen, alcohol (Reed & Beatty 1980, Sato *et al.* 1981, Altomare *et al.* 1984), and in a number of animal studies acute and chronic ethanol consumptions have been reported to cause hepatic GSH depletion (Guerri & Grisoliz 1980, Shaw *et al.* 1981) and alterations of hepatic and biliary GSH concentrations (Vendemiale *et al.* 1984).

In spite of abundant literature on GSH studies in animal species, little has been established about GSH levels during chronic liver diseases in humans, mainly because of varying criteria for patients and controls selection and different assay methods which may not distinguish GSH and mixed disulfides (Poulsen *et al.* 1981, Hissen & Hilf 1976).

Our group has recently carried out two studies in humans to evaluate hepatic GSH concentrations in patients with alcoholic and non-alcoholic liver diseases.

8.5.2 HEPATIC GSH LEVELS DURING CHRONIC LIVER INJURY

In our first study (Jewell *et al.* 1986) 30 male patients (28–54 years) were selected. They were divided into two groups:

(1) 20 chronic alcoholics, who conformed to the following standards: history of alcohol abuse (>150 g/day for 3 yr until admission); good nutritional status; no regular ingestion of other drugs during the last 3 months; no other major pathologies;

(2) 10 control subjects selected from consenting male patients admitted to the Department of Surgery for uncomplicated abdominal procedures. These patients showed infrequent and minor alcohol consumption (<40 g/day, <3 times/week); good nutritional status; normal liver function tests and histology.

GSH and GSSG were measured in liver biopsies from all patients by high-performance liquid chromatography (HPLC) as previously described (Reed *et al.* 1980). Results were also correlated with independent histology reports and blood chemistry values from the same subjects.

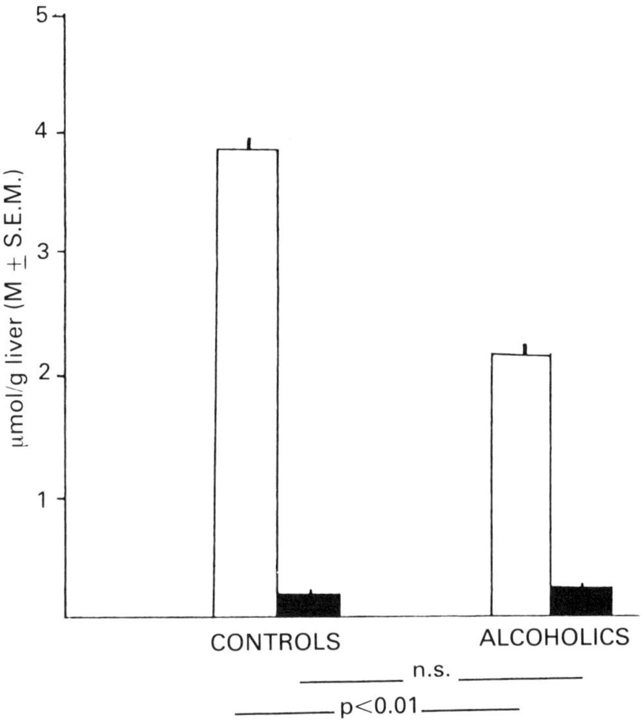

Fig. 1.—GSH (□) and GSSG (■) concentrations in hepatic tissue from control ($n = 10$) and alcoholic patients ($n = 20$). Results are expressed as mean ± SEM.

The glutathione values obtained from hepatic samples of the alcoholic group were found significantly lower than the controls (Fig. 1). This decrease was due to loss of GSH as the GSSG concentrations was found to be similar in both groups. The relationship between GSH levels and the progression of alcoholic liver injury was investigated by dividing alcoholic patients into two subgroups (on the basis of the degree of microscopic alterations) as follows:

(A) patients with no histological changes or steatosis only;
(B) patients with hepatitis or fibrosis.

No difference was observed in GSH levels between these subgroups (Fig. 2), suggesting that GSH is a poor index for discrimination between mild vs advanced liver injury, whereas it may represent an early marker of alcohol-induced liver impairment.

Our second experiment focused on hepatic GSH levels also in patients with mixed-aetiology liver diseases (Altomare *et al.* submitted). We studied 35 selected chronic alcoholic patients, 20 patients with non-alcoholic liver diseases (chronic active hepatitis, $n = 7$; chronic persisting hepatitis, $n = 3$; steatosis, $n = 2$; cirrhosis, $n = 8$), and 15 appropriate control subjects.

Hepatic GSH and GSSG were measured in liver biopsies from all patients by HPLC according to the method of Reed *et al.* (1980).

Also, in this study, alcoholic and non-alcoholic patients reported a significant decrease of hepatic glutathione in respect to control subjects (Fig. 3). Even if GSSG

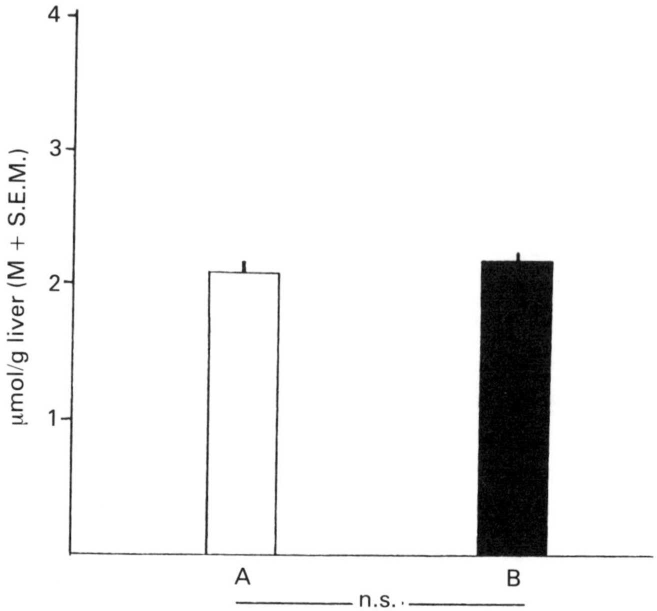

Fig. 2.—Total hepatic GSH concentration in two subgroups of alcoholics dvided on the basis of the degree of microscopic alterations; A: patients with no histological damage or steatosis only ($n = 11$); B: patiens with hepatitis and/or fibrosis ($n = 9$).Results are expressed as mean + SEM.

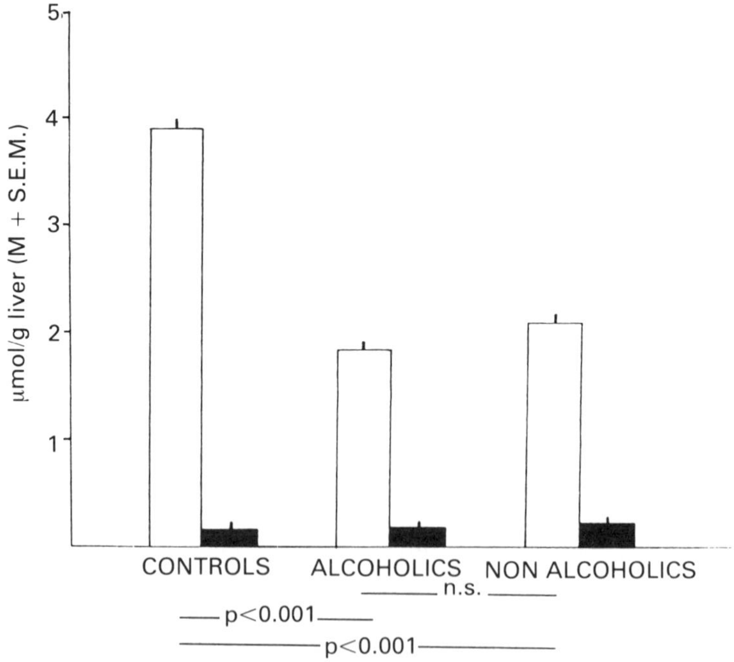

Fig. 3.—Hepatic GSH (□) and GSSG (■) concentrations in:
—control subjects ($n = 15$)
—alcoholic patients ($n = 35$)
—patients with non-alcoholic liver disease ($n = 20$)
Results are expressed as mean ± SEM.

concentration was comparable in the three groups, alcoholic and non-alcoholic patients showed higher GSSG level (as percentage of total) compared to controls (controls: $4.4 \pm 0.2\%$ of total GSH mean $\pm$ SEM; alcoholic patients: 8.2 ± 0.3, $p < 0.001$; non-alcoholic patients: 8.5 ± 0.8, $p < 0.001$).

8.5.3 CONCLUSIONS

The results reported in these studies support the hypothesis that several ethanol and non-ethanol mediated mechanisms may lead to the reduction of hepatic glutathione levels in patients with chronic liver diseases.

Decrease in GSH levels, during alcohol consumption, could indeed result via several mechanisms: binding to acetaldehyde; scavenging of free radicals; oxidation to GSSG by glutathione peroxidase (Lieber 1984). In addition, other non-alcohol-related mechanisms could lead to GSH depletion, including an impairment of transulfuration pathway during cirrhosis (Horowitz *et al.* 1981). In conclusion, it would be of interest to evaluate the efficacy of pharmacological administration of glutathione and glutathione precursors in the restoration of normal GSH hepatic levels during chronic liver diseases, and to assess whether interventions that restore GSH concentrations in the liver can alter the progression of hepatic damage.

REFERENCES

Altomare, E., Leo, M. A., Sato, C., Vendemiale, G., & Lieber, C. S. (1984). Interaction of ethanol with acetaminophen metabolism in the baboon. *Biochem. Pharmacol.* **33,** 2207–2214.

Comporti, M. (1985). Biology of disease. Lipid peroxidation and cellular damage in toxic liver injury. *Lab. Invest.* **53,** 599–623.

Di Luzio, N. R. (1966). A mechanism of the acute ethanol-induced fatty liver and the modification of liver injury by antioxidants. *Lab. Invest.* **15,** 50–58.

Ekstrom, G. & Ingelman-Sundberg, M. (1986). Mechanism of lipid peroxidation dependent upon cytochrome P-450 LM2. *Eur. J. Biochem.* **158,** 195–201.

Guerri, C. & Grisolia, S. (1980). Changes in glutathione in acute and chronic ethanol intoxication. *Pharmac. Biochem. Behav.* **13 (suppl. 1**), 53–61.

Hissen, P. J. & Hilf, R. (1976). A fluorometric method for determination of oxidized and reduced glutathione in tissues. *Anal. Biochem.* **74,** 214–226.

Horowitz, J. H., Rypins, E. B., Enderson, J. M., Heymsfield, S. B., Moffit, S. D., Bain, R. P., Chawla, R. K., Bleier, J. C., & Rudman, D. (1981). Evidence for impairment of transulfuration pathway in cirrhosis. *Gastroenterology* **81,** 668–675.

Jewell, S. A., Di Monte, D., Gentile, A., Guglielmi, A., Altomare, E., & Albano, O. (1986). Decreased hepatic glutathione in chronic alcoholic patients. *J. Hepatol.* **3,** 1–6.

Kaplowitz, N. (1981). The importance and regulation of hepatic glutathione. *Yale. J. Biol. Med.* **54,** 497–502.

Poulsen, H. E., Ranek, L., & Andresen, P. B. (1981). The hepatic glutathione content in liver diseases. *Scand. J. Clin. Lab. Invest.* **41,** 573–576.

Reed, D. J., Babson, J. R., Beatty, P. W., Brodie, A. E., Ellis, W. W., & Potter, D. W. (1980). High performance liquid chromatography analysis of nanomole levels of glutathione, glutathione disulfide, and related thiols and disulfides. *Anal. Biochem.* **106,** 55–62.

Reed, D. J. & Beatty, P. W. (1980). Biosynthesis and regulation of glutathione. Toxicological implications. *Rev. Biochem. Toxicol.* **2,** 213–242.

Sato, C., Matsuda, Y., & Lieber, C. S. (1981). Increased hepatotoxicity of acetaminophen after chronic ethanol consumption in the rat. *Gastroenterology* **80,** 140–148.

Shaw, S., Jayatilleke, E., Ross, W. A., Gordon, E. R., & Lieber, C. S. (1981). Ethanol-induced lipid peroxidation: potentiation by long-term alcohol feeding and atenuation by methionine. *J. Lab. Clin. Med.* **98,** 417–424.

Vendemiale, G., Jayatilleke, E., Shaw, S., & Lieber, C. S. (1984). Depression of biliary glutathione excretion by chronic ethanol feeding in the rat. *Life Sci.* **34,** 1065–1073.

8.6 Protective role of S-adenosylmethionine during chronic liver injury and rationale for therapy

G. Vendemiale, E. Altomare, T. Trizio, I. Grattagliano, P. Portincasa, & O. Albano†

It is well established that methionine can provide a significant source of sulfur incorporated into glutathione (GSH) through S-adenosylmethionine (SAM) formation via the transulfuration pathway.

Patients with chronic liver disease exhibit a significant decrease in hepatic GSH content in association with an impairment of transulfuration pathway and a reduction of SAM-synthetase activity and SAM levels.

To evaluate the effect of long-term SAM treatment on hepatic GSH levels during chronic liver injury we measured GSH in liver biopsies of patients with alcoholic and non-alcoholic liver diseases before and after 6 months' SAM administration (1.2 g/day p.o.) and in a group of placebo-treated patients.

SAM treatment resulted in a significant increase of hepatic GSH levels in patients with both alcoholic and non-alcoholic liver disease compared to the placebo treated patients.

The results indicate that SAM administration may exert an important role in hepatic protective mechanism during chronic liver injury.

8.6.1 INTRODUCTION

A number of studies have pointed out the biologic and pharmacologic role of S-adenosylmethionine (SAM) which is known to be involved in transmethylation, transulfuration, and aminopropylation reactions (Salvatore *et al.* 1977, Usdin *et al.* 1982).

Also, it has been shown that SAM has an active role in the transformation of phosphatidylethanolamine to phosphatidylcholine (PC) (Rama-Sastry *et al.* 1981).

Furthermore, Reed & Orrenius (1977) have observed that the sulfur atom of methionine, an essential sulfur-containing aminoacid, precursor of SAM, makes a significance contribution to glutathione (GSH) synthesis through S-adenosylmethionine and cysteine formation with the transulfuration pathway (Fig. 1), and the importance of GSH levels for the normal liver functioning is well established (Reed & Fariss 1984).

In a recent study Horowitz *et al.* (1981) reported an impairment of transulfuration pathway in patients with liver cirrhosis. Since, in that study, after an oral methionine

† Institute of Clinica Medica I, University of Bari, Bari, Italy

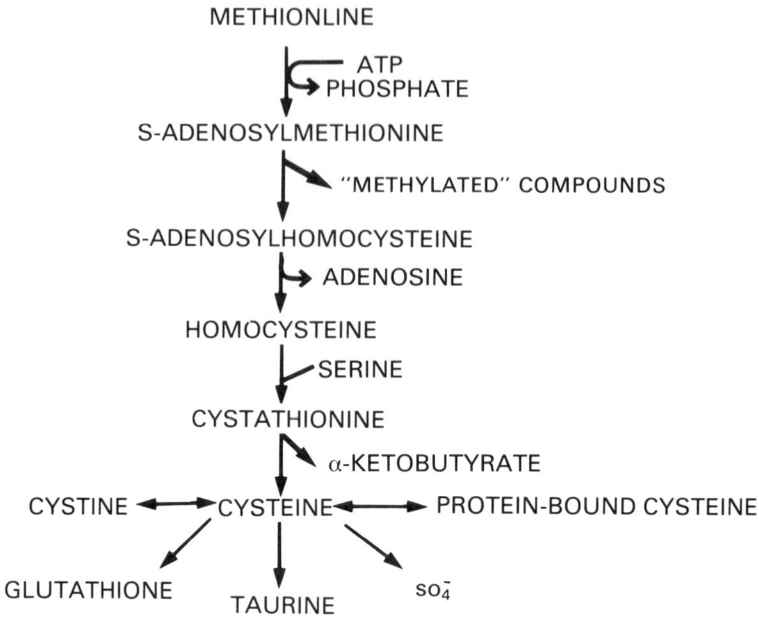

Fig. 1.—Methionine catabolism and the transulfuration pathway

load, cirrhotic patients exhibited higher methionine levels, compared to controls, without accumulation of intermediates of the pathway, it was suggested that the rate-limiting block should occur early, probably in the conversion of methionine to S-adenosylmethionine. This observation has been recently confirmed by Duce *et al.* (1987) who reported that SAM-synthetase activity in alcoholic and post-hepatitic cirrotic patients is indeed reduced. This prompted us to study the effect of SAM administration on hepatic reduced (GSH) and oxidized glutathione (GSSG) in patients with chronic liver diseases.

8.6.2 EFFECTS OF S-ADENOSYLMETHIONINE ON HEPATIC GLUTATHIONE IN PATIENTS WITH ALCOHOLIC AND NON-ALCOHOLIC LIVER DISEASES

In a preliminary study, liver GSH was measured in liver biopsies from a group of 9 patients with chronic liver diseases (5 alcoholics) before and after 6 months of SAM treatment (1.2 g/daily p.o.). Liver GSH was measured by high-pressure liquid chromatography (HPLC) according to the method of Reed *et al.* (1980). Patients liver GSH content was compared (before starting SAM administration) to a well-selected group with no liver injury (10 subjects) and was found to be significantly reduced (2.4 ± 0.1 μmol/g. liver vs 4.1 ± 0.1, mean $\pm$ SEM, $p < 0.001$). Total hepatic GSH content showed significant increases after SAM treatment when compared to values before therapy (3.7 ± 0.1 μmol/g. liver vs 2.4 ± 0.1, mean $\pm$ SEM, $p < 0.001$). No difference was found for liver GSSG concentration (0.2 ± 0.007 μmol/g. liver vs 0.2 ± 0.01, mean $\pm$ SEM, n.s.), suggesting that the increase was due to the reduced form (Vendemiale *et al.* 1986).

Next, we studied 24 patients divided as follows:

(A) 9 patients with alcoholic liver disease, who received SAM, 1.2 gr./day p.o. for 6 months;
(B) 7 patients with non-alcoholic liver disease treated as above;
(C) 8 patients with alcoholic liver disease who received a placebo treatment according to the same regimen.

The alcoholic patients (all males, age 30–56 yr) conformed to the following criteria of inclusion:

- history of alcohol abuse ($\geqslant$150 g/day) for at least 3 yr until hospitalization;
- good nutritional status as assessed by dietary history, lack of weight loss, normal anthropometric data, normal total protein and albumin levels, normal creatinine clearance;
- no regular ingestion of other drugs ($\geqslant$1 month).

Patients with non-alcoholic liver disease (5 males, 2 females, age 42–51 yr) did not report a major alcohol consumption (less than 40 g/day and than 3 times/week). These patients were included in this group on the basis of: clinical history, biochemical liver function tests, liver histology.

All patients underwent Menghini biopsy (during laparoscopy or guided by ultrasonography) 3–4 day after admission.

GSH and GSSG were measured in liver tissue as previously described (Reed *et al.* 1980).

Also, in this case, patients' liver GSH content was found significantly decreased (before starting the study) when compared to a well-selected group without liver injury (controls: 4.1 ± 0.1 μmol/g liver, mean $\pm$ SEM; group A: 2.5 ± 0.2, $p < 0.001$; group B: 2.7 ± 0.2, $p < 0.001$; grup C: 2.4 ± 0.1, $p < 0.001$).

Fig. 2 shows the hepatic content of reduced and oxidized GSH in patients with alcoholic liver disease treated with SAM. An increased level of GSH was observed after the treatment period, whereas GSSG concentration did not show any difference.

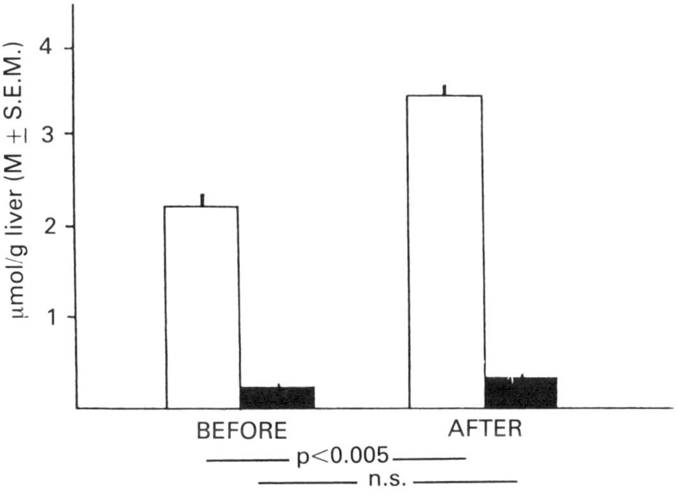

Fig. 2.—Hepatic reduced (□) and oxidized (■) glutathione in 9 patients with alcoholic liver diseases before and after SAM treatment (1.2 g/daily p.o. for 6 months). Results are expressed as mean $\pm$ SEM.

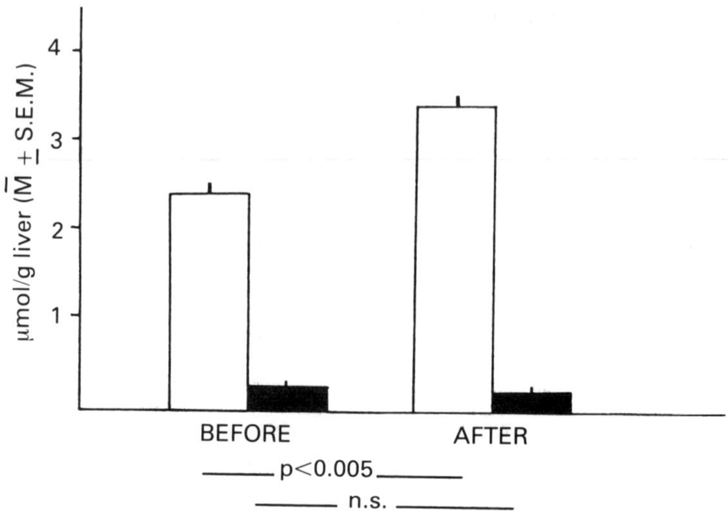

Fig. 3.—Hepatic reduced (□) and oxidized (■) glutathione in 7 patients with non-alcoholic liver diseases before and after SAM treatment (1.2 g/daily p.o. for 6 months). Results are expressed as mean ± SEM.

Similar results were observed for GSH levels of patients with non-alcoholic liver disease receiving the SAM treatment (Fig. 3), whereas alcoholic patients treated with placebo did not report any change in liver glutathione content after the 6-month period (Fig. 4).

8.6.3 CONCLUSIONS

It is well known that normal liver GSH levels (and normal GSH/GSSG ratio) are extremely important in a number of protective and physiological processes, including

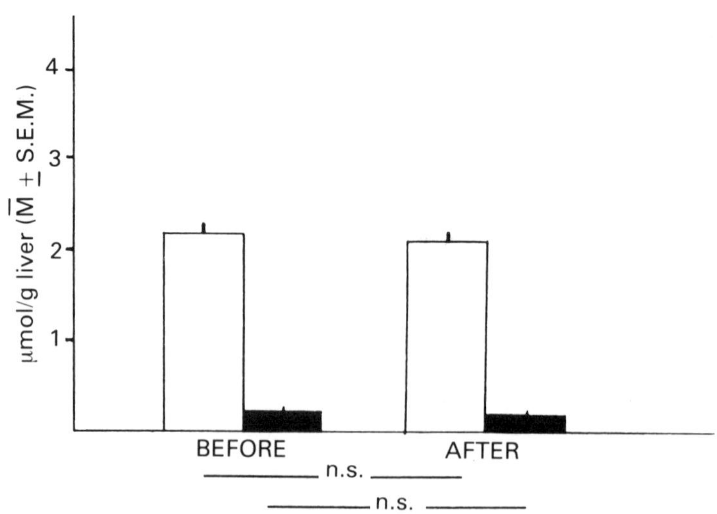

Fig. 4.—Hepatic reduced (□) and oxidized (■) glutathione in 8 patients with alcoholic liver diseases before and after a placebo treatment. Results are expressed as mean ± SEM.

detoxification reactions of electrophilic substances, reduction of peroxides and radicals, maintenance of redox state, protein synthesis, and microtubular function (Kaplowitz 1981).

The reported reduction of SAM-synthetase activity in cirrhotic patients (Horowitz *et al.* 1981) may well account for the observed decrease of GSH levels in these patients since it has been shown that the sulfur atom of methionine may provide (through the transulfuration pathway) approximately one half of GSH synthesised (Reed & Orrenius 1977).

In our studies we observed a significant increase of hepatic total GSH concentration in patients with chronic liver disease, treated with S-adenosylmethionine; this increase represents most likely the result of the restoration of the deficiency of SAM in cirrhosis due to the reduction of SAM-synthetase activity.

In conclusion the reported results indicate that SAM may play an important role in hepatic protective mechanisms during chronic liver injury.

REFERENCES

Duce, A. M., Ortiz, P., Cabrero, C., & Mato, J. M. (1987) S-adenosylmethionine synthetase and phospholipid methyl-transferase are inhibited in human cirrhosis. *Hepatology* (in press)

Horowitz, J. H., Rypins, E. B., Henderson, J. M., Heymsfield, S. B., Moffit, S. D., Bain, R. P., Chawla, R. K., Bleier, J. C., & Rudman, D. (1981) Evidence for impairment of transulfuration pathway in cirrhosis. *Gastroenterology* **81,** 668–675

Kaplowitz, N. (1981) The importance and regulation of hepatic glutathione. *Yale J. Biol. Med.* **54,** 497–502

Pascale, R., Pirisi, L., Daino, L., Zanetti, S., Satta, A., Bartoli, E., & Feo, F. (1982) Role of phosphatidylethanolamine methylation in the synthesis of phosphatidylcoline by hepatocytes isolated from choline-deficient rats. *FEBS Lett.* **145,** 293–297

Rama-Sastry, B. V., Stathan, C. N., Axelrod, J., & Hirata, F. (1981) Evidence for two methyltransferases involved in the conversion of phosphatidylethanolamine to phosphatidylcholine in the rat liver. *Arch. Biochem. Biophys.* **211,** 762–773

Reed, D. J., Babson, J. R., Beatty, P. W., Brodie, A. E., Ellis, W. W., & Potter, D. W. (1980) High performance liquid chromatography analysis of nanomole levels of glutathione, glutathine disulfide, and related thiols and disulfides. *Anal. Biochem.* **106,**55–62

Reed, D. J. & Fariss, M. W. (1984) Glutathione depletion and susceptibility. *Pharmacol. Rev.* **36,** 259–333

Reed, D. J. & Orrenius, S. (1987) The role of methionine in glutathione biosynthesis by isolated hepatocytes. *Biochem. Biophys. Res. Commun.* **77,** 1257–1264

Salvatore, F., Borek, E., Zappia, V., Williams-Ashman, H. G., & Schlenk, F. (eds) (1977) *The biochemistry of adenosylmethionine*, Columbia Univ. Press, New York

Usdin, E., Borchardt, R. T., & Creveling, C. R. (eds) (1982) *Biochemistry of S-adenosylmethionine and related compounds.* Macmillan and Co., London

Vendemiale, G., Altomare, E., Trizio, T., Salerno, M. T., Stufano, N., Palasciano, G., & Albano, O. (1986) Effect of S-adenosylmethionine on hepatic glutathione in patients with liver injury. *Dis. Di. Sci.* (*suppl.*) **31,** 929

8.7 Protein-ubiquinone interactions in mitochondrial cytochrome c reductase

M. Lorusso, D. Boffoli, T. Cocco, & S. Papa†

The effect of papain digestion on polypeptides and enzymatic activities of mitochondrial b-c_1 complex is reported. The results obtained indicate:

(1) the protein complex shows a different susceptibility to proteolysis depending on the redox state of the metal redox centres;
(2) the reductase activity of the oxidized form of the enzyme is only slightly inhibited by papain, whereas digestion of the ascorbate-reduced enzyme results in a more substantial inhibition of the activity;
(3) the reductase activity decreases along with the digestion of the Fe-S protein and the suppression of the antimycin-sensitive ubisemiquinone radical (SQ_c).

It is suggested that the Fe-S protein is involved, possibly together with other complex subunits, in the stabilization of SQ_c.

8.7.1 INTRODUCTION

Two roles have so far been recognized for mitochondrial ubiquinone (CoQ or UQ_{10}). One of these is concerned with energy conversion in coupling membranes, the other with its ability to act, in the reduced form, as antioxidant and thus to scavenge superoxide or oxygen radicals (Beyer *et al.* 1986). Owing to its higher lipophilicity with respect to other antioxidants such as α-tocopherol or glutathione and its ready re-reducibility by mitochondrial respiration within the membrane, ubiquinone would be preferred as antioxidant drug when poisoning or failure of oxidation pathways will occur (Crane 1986).

In this paper we shall focus on the role of ubiquinone as electron carrier between and/or within the protein complexes in the inner mitochondrial membrane. Kroger & Klingenberg (1973) have shown that ubiquinone functions as an homogenous pool connecting the reduction and the oxidation enzymes in the membrane bilayer. However, semiquinone species have been detected in succinate cytochrome c reductase (complex II) and in ubiquinol-cytochrome c reductase (b-c_1 complex, complex III), most likely stabilized by binding to specific enzyme protein subunits. A protein (QP_s) which is apparently involved in the binding of the semiquinone (SQ_s) (Yu *et al.* 1978) and converts soluble succinate dehydrogenase into succinate-ubiquinone oxido-reductase has been isolated and characterized. Furthermore, a 14–15 kDa protein

† Institute of Medical Biochemistry and Chemistry, University of Bari, Bari, Italy

(QP_c) has been isolated from beef-heart b-c_1 complex (Wang & King, 1982) which appears to be involved in the binding of SQ_c and is essential for the cytochrome c reductase activity.

Coupled to the electron transfer in the b-c_1 complex, a proton pumping activity with an overall H^+/e^- stoichiometry of 2 has been clearly documented both in the native and in the reconstituted system (Papa *et al.* 1983). The mechanism of electron flow within the complex and of coupled proton translocation is unknown. In addition, the precise role of semiquinone in the enzymatic activities of the complex and the identity of the SQ_c-stabilizing subunits are also to be settled. Our group (Papa *et al.* 1983) has developed a model, denominated Q-gated proton pump (Fig. 1) in which

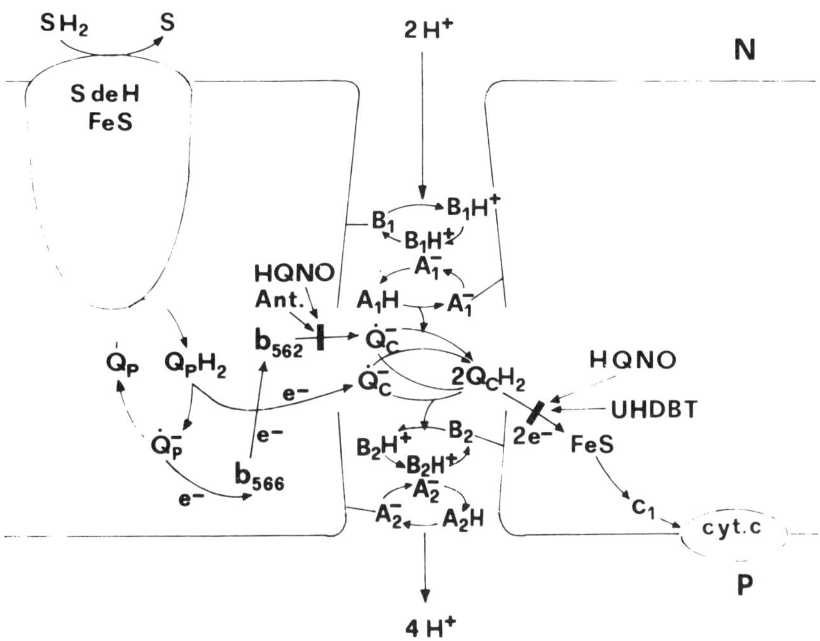

Fig. 1.—Q-gated proton pump model of ubiquinol-cytochrome c reductase.

quinone molecules are thought to be tightly bound to proteins, without any significant exchange at the steady state with the quinone of the pool, and to provide a split pathways for sequential transfer of the two electrons of a quinol molecule to cytochrome c. In addition, apoproteins of the complex are considered to be involved in the proton translocating activity. Accordingly, proton translocation coupled to oxido-reduction of the quinone system, rather than deriving from specific mobilities of Q and QH_2 (Q-cycle, Mitchell 1976) or SQ_c (SQ-cycle, Wikström & Krab 1986) across the membrane is thought instead to be imposed on the catalytic process of the system by proteins which provide asymmetric pathways for proton conduction between aqueous phases and bound quinone molecules.

We would like to mention the effect of papain digestion on polypeptide subunits and on the enzymatic properties of the b-c_1 complex. The protein complex shows a different susceptibility to proteolysis, depending on the redox state of the metal redox centres. This would suggest a gross conformational change accompanying the respiratory oxido-reduction cycle. The results also show that special quinone molecules firmly bound as prosthetic groups to apoproteins, play a fundamental role in electron transport and energy transfer activities in the b-c_1 complex.

8.7.2 MATERIALS AND METHODS

The b-c_1 complex was isolated from beef-heart mitochondria as described by Rieske (1967) and characterized by Papa *et al.* (1983).

8.7.2.1 Papain treatment

b-c_1 complex (30 mg protein/ml), dissolved in 100 mM KCl, 20 mM Hepes (pH 8) and 50 μM EDTA, was incubated, for intervals indicated in the legends to the figures with papain at a concentration of 1 mg papain/20 mg proteins at 18°C in aerobiosis. After incubation, aliquots were diluted 200 times with 100 mM KCl, 20 mM Hepes (pH 7.2), 100 μM EDTA and 0.02% Tween 80, and immediately assayed for enzymatic activity. For SDS-Page, aliquots of the enzyme solution were added to 10% trichloro-acetic acid. After centrifugation the pellets were solubilized in 5% SDS, 15% glycerol, 50 mM Tris (pH 6.8), 2% mercaptoethanol, 0.003% bromo-phenol-blue, and subjected to electrophoresis.

8.7.2.2 Measurement of cytochrome c reductase activity

The duroquinol-cytochrome-c reductase activity was measured spectrophotometrically at 550–540 nm in the same mixture also containing 1 mM KCN, 8 μM ferricytochrome c, and 33 μM duroquinol.

8.7.2.3 Electrophoretic analysis of the b–c_1 complex

SDS-Page analysis of the b-c_1 complex was performed according to Schagger *et al.* (1985) using Tris-Tricine buffer system at pH 6.8. Gels were stained and destained as described by Weber & Osborn (1969).

8.7.2.4 EPR measurements

For EPR measurements samples poised anaerobically to 100 mV in the presence of mixtures of redox mediators were transferred into pre-cooled EPR-tubes and immediately frozen.

8.7.3 RESULTS

When subjected to SDS-Page cytochrome c reductase appears to contain eleven polypeptides: the two higher molecular mass polypeptides represent core protein I and II, the 30 kDa band comprises, in the present experimental conditions, the apoprotein of b cytochromes and the cytochrome c_1, the 25 kDa subunit represents the Rieske Fe-S protein. In addition there appear up to six low molecular mass polypeptides.

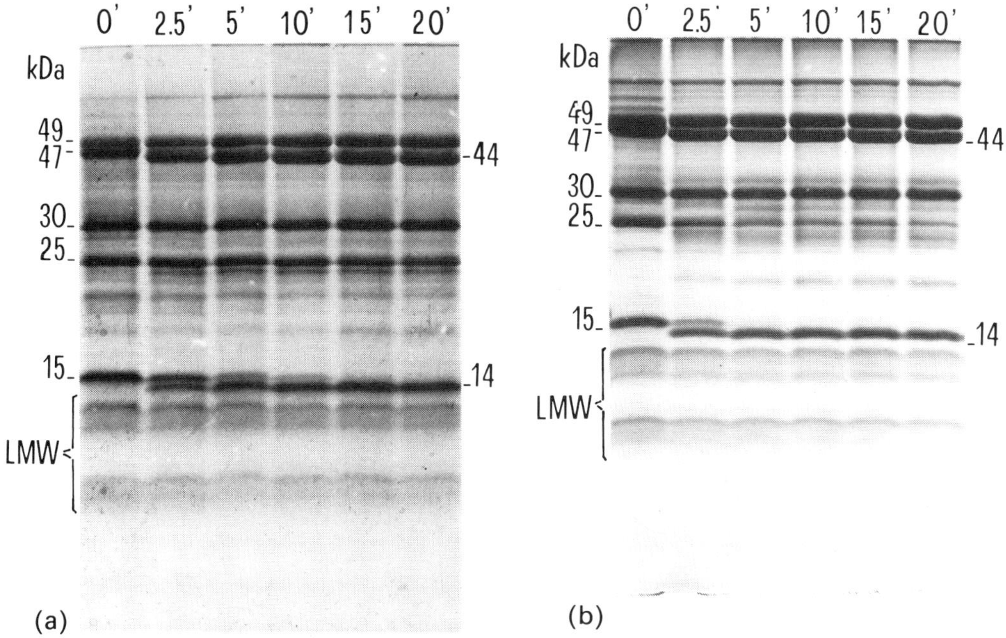

Fig. 2.—Coomassie-blue stained gels of b-c_1 complex: effect of papain digestion on electrophoretic mobility. b-c_1 complex in oxidized (2a) or ascorbate reduced form (2b) was incubated with papain as described under *Materials and methods*.

Fig. 2 illustrates the time course of papain digestion of subunits of the b-c_1 complex. With the oxidized enzyme (2a) there occurs a partial digestion of core protein II, with a loss of a 3 kDa fragment, which is completed in 5 min incubation. The 15 kDa subunit also undergoes digestion to a 14 kDa product, the process being completed in 20 min. At longer incubation times also the Fe-S protein is digested as revealed by the attenuation of the 25 kDa band (see below).

When the b-c_1 complex is supplemented with ascorbate (2b), which induces full reduction of both the Fe-S centre and cytochrome c_1, the 15 kDa protein and the FeS protein are more rapidly digested by papain. The partial digestion of core protein II remains the same as with the fully oxidized enzyme. In either the oxidized or in the partially reduced b-c_1 complex, no other subunits are digested by papain within 20 min.

Fig. 3 shows the effect of papain digestion on cytochrome c reductase activity of oxidized and ascorbate-reduced b-c_1 complex. Whilst papain digestion of the oxidized b-c_1 complex results in a small inhibition of the reductase activity, digestion of the reduced enzyme results in a more substantial inhibition. It is interesting to note that, in both cases, the digestion of the FeS protein, as estimated from the integration of the corresponding densitometric band, strictly correlates with the inhibition of the reductase activity.

Fig. 4 shows an experiment in which the b-c_1 complex is poised at 100 mV and the antimycin-sensitive semiquinone (SQ_c) signal is recorded by EPR measurements. Papain treatment of the complex results in a suppression of the SQ_c signal, which again parallels the inhibition of the electron transfer activity.

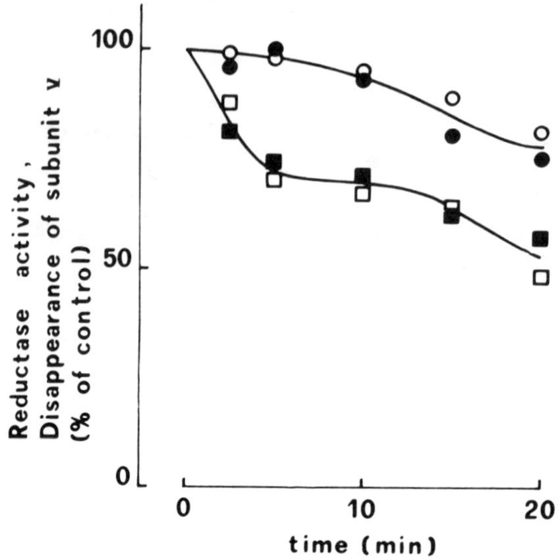

Fig. 3.—Effect of papain digestion on reductase activity and on Fe-S protein electrophoretic band of b-c_1 complex. b-c_1 complex was incubated with papain in oxidized (○, ●) or ascorbate-reduced form (□, ■). Reductase activity of oxidized (●) and reduced (■) enzyme was measured as described under *Materials and methods*. The band correspond to Fe-S subunit of the oxidized (○) or reduced (□) enzyme was integrated and the integrals reported as percentage of the control band.

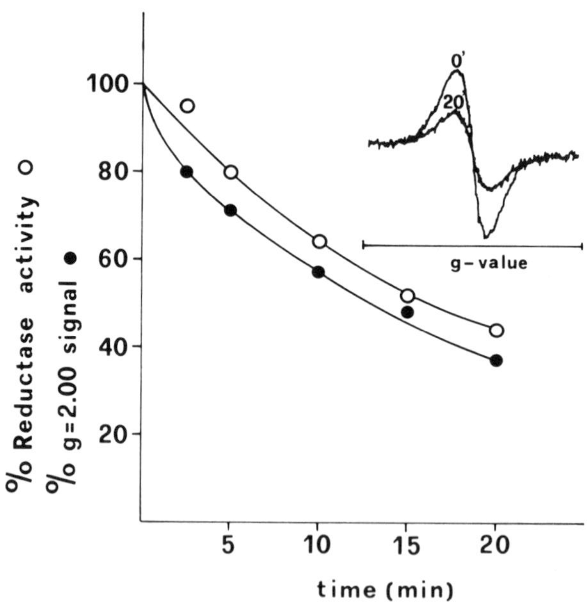

Fig. 4.—Effect of papain digestion on the height of $g = 2.00$ EPR signal of SQ_c and reductase activity of b-c_1 complex. The b-c_1 complex, poised at 100 mV in anaerobiosis, was incubated with papain. Samples for EPR analysis and measurements of cytochrome c reductase activity were withdrawn at the intervals indicated. For experimental conditions see also under *Materials and methods*. The conditions of E.P.R. spectroscopy were: power 10 μW, modulated amplitude 12.5 G, temperature $-136°$C, microwave frequency 9.32 GHz.

8.7.4 DISCUSSION

We have previously shown (Lorusso *et al.* 1985) that selective digestion of core protein II and the 15 kDa subunit of the b-c_1 complex is accompanied by decoupling of proton pumping with little, if any, inhibition of the rate of electron flow. When the incubation time is prolonged, a significant inhibition of the electron flow takes place, which parallels the proteolytic digestion of the Fe-S protein. Upon reduction of the high-potential redox centres, namely Fe-S centre and cytochrome c_1, by ascorbate, a more substantial inhibition of the rate of electron flow is observed, which again follows the time course of the digestion of the Fe-S protein. The observation that papain digestion of polypeptide subunits of the b-c_1 complex is also affected by ascorbate reduction of the enzyme shows that redox transitions within the complex result in a gross conformational change of the complex (see also Das Gupta *et al.* 1979). Under these conditions, the antimycin-sensitive ubisemiquinone radical (SQ_c) content decreases along with the digestion of the Fe-S protein. This would indicate that the Fe-S protein is involved in the stabilization of SQ_c.

Evidence has been presented showing involvement of a 14–15 kDa subunit (QP_c), isolated from the mitochondrial b-c_1 complex, in the formation of SQ_c (Wang & King, 1982, Yu *et al.* 1977). It is possible that the removal of 1 kDa fragment affected by papain suppresses direct binding of SQ_c to that protein. Core protein II can also be involved in the stabilization of semiquinone species (Lorusso *et al.* 1987). Thus more than one protein appears to contribute to form a ubiquinone reaction pocket in the b-c_1 complex. This could also involve the protein(s) that bind(s) antimycin (Yu & Yu, 1980, Van Keulen & Berden 1985), an inhibitor which suppresses SQ_c formation (Ohnishi & Trumpover 1980) and blocks the electron transfer activity.

ACKNOWLEDGEMENT

The help and support of Drs S. Meinhardt and T. Ohnishi in Philadelphia in the performance of E.P.R. experiments are gratefully acknowledged.

REFERENCES

Beyer, R. E., Nordenbrand, K., & Ernster, L. (1986) The role of coenzyme Q as a mitochondrial antioxidant: a short review. In: *Biomedical and clinical aspects of coenzyme Q* (eds Folkers, K. & Yamamura, Y.), Elsevier Sci. Publishers, Amsterdam, Vol. 5, pp. 17–24.

Crane, F. L. (1986) Physiological coenzyme Q function and pharmacological reaction. In: *Biomedical and clinical aspects of coenzyme Q* (eds Folkers, K. & Yamamura, Y.), Elsevier Sci. Publishers, Amsterdam, Vol. 5, pp. 3–14.

Das Gupta, U., Wharton, D. C., & Rieske, J. S. (1979) Detection of conformational changes in complex III of the respiratory chain by Maleimido Spin Label. *J. Bioenerg. Biomembr.* **11,** 79–95.

Kroger, A. & Klingenberg, M. (1973) Further evidence for the pool function of ubiquinone as derived from the inhibition of the electron transport by antimycin. *Eur. J. Biochem.* **39,** 313–323.

Lorusso, M., Gatti, D., Marzo, M., & Papa, S. (1985) Effect of papain digestion on redox-linked proton translocation in b-c_1 complex from beef-heart reconstituted into liposomes. *FEBS Lett.* **182,** 370–374.

Lorusso, M., Gatti, D., Marzo, M., Boffoli, D., Cocco, T., & Papa, S. (1987) Chemical modification studies of beef-heart mitochondrial b-c_1 complex. Effect of modification by ethoxyformic anhydride. *Eur. J. Biochem.* **162,** 231–238.

Mitchell, P. (1976) Possible molecular mechanism of the proton-motive function of cytochrome system. *J. Theor. Biol.* **62,** 327–367.

Ohnishi, T. & Trumpower, B. L. (1980) Differential effects of antimycin on ubisemiquinone bound in different environments in isolated succinate-cytochrome c reductase complex. *J. Biol. Chem.* **255,** 3278–3284.

Papa, S., Lorusso, M., Boffoli, D., & Bellomo, E. (1983) Redox-linked proton translocation in the b-c_1 complex from beef-heart mitochondria reconstituted into phospholipid vesicles. General characteristics and control of electron flow by $\Delta\mu H^+$. *Eur. J. Biochem.* **137,** 405–412.

Rieske, J. S. (1967) Preparation and properties of reduced coenzyme Q-cytochrome c reductase (complex III) of the respiratory chain. In: *Methods Enzymol.* (eds Estabrook, R. W. & Pulmann, M. E.), Vol. **10,** 239–245.

Schagger, H., Borchart, U., Aquila, H., Link, T. A., & Von Jagow, G. (1985) Isolation and amino acid sequence of the smallest subunit of beef-heart b-c_1 complex. *FEBS Lett.* **190,** 89–94.

Van Keulen, M. A. & Berden, J. A. (1985) Antimycin binds to a small subunit of the ubiquinol: cytochrome c reductase. *Biochim. Biophys. Acta* **808,** 32–38.

Weber, K. & Osborn, M. (1969) The reliability of molecular weight determination by dodecil-sulfate-Polyacrylamide gel electrophoresis. *J. Biol. Chem.* **244,** 4406–4412.

Wang, T. Y. & King, T. E. (1982) Isolation of QP-C and reconstitution of the QH_2-C reductase. *Biochem. Biophys. Res. Commun.* **104**, 591–596.

Wei, Y., Scholes, C. P., & King, T. E. (1981) Ubisemiquinone radicals from the cytochrome b-c_1 complex of the mitochondrial electron transport chain. Demonstration of QP-S radical formation. *Biochem. Biophys. Res. Commun.* **99,** 1411–1419.

Wikström, M. & Krab, K. (1986) The semiquinone cycle. A hypothesis of electron transfer and proton translocation in cytochrome bc-type complexes. *J. Bioenerg. Biomembr.* **18,** 181–193.

Yu, L., Yu, C. A., & King, T. E. (1978) The indispensability of phospholipid and ubiquinone in mitochondrial electron transfer from succinate to cytochrome c. *J. Biol. Chem.* **253,** 2657–2663.

Yu, C. A. & Yu, L. (1980) Identification of ubisemiquinone binding proteins in ubiquinol–cytochrome c reductase by Arylazido ubiquinone derivative. *Biochem. Biophys. Res. Commun.* **96,** 286–292.

8.8 Antibacterial activity against *Salmonella typhi* exerted by human peripheral blood lymphocytes from subjects belonging to an endemic area for salmonellosis

Pia P. Grassi†, Angela B. Maffione†, Annamaria Catino†, Luciano Nencioni‡, Emilio Jirillo†, & Aldo Tagliabue†

Human peripheral blood lymphocytes from endemic individuals display anti *Salmonella typhi* activity which is many folds higher than that noted in non-endemic people. CD4+ cell armed by IgA and CD8+ cells armed by IgG are the effectors of the above activity, while natural killer cells and macrophages do not play any role in this immune function.

Recently, Tagliabue *et al.* (1985) have described an antibody-dependent cellular cytotoxicity (ADCC) against enteropathogenic bacteria, which is performed by CD4+ lymphocytes armed by IgA. On this basis, it was of interest to evaluate anti *Salmonella typhi* ADCC in individuals from an endemic area for salmonellosis (Bari, Italy). In fact, *S. typhi* has been shown to bind to human peripheral blood lymphocytes (PBL) in typhoid patients from the same area (Jirillo & Antonaci 1985), this suggesting a close relationship between *Salmonella* and lymphocytes.

In the present paper, we shall demonstrate that endemic individuals possess anti-*S. typhi* activity which is more elevated than that observed in non-endemic donors (Siena, Italy) and is sustained by both CD4+ and CD8+ cells armed by IgA and IgG, respectively.

In preliminary experiments, it was evident that endemic peripheral blood mononuclear cells (PBMC) displayed ADCC against *S. typhi* strain Ty2 which at elevated effector/target ratios (e.g. 25–6) was still higher (about 40%) when compared to that exhibited by non-endemic PBMC (less than 5%). Therefore, in a separate set of experiments, efforts have been made to identify the effectors of such an activity. Removal of monocytes by plastic adherence or of natural killer (NK) cells by complement-mediated lysis in the presence of the HNK-1 monoclonal antibody (Mo Ab) (Abo & Balch 1981) from PBL did not modify the activity described above.

Therefore, T cells from endemic subjects obtained by the E-rosette technique were enriched in CD4+ and CD8+ cells. Purified cell suspensions were recovered after

† Immunologia Medica, University of Bari, Medical School, Policlinico, 70124 Bari, Italy
‡Sclavo Research Center, 53100 Siena, Italy

complement-mediated lysis in the presence of OKT8+ and OTK4+ Mo Ab according to the method of Wählin & Perlmann (1983). Interestingly, in experiments conducted by using these two purified populations both CD4+ and CD8+ cells exerted anti-*S. typhi* activity with a similar degree of efficacy.

Finally, investigation was made in order to determine the antibody class(es) which could arm the effector cells. Therefore, blocking experiments were performed pretreating CD4+ and CD8+ lymphocytes with $F(ab')_2$ fragments of goat anti-human serum IgA (alpha chain specific) and of goat anti-human IgG (Fc gamma fragment specific). Results show that CD4+ cells are armed by IgA, and CD8+ cells are armed by IgG to perform antibacterial activity.

Humoral response to lipopolysaccharide from *S. typhi* was evaluated in endemic vs non-endemic subjects. Only a moderate increase of IgM and a decrease of IgG were noted in endemic individuals as assessed by ELISA.

The overall data indicate that in subjects from an endemic area a more efficient mechanism against enteropathogenic bacteria has been developed under conditions of antigenic pressure. In fact, besides CD4+ cells armed by IgA, CD8+ lymphocytes armed by IgG also participate to the antibacterial function.

In conclusion, antibacterial activity exerted by human PBL represents a novel physiological activity by which these cells protect the host.

ACKNOWLEDGEMENTS

This paper was supported in part by grants from Ministero Pubblica Istruzione and Regione Puglia, Italy.

REFERENCES

Abo, T. & Balch, C. M. (1981). A differentiation antigen of human NK and K cells identified by a monoclonal antibody (HNK-1), *J. Immunol.* **127,** 1024–1029.

Jirillo, E. & Antonaci, S. (1985). Spontaneous adherence of *Salmonella typhosa* to human peripheral blood lymphocytes in typhoid fever, *Infection* **13,** 157.

Tagliabue, A., Villa, L., Boraschi, D., Peri, G., De Gori, V., & Nencioni, L. (1985). Natural anti bacterial activity against *Salmonella typhi* by human T4+ lymphocytes armed with IgA antibodies, *J. Immunol.* **135,** 4178–4182.

Wählin, B. & Perlmann, P. (1983). Characterization of human K cells by surface antigens and morphology at the single cell levels, *J. Immunol.* **131,** 2340–2347.

Part 9
Cardiovascular disease

9.1 Role of serotonin in cardiovascular diseases

Jan M. Van Nueten†

(1) The endogenous substance serotonin can be released from aggregating platelets (e.g. in cardiovascular pathological conditions such as hypertension and atherosclerosis) in sufficient concentrations to affect local vascular functions in a number of ways. Serotonin itself will cause further platelet aggregation by direct action on platelets, or by an amplifying effect on aggregation induced by other substances, both effects of serotonin being mediated by 5-HT_2 serotonergic receptors. In the vasculature it causes either constriction or dilatation, and consequently either an increase or a decrease in blood pressure.
(2) Vasoconstriction is due to a direct action of the endogenously released monoamine on smooth muscle or to potentiation ('amplification') of the effect of other endogenous vasoconstrictors. Both the vasoconstrictor (in most blood vessels) and the hypertensive effects of serotonin are mediated by 5-HT_2 serotonergic receptors. Serotonin can also induce vasodilatation by a direct effect on smooth muscle, by inhibition of adrenergic neurotransmission, or by release of a vasodilator substance (EDRF = endothelium derived relaxing factor) from the endothelium. The latter effect is mediated by 5-HT_1 serotonergic receptors.
(3) Blood vessels will become hypersensitive to the vasoconstrictor effects of serotonin in cardiovascular diseases. This will be particularly the case when the vascular endothelium is damaged (e.g. in atherosclerosis), and in blood vessels from the elderly or from hypertensive animals and patients. Interaction of serotonin released from aggregating platelets with other endogenous vasoactive substances may play a crucial role in these conditions. Vascular hyperreactivity associated with impairment of platelet function (e.g. accelerated activation, decreased uptake of serotonin) and decreased degradation of serotonin by the endothelium may then lead to an increase in peripheral vascular resistance resulting in further impairment of tissue perfusion or in high blood pressure.
(4) The 5-HT_2 serotonergic antagonist ketanserin counteracts the platelet aggregating and vasoconstrictor effects of serotonin and reduces hypersensitivity, both *in vitro* and *in vivo*. The pronounced chronic antihypertensive efficacy of ketanserin in particular in the elderly suggests an important role for serotonin in the pathology of the aging vascular system.

9.1.1 INTRODUCTION

The role of the cardiovascular system is to ensure a continuum supply of nutrients and oxygen to the cells and a continuous wash-out of waste products from the tissue cells. If this can no longer be assured, tissue ischemia and dysfunction become unavoidable and will lead to deterioration of the organism. The appropriate blood stream to the tissues is controlled by changes in wall tension and diameter of the precapillary blood vessels, which helps to determine both peripheral vascular resistance and fuid exchanges at the capillary level. Although active changes in

† International Research Council, Janssen Research Foundation, B-2340 Beerse, Belgium

diameter of the blood vessels are controlled mainly by the sympathetic tone, they can be modulated by a number of endogenous substances including those formed or released in the vicinity of the vascular smooth muscle cells (Shepherd & Vanhoutte 1979).

One of these substances is serotonin, identified as a gut-stimulating substance from enterochromaffin cells (Erspamer & Asero 1952) and as a vasoconstrictor agent present in serum after blood has clotted (Page 1954). Blood platelets are the main source of serotonin available to the blood vessel wall, which when they aggregate release serotonin along with other vasoactive substances such as thromboxane A_2. In addition, some blood vessels are innervated by serotonergic neurons, releasing serotonin during stimulation (Edvinsson *et al.* 1983). The effects of serotonin on the cardiovascular system are complex, and their multiplicity is well established (Page 1954). Recently, specific serotonergic antagonists such as ketanserin became available, thus stimulating a revival in fundamental studies on serotonin (Van Nueten *et al.* 1981, Janssen 1985). Platelet-vessel wall interaction, related in particular to the release of serotonin and other endogenous substances, may be of crucial significance in the aetiology of some cardiovascular diseases (Van Nueten *et al.* 1985).

The present paper discusses the experimental and clinical evidence for a possible role of serotonin in a number of cardiovascular pathological conditions including hypertension and diseases related to impaired tissue perfusion.

9.1.2 PLATELET AGGREGATION

Whereas aggregating platelets are the peripheral source of serotonin for the cardiovascular system, the monoamine itself induces further aggregation of platelets. Although serotonin by itself induces only a weak reaction in normal human platelets, patients with cardiovascular diseases may have irreversible platelet aggregation in response to serotonin. Such aggregation is inhibited by ketanserin (Fig. 1) (De Crée *et al.* 1985a, Van Nueten *et al.* 1987).

Serotonin also strongly potentiates ('amplifies') aggregation of platelets induced by low concentrations of other agonists. These amplifying effects of serotonin on platelets are prevented or inhibited by ketanserin, indicating that 5-HT_2 serotonergic receptors are involved (De Clerck *et al.* 1982).

Such serotonin-induced (direct or amplifying) aggregation may greatly contribute to the mechanical obstruction of blood vessels by the formation of a thrombus. Platelet aggregation and subsequent thrombotic obstruction were observed in canine coronary arteries damaged by mechanically-induced stenosis. The antithrombotic effects of ketanserin in this model substantiate the hypothesis for a contribution of endogenously released serotonin in this pathological event (Bush *et al.* 1984). Release of serotonin leading to pulmonary vasoconstriction and bronchoconstriction is observed during experimental embolization induced in dogs by autologous clot injected intravenously. The cardiopulmonary consequences of pulmonary embolism include pulmonary hypertension, increase of pulmonary vascular resistance, and hypoxaemia. The 5-HT_2-serotonergic antagonist ketanserin reverses these phenomena and induces vascular recruitment (Fig. 2) (Huval *et al.* 1983).

9.1.3 VASCULAR TISSUE

Serotonin has different, and even opposite, actions on the cardiovascular system: it

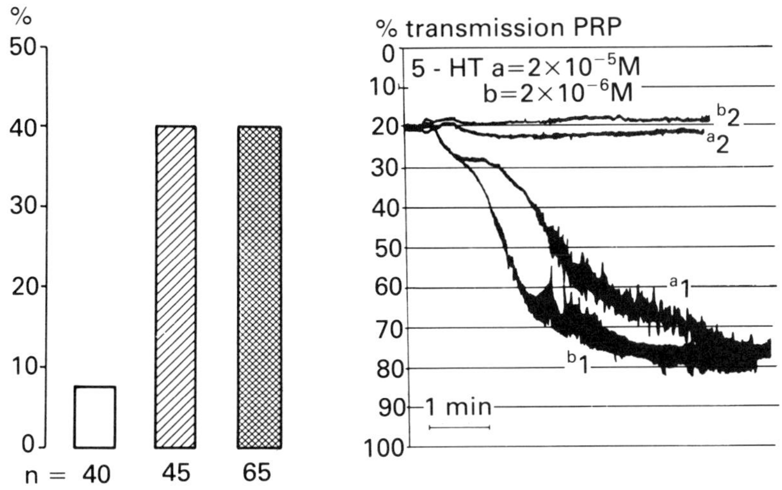

Fig. 1.—(Left) The % incidence of serotonin (2×10^{-6} M)-induced irreversible platelet aggregation in (left to right) 40 normal volunteers, in 45 patients with acute myocardial infarction, and 65 patients with peripheral arterial obstructive disease (De Crée *et al.* 1985a, by courtesy of Birkhäuser Verlag, Basel). (Right) Irreversible platelet aggregation measured as % light transmission induced by serotonin in a patient with acute mycoardial infarction (a_1 and b_1). A single oral dose of 60 mg ketanserin abolishes this effect (a_2 and b_2) (data from De Crée *et al.* 1985a, Van Nueten *et al.* 1987, by courtesy of Raven Press).

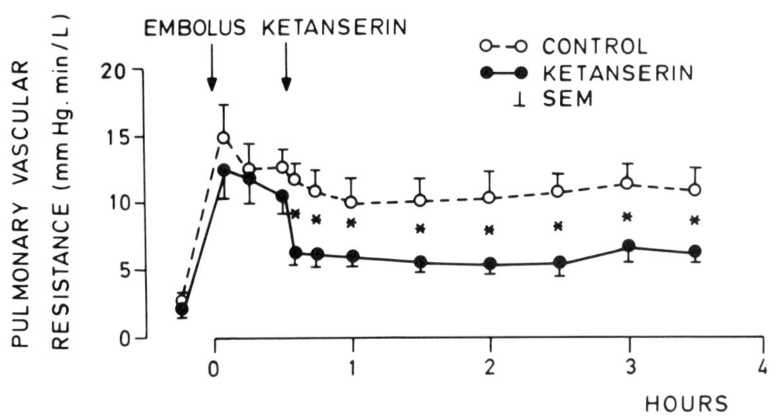

Fig. 2.—The cardiopulmonary consequences of pulmonary embolism induced in dogs by an intravenously injected autologous clot include pulmonary hypertension, increase of pulmonary vascular resistance, and hypoxaemia. Ketanserin (0.15 mg/kg i.v.) reverses these phenomena (Huval *et al.* 1983, by courtesy of J. B. Lippincott Company).

can cause either an increase or a decrease in systemic blood pressure; it can induce peripheral vasoconstriction or vasodilatation, depending on various conditions. This complexity is due to the fact that serotonin can act on different cell types of one tissue (e.g. on smooth muscle or on endothelial cells of the blood vessel wall), or on different subtypes of serotonergic receptors (e.g. in vascular smooth muscle, on 5-HT_1 or 5-HT_2 receptors).

9.1.3.1 Direct vasoconstrictive effects

In most arterial and venous smooth muscles serotonin induces contractions through activation of 5-HT_2 serotonergic receptors. Platelets aggregating in the vicinity of vascular smooth muscle, release serotonin in amounts sufficient to cause vasoconstriction (Van Nueten *et al.* 1985). Vasoconstrictor responses to serotonin either exogenous or released from aggregating platelets, are inhibited by ketanserin (Fig. 3) (Vanhoutte & Cohen 1983, De Clerck & Van Nueten 1982, Van Nueten 1985).

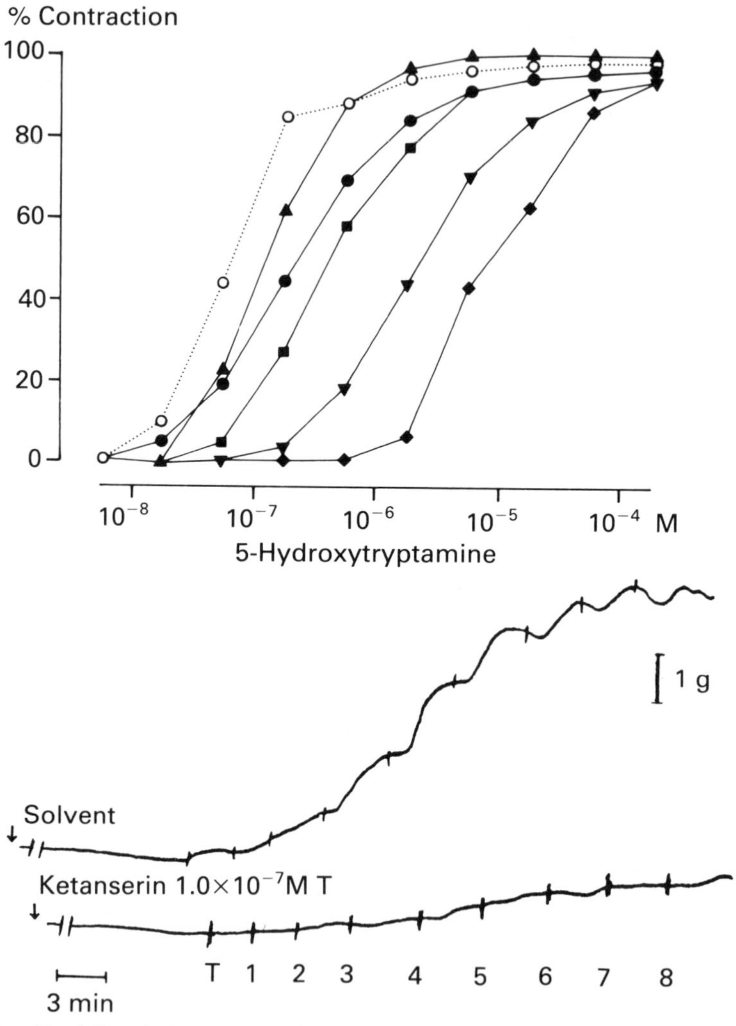

Fig. 3.—(Top) Cumulative concentration-response curves to serotonin (5-hydroxytryptamine) under control conditions and in the presence of ketanserin (mean values of 5–6 experiments; incubation time: 30 min) on the isolated rabbit pulmonary artery. Ketanserin (○ control, ▲ 4×10^{-10} M; ● 1.6×10^{-9} M; ■ 6.3×10^{-9} M; ▼ 2.5×10^{-8} M; ◆ 1×10^{-7} M) causes a concentration-dependent parallel shift of the right, indicating competitive antagonism (Van Nueten 1985, by courtesy of Raven Press). (Bottom) Typical experiment showing contractions, of an isolated rabbit pulmonary artery, evoked by aggregating rat platelets (upper) and its inhibition by ketanserin (incubation time: 30 min), indicating that these contractions are due to released serotonin. T: Thrombin (0.5 N.I.H. Units/ml); 1, 2, . . ., 8: platelets (2.5×10^6, 5×10^6, 10^7, 2×10^7, 3×10^7, 4×10^7, 5×10^7, 6×10^7 platelets/ml).

9.1.3.2 Amplifying effects

A threshold concentration of serotonin augments ('amplifies') the vasoconstrictor effects of other neurohumoral mediators. Thus, the monoamine amplifies vasoconstriction induced by angiotensin II, histamine, noradrenaline, prostaglandin $F_{2\alpha}$, and thromboxane A_2. Such amplification has also been demonstrated when platelets aggregate, and thus release vascoactive substances (e.g. serotonon), in the presence of minute amounts of vasoactive substances such as noradrenaline released from sympathetic nerve endings (Fig. 4). Amplifying effects have been observed in many isolated vascular tissues and beds, including human vessels, and also *in vivo* in various species including the human. It is more pronounced in hypertensive animals (de la Lande *et al.* 1966, Myers *et al.* 1985, Scroop & Walsh 1968, Van Nueten *et al.* 1985).

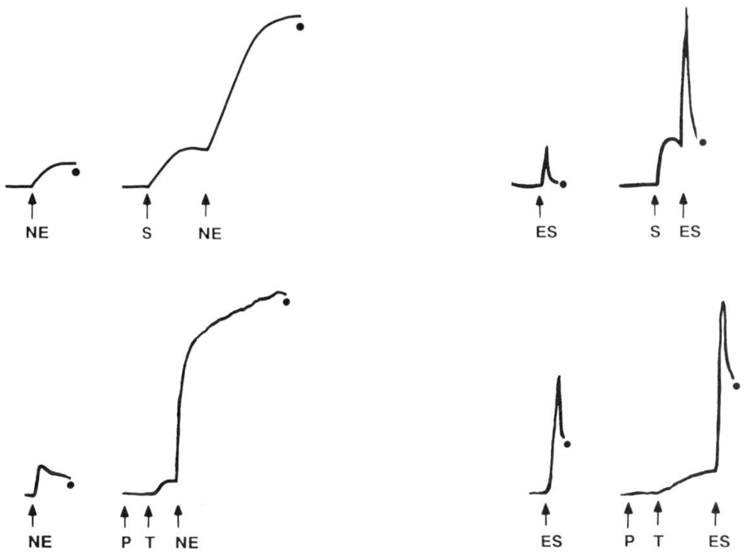

Fig. 4.—Amplifying effects of serotonin (S) in vascular tissues; typical experiments on isolated femoral artery segments of the rabbit. (Left) Small amounts of exogenous serotonin (upper panel) or of rat platelets (P) stimulated with thrombin (T) (lower panel) potentiate ('amplify') the contractile responses to exogenous noradrenaline (N). (Right) Similar amplifying effects are produced on vasoconstrictor responses to electrical stimulation (ES) of the periarterial sympathetic nerves.

9.1.3.3 Vasodilatation

The vasodilator effect of serotonin has been observed mainly in the intact organism. It can be demonstrated on isolated blood vessels with an elevated tone. In most blood vessels the serotonin-induced vasodilatation is observed when the endothelium is still present. In precontracted coronary arteries serotonin released from aggregating platelets causes opposite, vasodilator or vasoconstrictor responses, depending on the presence or absence of endothelium (Cohen *et al.* 1983). In the dog, 2–3 weeks after the superficial femoral artery has been occluded, vasodilatation normally induced by serotonin becomes vasoconstriction, with a reduction in calf blood flow (Hollenberg 1985). The receptor mediating this endothelium-dependent relaxation may belong to the 5-HT_1 serotonergic subtype (Cohen *et al.* 1983). This explain why, in the intact vascular bed, still provided with a functional endothelium, the 5-HT_2 serotonergic antagonist ketanserin not only prevents vasoconstriction, but can unmask, or even potentiate, vasodilator responses to serotonin (Van Nueten *et al.* 1981, Cocks & Angus 1983, Vanhoutte 1987).

9.1.4 SEROTONIN AND VASCULAR DISEASE

9.1.4.1

Small amounts of vasoactive neurohumoral mediators continuously circulating in the vascular beds may, in the presence of an amplifying agent such as endogenously released serotonin, produce vasoconstriction and even vasospasms. They will eventually result in pathological manifestations (e.g. cerebral vasospasms, Raynaud's phenomenon, obstructive vascular disease), due to impairment of regional circulation and deficient tissue perfusion (Vanhoutte 1983, 1987, Van Nueten *et al.* 1987).

Amplifying effects of serotonin will be of consequence, in particular when there is an enhanced release of serotonin from platelets and a simultaneous vascular hyperreactivity to serotonin as observed in a number of acute and chronic pathological conditions. Supersensitivity to serotonin may be one of the causes, or it may at least be involved in the maintenance of cardiovascular dysfunction attributable to serotonin. For instance, in hypertensive animals and man (Fig. 5), and in

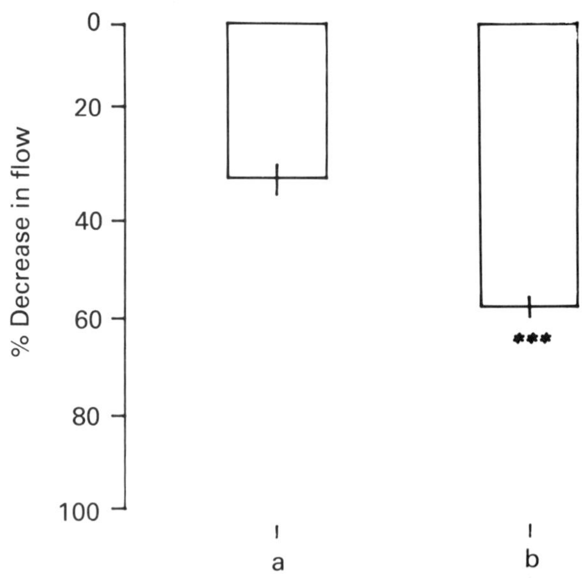

Fig. 5.—% decrease in forearm blood flow caused by an infusion of serotonin (8 μg/min) in (a) human volunteers ($n = 17$) and (b) hypertensive patients ($n = 20$; *** $p < 0.05$; Students t-test, based on data from Doyle *et al.* 1959).

atherosclerotic animals, increased vasoconstriction to serotonin has been observed, and isolated vascular preparations taken from hypertensive animals are more sensitive to the vasoconstrictor action of the monoamine. Also, cutaneous arteries at autopsy from patients who suffered from cardiac disease and varicose veins are more sensitive to the vasoconstrictor effect of serotonin (Haeusler & Finch 1972, Collis & Vanhoutte 1977, Doyle *et al.* 1959, Myers *et al.* 1985, Kalsner & Richards 1984, Heistad *et al.* 1984).

Old age is a predisposing factor leading to enhancement of the vasoconstrictor response to serotonin. Experiments on perfused kidneys of normotensive and spontaneously hypertensive rats have demonstrated that both the direct vasoconstrictor action of serotonin, and its amplifying effect on norepinephrine-induced vasoconstriction are more pronounced in older than in younger animals (De Mey & Vanhoutte 1981, Janssens & Van Nueten 1986).

In a number of pathological conditions (e.g. hypertension, atherosclerosis) vascular hyperreactivity for the vasoconstrictor effect of serotonin is associated with damage of the endothelium, resulting in a reduced release of endothelium derived relaxing factor (Vanhoutte 1987). This, together with an augmented release of serotonin (e.g. in old age), may lead to an increase in peripheral vascular resistance resulting in further impairment of tissue perfusion or in high blood pressure.

9.1.4.2 Hypertension

Earlier observations have suggested that serotonin may be implicated in the pathogenesis of essential hypertension or of its vascular complications (Page 1954, see also Vanhoutte 1985). Vascular tissue from hypertensive patients becomes hyperreactive to the vasoconstrictor component of the effect of serotonin. Under normal, physiological conditions, little serotonin circulates in the plasma, since it is avidly taken up by platelets and rapidly destroyed by the monoamino-oxydase in the endothelium. However, in hypertensive patients, the ability of platelets to bind serotonin is diminished, and the endothelium may become dysfunctional resulting in a prolonged exposure of vascular tissues to serotonin (Vanhoutte 1985). Moreover,

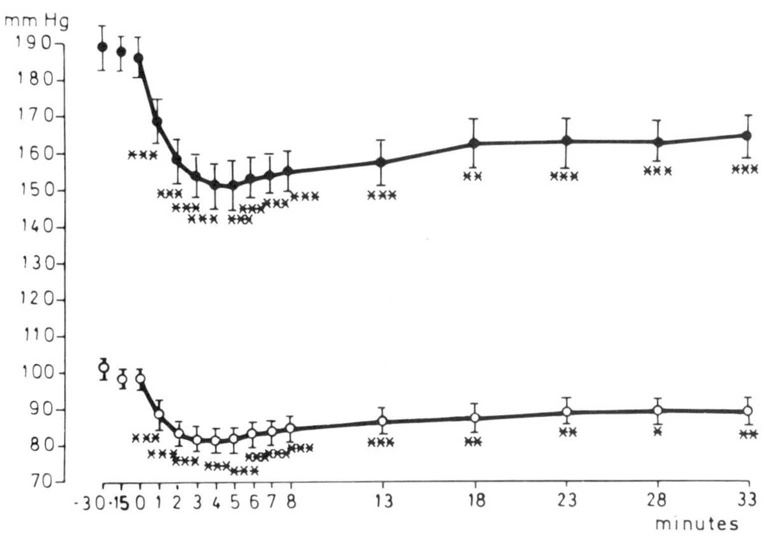

Fig. 6.—Mean systolic (●) and diastolic (○) blood pressure in hypertensive patients is reduced by treatment with ketanserin 10 mg i.v. (De Crée *et al.* 1981, by courtesy of Angiology Research Foundation).

in these patients, platelets are more sensitive to aggregating agents, including serotonin, and platelet release reaction is augmented as shown by increased plasma levels of β-thromboglobulin (Kjeldsen *et al.* 1983).

The 5-HT_2 serotonergic antagonist ketanserin lowers blood pressure both in hypertensive animals and in hypertensive patients (Fig. 6). The peripheral blockade of 5-HT_2 receptors leading to inhibition of both direct and amplifying vascular effects of serotonin, is suggested as the main mode of the hypotensive action of ketanserin, although the alpha-adrenergic blockade observed at higher doses of ketanserin may contribute to its effect (De Crée *et al.* 1981, Wenting *et al.* 1984). The blood pressure lowering effect of ketanserin (40 mg b.i.d.) is more pronounced in subjects over 55 years (Fig. 7), which may be related to the findings that aged vascular tissue becomes more sensitive to the vasoconstrictor effects of serotonin (De Crée *et al.* 1985b, Janssens & Van Nueten 1986).

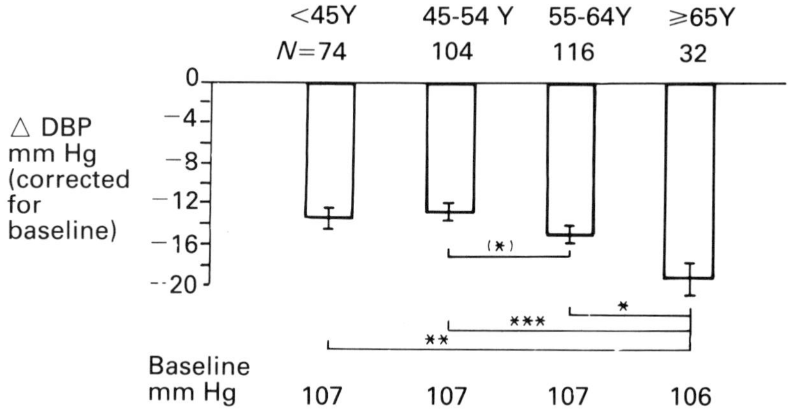

Fig. 7.—The blood pressure lowering effect of chronic treatment of hypertensive patients with ketanserin 40 mg b.i.d. oraly for 3 months increases as a function of age; DBP: decrease of diastolic blood pressure (modified from Van Nueten *et al.* 1987).

ACKNOWLEDGEMENTS

The author thanks Dr W. Janssens and Dr J. Schuurkes for editorial assistance, Dr J. De Crée for providing the data from his studies and L. Geentjens, J. Kuyps, and W. De Ridder for their help in preparing the manuscript. Part of this study was supported by a grant from I.W.O.N.L.

REFERENCES

Bush, L. R., Campbell, W. B., Kern, K., Tilton, G. D., Apprill, P., Ashton, J., Schmitz, J., Buja, L. M., & Willerson, J. T. (1984) The effects of alpha$_2$-adrenergic and serotonergic receptor antagonists on cyclic blood flow alterations in stenosed canine coronary arteries, *Circ. Res.* **55,** 642–652.

Cocks, T. M. & Angus, J. A. (1983) Endothelium-dependent relaxation of coronary arteries by noradrenaline and serotonin, *Nature* **305,** 627–630.

Cohen, R. A., Shepherd, J. T., & Vanhoutte, P. M. (1983) Inhibitory role of the endothelium in the response of isolated coronary arteries to platelets, *Science* **221,** 273–274.

Collis, M. G. & Vanhoutte, P. M. (1977) Vascular reactivity of isolated perfused kidneys from male and female spontaneously hypertensive rats, *Circ. Res.* **41,** 759–767.

De Clerck, F. & Van Nueten, J. M. (1982) Platelet-mediated vascular contractions: inhibition of the serotonergic component by ketanserin, *Thromb. Res.* **27,** 713–727.

De Clerck, F., David, J. L., & Janssen, P. A. J. (1982) Inhibition of 5-hydroxytryptamine-induced and -amplified human platelet aggregation by ketanserin (R 41 468), a selective 5-HT_2 receptor antagonist, *Agents Actions* **12,** 388–397.

De Crée, J., Leempoels, J., De Cock, W., Geukens, H., & Verhaegen, H. (1981) The antihypertensive effects of a pure and selective serotonin-receptor blocking agent (R 41 468) in elderly patients, *Angiology* **32,** 137–144.

De Crée, J., Leempoels, J., Demoen, B., Roels, V., & Verhaegen, H. (1985a) The effect of ketanserin, a 5-HT_2-receptor antagonist on 5-hydroxytryptamine-induced irreversible platelet aggregation in patients with cardiovascular diseases, *Agents Actions* **16,** 313–317.

De Crée, J., Hoing, M., De Ryck, M., & Symoens, J. (1985b) The acute antihypertensive effect of ketanserin increases with age, *J. Cardiovasc. Pharmacol.* **7,** S126–S127.

de la Lande, I. S., Cannell, V. A., & Waterson, J. C. (1966) The interaction of serotonin and noradrenaline on the perfused artery, *Br. J. Pharmacol.* **28,** 255–272.

De Mey, C. & Vanhoutte, P. M. (1981) Effect of age and spontaneous hypertension on the tachyphylaxis to 5-hydroxytryptamine and angiotensin II in the isolated rat kidney, *Hypertension* **3,** 718–724.

Doyle, A. E., Fraser, J. R. E., & Marshall, R. J. (1959) Reactivity of forearm vessels to vasoconstrictor subtances in hypertensive and normotensive subjects. *Clin. Sci.* **18,** 441–454.

Edvinsson, L., Deguerce, A., Duverger, D., Mackenzie, E. T., & Scatton, B. (1983) Central serotonergic nerves project to the pial vessels of the brain, *Nature* **306,** 55–57.

Erspamer, V. & Asero, B. (1952) Identification of enteramine, the specific hormone of the enterochromaffin cell system, as 5-hydroxytrptamine, *Nature* **169,** 800–801.

Haeusler, G. & Finch, L. (1972) Vascular reactivity to 5-hydroxytryptamine and hypertension in the rat, *Naunyn Schmiedebergs Arch. Pharmacol.* **272,** 101–116.

Heistad, D. D., Armstrong, M. L., Marcus, M. L., Piegors D. J., & Mark, A. L. (1984) Augmented responses to vasoconstrictor stimuli in hypercholesterolemic and atherosclerotic monkeys, *Circ. Res.* **54,** 711–718.

Hollenberg, N. K. (1985) Segmental vascular responses to serotonin. In: *Serotonin and the cardiovascular system* (ed by Vanhoutte, P. M.), Raven Press, New York, pp. 165–170.

Huval, W. V., Lelcuk, S., Shepro, D., & Hechtman, H. B. (1984) Role of serotonin in patients with acute respiratory failure. *Ann. Surg.* **200**(2), 166–172.

Janssen, P. A. J. (1985) Pharmacology of potent and selective S_2-serotonergic antagonists. *J. Cardiovasc. Pharmacol.* **7,** S2–S11.

Janssens, W. J. & Van Nueten, J. M. (1986) The direct and amplifying effects of serotonin are increased with age in the isolated perfused kidney of Wistar and spontaneously hypertensive rats, *Naunyn Schmiedebergs Arch. Pharmacol.* **334,** 327–332.

Kalsner, S. & Richards, R. (1984) Coronary arteries of cardiac patients are hyperreactive and contain stores of amines: a mechanism for coronary spasm, *Science* **223,** 1435–1437.

Kjeldsen, S., Gjesdal, K., Eide, I., Aakeson, I., Amundsen, R., Foss, O. P., & Leren, P. (1983) Increased β-thromboglobulin in essential hypertension: interactions between arterial plasma adrenaline, platelet function and blood lipids, *Acta Med. Scand.* **213,** 369–373.

Myers, J. H., Mecca, T. E., & Webb, R. C. (1985) Direct and sensitizing effects of serotonin agonists and antagonists in vascular smooth muscle, *J. Cardiovasc. Pharmacol.* **7,** S44–S48.

Page, I. H. (1954) Serotonin (5-hydroxytryptamine), *Physiol. Rev.***34,** 563–588.

Scroop, G. C. & Walsh, J. A. (1968) Interactions between angiotensin, noradrenaline and serotonin on the peripheral blood vessels in man, *Aust. J. Exp. Biol. Med. Sci.* **46,** 573.

Shepherd, J. T. & Vanhoutte, P. M. (1979) In: *The human cardiovascular system. Facts and concepts.* Raven Press, New York, pp. 351.

Vanhoutte, P. M. (1983) 5-Hydroxytryptamine and vascular disease, *Fed. Proc.* **42,** 233–237.

Vanhoutte, P. M. (1985) In: *Serotonin and the cardiovascular system.* Raven Press, New York, pp. 1–288.

Vanhoutte, P. M. (1987) Serotonin and the vascular wall, *Int. J. Cardiol.* **14,**189–203.

Vanhoutte, P. M. & Cohen, R. A. (1983) The elusory role of serotonin in vascular function and disease. *Biochem. Pharmacol.* **32,** 3671–3674.

Van Nueten, J. M. (1985) Serotonin and the blood vessel wall, *J. Cardiovasc. Pharmacol.* **7,** S49–S51.

Van Nueten, J. M., Janssen, P. A. J., Van Beek, J., Xhonneux, R., Verbeuren, T. J., & Vanhoutte, P. M. (1981) Vascular effects of ketanserin (R 41 468), a novel antagonist of 5-HT_2 serotonergic receptors, *J. Pharmacol. Exp. Ther.* **218,** 217–230.

Van Nueten, J. M., Janssens, W. J., & Vanhoutte, P. M. (1985) Serotonin and vascular reactivity, *Pharm. Res. Commun.* **17,** 585–608.

Van Nueten, J. M., Janssen, P. A. J., Symoens, J., Janssens, W. J., Heykants, J., De Clerck, F., Leysen, J. E., Vancauteren, H., & Vanhoutte, P. M. (1987) Ketanserin. In: *New cardiovascular drugs 1987* (ed Scriabine, A.), Raven Press, New York, pp. 1–56.

Wenting, G. J., Woittiez, A. J., Man in't Veld, A. J., & Schalekamp, M. A. D. H. (1984) 5-HT, alpha-adrenoceptors, and blood pressure. Effects of ketanserin in essential hypertension and autonomic insufficiency, *Hypertension* **6,** 100–109.

9.2 Metabolism of catecholamines in uraemia

Vito M. Campese†

In this paper the abnormalities of catecholamine metabolism in uremia are reviewed. Plasma concentrations of norepinephrine (NE) are usually increased in uraemia. Studies *in vivo* have shown that this derangement may be partially due to increased release; however, experiments *in vitro* have suggested a decrease in NE release from brain synaptosomes of uremic rats. The major defect in NE metabolism in uraemia appears to be a decrease in NE uptake and degradation.

Several abnormalities of autonomic nervous system function have been described in uraemia (Goldberger *et al.* 1971, Soriano & Eisinger 1972, Campese *et al.* 1981, Pickering *et al.* 1972, Lazarus *et al.* 1973, Kersh *et al.* 1974, Campese *et al.* 1982, Atuk *et al.* 1976, Lake *et al.* 1979). The role of these abnormalities in the cardiovascular derangements, such as hypertension, commonly observed in uraemic patients, is in large part unknown.

Much of the confusion derives from the fact that the methods to directly measure the activity of the sympathetic nervous system are not available in man, and that most of the studies have relied on indirect indices of sympathetic nervous system activity. Since the development of highly sensitive and specific radioenzymatic assays for the measurement of catecholamines, the determination of free norepinephrine (NE) in the plasma has been the most widely used indirect index of sympathetic nervous system activity. It should be pointed out, however, that the amount of NE reaching the blood is only a minute fraction of the total amount released into the synaptic clefts, and blood NE does not only reflect the rate of release from the sympathetic nerve ending, but also the rate of re-uptake into the nerve endings or into extraneuronal cells, the density, distribution, and width of the neuroeffector junctions, and the rate of clearance.

9.2.1 PLASMA LEVELS OF CATECHOLAMINES IN URAEMIC PATIENTS

Plasma concentrations of catecholamines are usually elevated in patients with chronic renal failure prior to the institution of dialysis treatment. In one study of 16 patients with

† Division of Nephrology, Department of Medicine, University of Southern California, Los Angeles, California, USA

mean creatinine clearance of 15 ml/min, plasma catecholamine levels (126 ± 11 ng/dl) were significantly ($p < 0.005$) greater than in normal subjects (48 ± 6 ng/dl) (Campese *et al.* 1981). In 21 nondialyzed patients with end-stage renal failure, we also showed that supine plasma NE (35 ± 3.6 ng/dl) and plasma epinephrine levels (3.3 ± 0.55 ng/dl) were significantly greater than in normal subjects (21 ± 0.9 ng/dl, and 2.5 ± 0.23 ng/dl, respectively (Campese *et al.* 1981). During upright posture, plasma NE levels were also signficantly greater ($p < 0.01$) in uraemic patients (97 ± 8.9 ng/dl) than in normal subjects (48 ± 2.4 ng/dl).

Less consistent are the data on plasma levels of catecholamines in patients on maintenance haemodialysis. In our laboratory, we found that supine plasma NE (24 ± 2.7 ng/dl) and epinephrine levels (2.1 ± 0.37 ng/dl) in 16 patients on chronic haemodialysis were not different from those in normal subjects (21 ± 0.9 and 2.5 ± 0.23 ng/dl, respectively) (Campese *et al.* 1981). Similarly, plasma levels of NE were not significantly different in dialysis patients from those in normal subjects during upright posture (55 ± 4.9 and 48 ± 2.4 ng/dl, respectively). Lake *et al.* (1979) also found no difference in basal plasma levels of NE between 60 normal subject (34 ± 2.3 ng/dl) and 20 age-matched dialysis patients (33 ± 3.0 ng/dl). On the contrary, other investigators have observed higher basal levels of NE and/or total catecholamines in patients on maintenance dialysis (Brecht *et al.* 1975, Henrich *et al.* 1977, McGrath *et al.* 1978). The reasons for these discrepancies are not obvious. They could be related to differences in age, or in serum potassium concentration, or in the sodium-volume state among the various patient populations or to the different methodology used to measure plasma catecholamines.

9.2.2 MECHANISMS RESPONSIBLE FOR THE ELEVATED LEVELS OF PLASMA CATECHOLAMINES IN URAEMIA

Since the levels of circulating catecholamines depend not only on the amount released from the sympathetic terminals, but also on the re-uptake, metabolism, and excretion, a rise in plasma catecholamines could be related to abnormality of any of those functions.

9.2.3 RELEASE OF NOREPINEPHRINE

Izzo *et al.* (1982), using metabolic turnover studies with cold NE have measured release rates and clearance rates of norepinephrine in 24 patients on maintenance haemodialysis and in 30 normal subjects. Plasma NE levels were not different between these two groups. However, when plasma NE levels were corrected for methylation index, they found that both plasma NE and epinephrine levels were increased in dialysis patients. They also found that the appearance rate and the clearance rate of NE were increased in uraemic patients. These turnover studies suggest that haemodialysis patients may display biochemical signs of sympathetic hyperactivity. Unfortunately, these investigators failed to give any clinical correlates of their biochemical findings. Furthermore, these data need confirmation with techniques using labelled NE, in concentrations substantially lower than those used for cold NE infusions.

Studies on isolated brain rat synaptosomes have shown that the release of NE in uraemic rats was significantly lower than in control rats (2 ± 0.2 vs 5.1 ± 0.47 pmol/mg protein/10 min, $p < 0.01$ (Smogorzewski *et al.* 1988).

Abnormalities in NE release could be limited only to some patients. Lilley *et al.* (1976), for example, measured plasma DBH activity in a group of patients with frequent haemodialysis hypotension, and, for comparison, in a group of patients with rare episodes of haemodialysis hypotension in an attempt to determine whether hypotension during haemodialysis was the result of abnormalities in the sympathetic nervous system activity. Plasma DBH activity was significantly higher in patients with haemodialysis hypotension than in the other group. Supine mean blood pressure before haemodialysis was also higher in patients with hypotension than in those without. These investigators suggested that haemodialysis hypotension may be the result of a lesion in the baroreceptors. They also suggested that the higher predialysis blood pressure in patients with frequent haemodialysis hypotension may be neurogenic in nature as reflected by the greater plasma levels of DBH activity, and it appears similar to the hypertension that follows baroreceptor deafferentation in experimental animals.

9.2.4 CONCENTRATION OF CATECHOLAMINE SYNTHETIC ENZYMES IN URAEMIA

Thyroxine hydroxylase, the rate-limiting enzyme of noradrenaline synthesis, was found to be significantly reduced in myocardial homogenates of uraemic rats (Hennemann *et al.* 1973).

Dopamine-β-hydroxylase (DBH), the enzyme that catalyses the conversion of dopamine to norepinephrine, was found to be significantly lower in dialysis patients than in normal subjects (Lake *et al.* 1979, Brecht *et al.* 1975, Henrich *et al.* 1977, McGrath *et al.* 1978, Izzo *et al.* 1982 Smogorzewski *et al.* 1988, Lilley *et al.* 1976, Hennemann *et al.* 1973, Aoki *et al.* 1975). This abnormality has been interpreted as reflecting a chronic decrease in sympathetic activity (Lake *et al.* 1979), and is, evidently, at variance with the finding of normal or elevated plasma levels of catecholamines in uraemic patients.

9.2.5 RE-UPTAKE OF NOREPINEPHRINE IN URAEMIA

A decreased neuronal uptake of NE along with decreased NE content in sympathetic nerve terminals have been demonstrated in uraemic rats (Hennemann *et al.* 1973).

We have recently studied the rat brain NE content and re-uptake in synaptosomes of uraemic and control rats.

Synaptosomes from rats with 21 days of chronic renal failure showed reduced NE content (11.0 ± 0.60 vs 13.6 ± 0.55 pmol/mg protein, $p < 0.01$), and uptake (87 ± 4.0 vs 110 ± 5.9 pmol/mg protein/50 min, $p < 0.01$) when compared to those from normal animals. Na^+-K^+ ATPase activity was also lower in uraemic synaptosomes compared with control rats (6.5 ± 0.81 vs 11.4 ± 0.76 μmol Pi/mg Protein/hr, $p < 0.01$) (Smogorzewski *et al.* 1988). Since the uptake of NE by brain synaptosomes requires energy and is dependent, directly or indirectly, on Na^+-K^+ ATPase activity (Fraser *et al.* 1985), it has been suggested that the decrease in NE uptake by brain synaptosomes in rats with renal failure may be due to reduced Na^+-K^+ ATPase activity (Ali *et al.* 1985).

A decrease in NE content in the brain of rats with chronic renal failure has also been shown by others (Ali *et al.* 1985).

9.2.6 CONCENTRATION OF CATECHOLAMINES DEGRADING ENZYMES IN URAEMIA

The activity of monoamine oxidase, the enzyme that catalyses the conversion of norepinephrine to 3,4-dihydroxymandelic acid (DOMA) and of normetanephrine to vanillylmandelic acid (VMA), was found to be increased in myocardial homogenates of uraemic rats, and the increments were directly related to the degree of renal failure (Hennemann *et al.* 1973). Similarly, platelet monoamine oxidase activity was found to be increased in uraemia (Kopple *et al.* 1975). On the contrary, the activity of COMT is reduced in the haemolyzed whole blood of uraemic patients (Atuk *et al.* 1976).

9.2.7 NOREPINEPHRINE CLEARANCE AND URINARY EXCRETION IN URAEMIA

The clearance of NE has been shown to be increased in two separate studies using the infusion of cold NE (Izzo *et al.* 1982, Schohn *et al.* 1985). This abnormality has been attributed to increased transepatic extraction and metabolism secondary to the high cardiac output commonly observed in anaemic haemodialysis patients (Axelrod & Weinshilbaum 1972, Kim *et al.* 1975). Urinary excretion of catecholamines or catecholamine metabolites was not impaired in patients with creatinine clearance above 19 ml/min (Darwish *et al.* 1984, Laederach & Weidman 1987) have shown a reduction in daily urinary excretion of catecholamines from 25 μg in normal subjects to 9 μg in 10 patients with chronic renal failure (mean creatinine clearance 15 ml/min) and to negligible levels in patients with end-stage renal failure.

9.2.8 VASCULAR RESPONSE TO INFUSED NOREPINEPHRINE IN URAEMIA

One important aspect to consider when evaluating the activity of the sympathetic nervous system is the relationship between concentrations of NE and vascular responsiveness. When we studied the effect of NE infusion into patients with terminal renal failure prior to any dialysis treatment, patients on maintenance haemodialysis, and in normal subjects (Campese *et al.* 1981), we found that in the predialysis patients, the changes in MBP with 100 ng/kg/min of NE were significantly lower ($p < 0.05$) than those observed in normal subjects. The changes in MBP in the dialysis patients were not different from those in normal subjects. Similarly, the decrements in heart rate were significantly smaller ($p < 0.05$) in the predialysis patients than in dialysis patients, and in normal subjects. The mechanisms responsible for this abnormality are complex. This could be related to downregulation of alpha-adrenergic receptors of the vascular smooth muscle in the presence of elevated plasma levels of NE (Meggs *et al.* 1986, Fadda *et al.* 1988). Rascher *et al.* (1982) have found diminished vascular response to NE in experimental chronic uraemia in the rat. They observed hyporesponsiveness to NE in the isolated perfused hindlimb and in aortic strips of uraemic rats. The hyporesponsiveness was specific for NE and not present for vasopressin or for potassium chloride. These data suggest that the reduced responsiveness to NE in uraemic rats may be due to downregulation of alpha-receptors.

A large body of evidence indicates that excessive levels of parathyroid hormone (PTH) in uraemia may be, at least partly, responsible for the decreased pressor response to NE. PTH is a vasodilator agent both *in vivo* and *in vitro* (Pang *et al.* 1980), and it blunts the pressor effect of both NE and angiotensin II in rats. This effect of PTH is completely abolished by pretreatment with indomethacin (Saglikes *et al.* 1985). Moreover, PTH increased the urinary excretion of PGF_{α} (the stable metabolite of prostacycline) in rat. These observations suggest that the modulating effect of PTH on the pressor response to NE may be mediated by prostaglandins. It is theoretically possible that the excessive PTH levels may stimulate production of prostaglandins and in turn reduce the pressor response to NE, in uraemic animals. This postulate is supported by studies in our laboratory showing that treatment of uraemic patients with indomethacin may improve or normalize the pressor response to NE (Collins *et al.* 1985).

REFERENCES

Ali, F., Tayeh, O., & Attalah, A. (1985) Plasma and brain catecholamines in experimental uremia: Acute and chronic studies. *Life Sci.* **37,** 1757–1764.

Aoki, K., Tazumi, K., & Takikawa, K. (1975) Serum dopamine-β-hydroxylase activity in essential hypertension and in chronic renal failure with hypertension. *Jap. Circul. J.* **39,** 1111–1114.

Atuk, N. O., Bailey, C. J., Turner, S., Peach, M. J., & Westervelt, F. B. (1976() Red blood cell catechol-*o*-methyl transferase, plasma catecholamines and renin in renal failure. *Trans. Am. Soc. Artif. Internal Organs* **22,** 195–200.

Axelrod, J. & Weinshilbaum, R. (1972) Catecholamines. *N. Engl. J. Med.* **287,** 237–242.

Brecht, H. M., Ernst, W., & Koch, K. M. (1975) Plasma noradrenaline levels in regular haemodialysis patients. *Proc. Eur. Dial. Transplant Ass.* **12,** 281–289.

Campese, V. M., Romoff, M. S., Levitan, D., Lane, K., & Massry, S. G. (1981) Mechanisms of autonomic nervous system dysfunction in uremia. *Kidney Int.* **20,** 246–253.

Campese, V. M., Procci, W. R., Levitan, D., Romoff, M. S., Goldstein, D. A., & Massry, S. G. (1982) Autonomic nervous system dysfunction and impotence in uremia. *Am. J. Nephrol.* **2,** 140–143.

Collins, J., Massry, S. G., & Campese, V. M. (1985) Parathyroid hormone and the altered vascular response to norepinephrine in uremia. *Am. J. Nephrol.* **5,** 110–113.

Darwish, R., Elias, A. N., Vaziri, N. D., Pahl, M., Powers, D., & Stokes, J. D. (1984) Plasma and urinary catecholamines and their metabolites chronic renal failure. *Arch. Int. Med.* **144,** 69–71.

Fadda, Z., Massry, S. G., El-Rafai, M., & Campese, V. M. (1988) Alpha adrenergic receptors in mesenteric arteries of rats with chronic renal failure. *Kidney Int.* **34,** 463–466.

Fraser, C. L., Sarnacki, P., & Arieff, A. I. (1985) Abnormal sodium transport in synaptosomes from brain in uremic rats. *J. Clin. Invest.* **75,** 2014–2023.

Goldberger, S., Thompson, A., Guha, A., Kramer, N., & Parrish, A. (1971) Autonomic nervous dysfunction in chronic renal failure. *Clin. Res.* **19,** 531A.

Hennemann, H., Hevendehl, G., Horler, E., & Heidland, A. (1973) Toxic sympathicopathy in uraemia. *Proc. Eur. Dial. Transplant Ass.* **10,** 166–170.

Henrich, W. L., Katz, F. H., Molinoff, P. B., & Schrier, R. W. (1977) Competitive effects of hypokalemia and volume depletion on plasma renin activity, aldosterone and catecholamine concentrations in hemodialysis patients. *Kidney Int.* **12,** 279–284.

Izzo, J. L., Izzo, M. S., Sterns, R. H., & Freeman, R. B. (1982) Sympathetic nervous system hyperactivity in maintenance hemodialysis patients. *Trans. Am. Soc. Artif. Internal Organs* **28,** 604–607.

Kersh, E. S., Kronfield, S. J., Unger, A., Popper, R. W., Cantor, S., & Cohn, K. (1974) Autonomic insufficiency in uremia as a cause of hemodialysis-induced hypotension. *New Engl. J. Med.* **290,** 650–653.

Kim, K. E., Onesti, G., & Swartz, C. D. (1975) Hemodynamics of hypertension in uremia. *Kidney Int.* **8,** S155–S162.

Kopple, J. D. & Marian, E. S. (1975) Monoamine oxidase, diamine oxidase and platelet serotonin in uremia. *Proc. 8th Ann. Contributors Conf. Artif. Kid. Prog. NIAMOD,* p. 53.

Laederach, K. & Weidmann, P. (1987) Plasma and urinary catecholamines as related to renal function in man. *Kidney Int.* **31,** 107–111.

Lake, C. R., Ziegler, M. G., Coleman, M. D., & Kopin, I. J. (1979) Plasma levels of norepinephrine and dopamine-β-hydroxylyase in CRF patients treated with dialysis. *Cardiovasc. Med.* **1979,** 1099–1111.

Lazarus, J. M., Hampers, D. L., Lowrie, E. G., & Merrill, J. P. (1973) Baroreceptor activity in normotensive and hypertensive uremic patients. *Circulation* **47,** 1015–1021.

Lilley, J. J., Golden, J., & Stone, R. A. (1976) Adrenergic regulation of blood pressure in chronic renal failure. *J. Clin. Invest.* **57,** 1190–1200.

McGrath, B. P., Ledingham, J. G. G., & Benedict, C. R. (1978) Catecholamines in peripheral venous plasma in patients on chronic hemodialysis. *Clin. Sci. Mol. Med.* **55,** 89–96.

Meggs, L., Ben-Ari, L., Gammon, D., *et al.* (1986) Effect of chronic uremia on the cardiovascular alpha$_1$ receptor. *Life Sci.* **39,** 169–179.

Pang, P. K. T., Tenner, T. E., Yee, J. A., Yang, M., & Janssen, H. F. (1980) Hypotensive action of parathyroid hormone preparations on rats and dogs. *Proc. Natl. Acad. Sci. USA* **77,** 675–678.

Pickering, T. G., Gribbin, B., & Oliver, D. O. (1972) Baroreflex sensitivity in patients on longterm haemodialysis. *Clin. Sci.* **43,** 645–657.

Rascher, W., Schomig, A., Kreye, V. A., & Ritz, E. (1982) Diminished vascular response to noradrenaline in experimental chronic uremia. *Kidney Int.* **21,** 20–27.

Saglikes, Y., Massry, S. G., & Campese, V. M. (1985) Evidence for a role of PTH in the reduced pressor response to norepinephrine in chronic renal failure. *Kidney Int.* **28,** 11–15.

Schohn, D., Weidmann, P., Jahn, H., Beretta-Piccoli, C. (1985) Norepinephrine-related mechanism in hypertension accompanying renal failure. *Kidney Int.* **28,** 814–822.

Smogorzewski, M., Campese, V. M., & Massry, S. G. (1988) Abnormal norepinephrine metabolism in brain synaptosomes of rats with chronic renal failure. Role of parathyroid hormone. *Kidney Int.* **33,** 385A.

Soriano, G. & Eisinger, R. P. (1972) Abnormal response to the Valsalva maneuver in patients on chronic hemodialysis. *Nephron* **9,** 251–256.

9.3 The role of calcium in muscle function and its regulation

Ernesto Carafoli†

Ca is a signalling element of general importance to all cells. In muscles, the key signalling function of Ca is the activation of troponin-C, which is essential for the contraction of myofibrils in skeletal and heart muscle, and of myosin light chain kinase, which is essential for the contraction of smooth muscles. The control of Ca within cells is performed by specific binding proteins, which are either soluble in the cytoplasm (e.g., calmodulin), organized in non-membranous structures (e.g., troponin-C), or intrinsic to membranes (e.g., ATPases, Na/Ca exchangers).

9.3.1 INTRODUCTION

Ca has been selected by evolution as a signalling agent to a large number of cellular functions, among them the generation of fuels, the synthesis and release of hormones, muscle and non-muscle motility, and a host of membrane-linked processes (see Carafoli 1987, for a recent comprehensive review). To heart cells, motility is of particular interest, although several aspects of the activity defined here as generation of fuels (i.e., regulation of metabolic pathways) are also of primary importance. The signalling function of Ca obviously demands its maintenance within cells at a very low free concentration, and ways and means to vary it rapidly and precisely in the different cell compartments to satisfy the requirements of the signalling function. The regulation of Ca within cells is performed by reversible complexation to specific proteins, either soluble, organized in non-membranous structures, or intrinsic to membranes. These proteins 'buffer' intracellular Ca at a level which is at least 10 000-fold lower than in the external spaces. The Ca-filtering function of the plasma membrane, which is based on the operation of membrane-intrinsic Ca binding proteins, is instrumental in the long-term maintenance of the Ca gradient. The latter is very convenient to the signalling function, since the very large inwardly directed Ca pressure at the plasma membrane ensures that even a minor increase in the Ca permeability of the plasma membrane will result in a significant swing in the intracellular concentration (i.e., in significant modulation of the signalling function).

† Laboratory of Biochemistry, Swiss Federal Institute of Technology (ETH), 8092 Zurich, Switzerland

9.3.2 THE HIGH AFFINITY Ca BINDING PROTEINS

Abundant information is available on the non-membranous high-affinity Ca binding proteins. Following the elucidation of the crystal structure of the muscle protein parvalbumin by Kretsinger and his associates (1973), a number of structural principles were established that preside over the complexing of Ca by parvalbumin. Based on these principles, extrapolations were made to other proteins that were also known to bind Ca with high affinity (see Kretsinger & Nelson, 1977, for a review). The parvalbumin principles demand that Ca-binding proteins of this type consist of repeat units made of two α-helices, oriented perpendicularly to each other, flanking a non-helical loop of 10–12 amino acids where Ca coordinates to 6–8 oxygen atoms of carboxylic side chains and, albeit less frequently, to carbonyl oxygens of the peptide backbone. The Ca-binding cavity has been evidently optimized by evolution, since only minimal variability is now tolerated in it: in fact, of the three helix–loop–helix units of parvalbumin, the first, termed A–B, does not bind Ca because of the amino acid substitutions in it. The parvalbumin model has become known as the EF-hand model, and has been shown to be compatible with the amino acid sequences of a number of other Ca-binding proteins; it has been directly demonstrated on the recently solved crystal structures of at least three other proteins (Szebenyi *et al.* 1981, Herzberg & James 1985, Babu *et al.* 1985).

The soluble Ca-binding proteins on the EF-hand group complex Ca, and in so doing obviously contribute to its buffering. They have, however, an additional function, which is in fact their main function. They express hydrophobic sites on their surface, and thus become capable of interacting with (enzyme) targets. Therefore, these proteins should be viewed essentially as processors of the Ca signal, rather as intracellular Ca buffers. That their Ca-buffering role is an accessory function is a plausible conclusion, also considering that their buffering function would be quantitatively limited by their amount in the cell. Bearing these caveats in mind, one can, nevertheless, attept to evaluate the total theoretical Ca-buffering capacity of the two most important Ca-binding proteins of this type, calmodulin and troponin C. The concentration of the former is lower in muscles than in other tissues, and it can be calculated that it could buffer approximately 8 μM Ca (Carafoli 1987). Troponin-C, on the other hand, is more concentrated in muscles than in other tissues; based on a measured content of 2 μM in heart, and 20 μM in skelelal muscles (Grand *et al.* 1979), it can be calculated that the buffering capacity of troponin-C could handle a maximum of 6 μM and 80 μM in heart and skeletal muscles, respectively (Carafoli 1987).

9.3.3 MEMBRANE TRANSPORT OF CALCIUM

The quantitative limitations in the Ca-buffering function described above do not apply to the case of another class of Ca-binding proteins, intrinsic to membranes. A membrane protein complexes Ca at one site of a membrane, delivers it across, and repeats the operation continuously, thus overcoming the problem of the possibly insufficient amount of protein available. Therefore, the membrane-intrinsic Ca-binding and transport proteins play the dominant role in the buffering of intracellular Ca. Normal (eukaryotic) cells possess several Ca-transporting systems, in the plasma membrane and in the membranes of the organelles (Fig. 1). There is no redundancy,

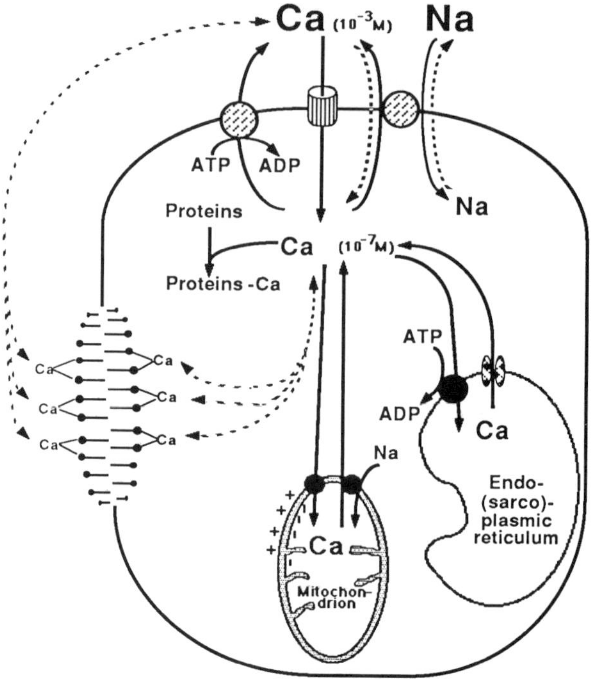

Fig. 1.—Ca transporting system in eukaryotic cells. The figure shows seven transporting systems; three in the plasma membrane (a Ca-ATPase, frequently referred to as the Ca-pump, a Na/Ca exchanger which normally imports Ca but sometimes also exports it, and a Ca channel); two in endo(sarco)plasmic reticulum (a Ca-ATPase and a still undefined release channel); two in the inner membrane of mitochondria (an electrophoretic uptake unporter and a Ca-releasing Na/Ca exchanger). The systems in the Golgi membranes and in the lysosomes have not been inserted in the figure, because they are still very poorly known. The soluble Ca-binding proteins of the cytosol and the acidic phospholipids of the plasma membrane have been included in the figure as participants in the Ca-buffering function.

however, since the various transporting systems operate with different kinetic properties, thus satisfying the variable demands of the functional cycle of cells. The latter sometimes requires rapid, precise, and high-affinity regulation of Ca, sometimes lower affinity and less rapid regulation (i.e., transport). As Fig. 1 indicates, eukaryotic cell membranes contain a minimum of seven (proteinaceous) Ca-transporting systems, which correspond to four basic transporting modes: ATPases, exchangers, channels, electrophoretic uniporters (Table 1). High-affinity Ca regulation depends obligatorily

Table 1—Ca transporting modes in cell membranes

Transporting mode	Membrane system	Ca affinity
ATPases	Plasma membrane Endo(sarco)plasmic reticulum (Golgi, lysosomes)	high
Exchangers (Na/Ca)	Plasma membrane Mitochondria	low
Channels	Plasma membrane Sarcoplasmic reticulum	low
Electrophoretic uniporters	Mitochondria	low

on ATPases, since only this transporting mode is capable of high-affinity interaction with Ca. When lower-affinity regulation is required, more options are open, and cells choose from amongst the other three modes.

9.3.4 Ca TRANSPORT IN THE PLASMA MEMBRANE

Fig. 2 shows the three Ca transporting systems of the plasma membrane: the Ca channel, the Na/Ca exchanger, and the Ca ATPase. The Ca channel is the system responsible for the controlled penetration of Ca into cells. Although known for almost

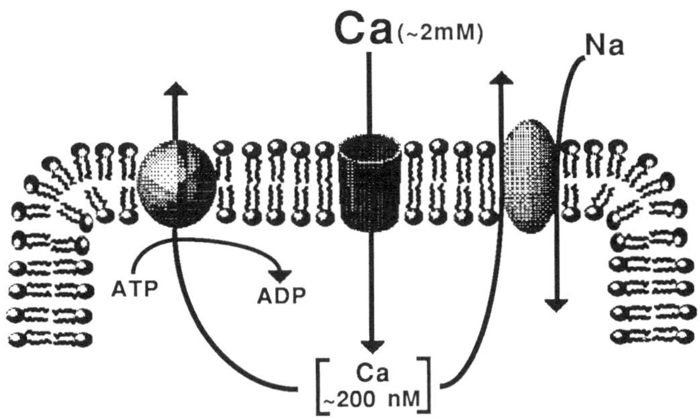

Fig. 2.—A scheme of the three plasma membrane Ca-transporting systems

three decades, the channel has been investigated at a molecular level only recently: the introduction of the patch-clamp technique has permitted the study of single channels, and has led to the precise definition of its kinetic parameters (see Reuter 1984, for a recent review). Patch-clamp recordings of currents through single channels have revealed a conductance of 15–25 pS, corresponding to the passage of about 3×10^6 Ca ions per sec. (Reuter *et al.* 1982). The density of the Ca channel is of the order of 0.1 to 1.0 per μm^2 in heart, but much higher in the T-tubular membranes of skeletal muscles. The channels are gated by the electrical potential across the plasma membrane, Ca currents becoming evident as the transmembrane potential increases from the resting level of -70 mV to about -40 mV (maximal Ca currents are seen at about 0 mV). The channels are blocked by several organic compounds, which are normally referred to as Ca antagonists (Fleckenstein 1983). The most important Ca antagonists are the dihydropyridines, which appear to block the channel from the lipid phase of the membrane. Work on Ca antagonists has greatly advanced knowledge on the Ca channel: one important recent development has been the determination of the primary structure of the dihydropyridine receptor of the T-tubular system (Tanabe *et al.* 1987). One interesting aspect of the Ca-channel is its sensitivity to adrenergic neurotransmitters: patch-clamp experiments have shown that cAMP enhances the opening probability of the channel (Reuter *et al.* 1982), a finding that offers obvious therapeutic possibilities in heart cells. It has recently been found that there are several Ca channel types, different in properties. Two have been identified by patch-clamp experiments in mammalian hearts (Nilius *et al.* 1985), the most common being the L-type, which is sensitive to dihydropyridines and whose openings produce currents of long duration. The T-type opens at more negative transmembrane potentials, is insensitive to dihydropyridines, and produces currents of shorter duration.

The Na/Ca exchanger is one of the two Ca-exporting systems of the plasma membrane (under some conditions it can also mediate the influx of Ca). It is a large-capacity, low-affinity system, particularly active in excitable tissues like heart. Most of the knowledge on the system indeed comes from work on heart, and the giant axon of the squid (see Blaustein & Nelson 1982, for a recent review). Early electrophysiological work has established that the system operates electrogenically, exchanging 3 Na for 1 Ca; thus, it does not only respond to the Na and Ca gradients, but also to the transmembrane electrical potential. More recent work using heart sarcolemmal vesicles (Reeves & Sutko 1979) has permitted determination of some essential kinetic parameters of the system, among them the affinity for Ca (K_m, 1–20 μM), and the maximal rate of Ca transport, which in heart corresponds to about 20 nmol per mg of sarcolemmal protein per sec. The low affinity of the system for Ca poses a problem, since it seems unlikely that the free Ca concentration in the cytosol will ever be as high as 10 μM. Although it is possible that the kinetic parameters of the exchanger in isolated vesicles are somewhat different from those in the intact tissue, the low affinity of the exchanger for Ca is difficult to reconcile with the demands of cell physiology. One lead, here, could be the activation of the exchanger by a kinase-linked phosphorylation process (Caroni & Carafoli 1983), which decreases the K_m(Ca) of the system to about 1 μM.

The Ca ATPase of the plasma membrane interacts with Ca with high affinity (K_m about 0.5 μM), but has low total transport capacity: in heart it corresponds to about 0.5 nmol per mg of membrane protein per sec. Given its high Ca affinity, the enzyme is qualified to export Ca from cells continuously, not only when its concentration in the cytosol has increased. Thus, the Ca ATPase is likely to play the most important role in maintaining the 10^4-fold gradient of Ca between cells and medium. The enzyme is an ATPase of the P-class, i.e., it forms an aspartyl phosphate during the reaction mechanism and is inhibited by vanadate (see Schatzmann 1982 for a review). It is a target of calmodulin stimulation: the interaction with calmodulin has been exploited to purify the ATPase on calmodulin columns: the purified enzyme is a single polypeptide of M_r 138,000, which can be reconstituted in liposomes with optimal transporting efficiency (Niggli *et al.* 1981). The liposomal system has permitted us to establish that the ATPase transports Ca with a 1:1 stoichiometry to ATP hydrolysis, i.e., it is less 'efficient' than the analogous enzyme of sarcoplasmic reticulum (see below). Of interest is the observation (Caroni & Carafoli 1981) that a cAMP-linked phosphorylation process stimulates the ATPase-mediated pumping of Ca. Since cAMP also stimulates the Ca channel activity (see above), the result of the cAMP-mediated protein phosphorylation reaction is apparently the overall increase of the plasma membrane Ca flux, rather than the unidirectional stimulation of any given transport reaction.

Work on the purified Ca ATPase has established that the enzyme can be stimulated by several treatments alternative to calmodulin, among them the exposure to acidic phospholipids and polyunsaturated fatty acids, and a controlled proteolytic treatment witha number of proteases. The physiological meaning of these alternative activations is not clear, but their role in the physiological modulation of the ATPase appears very possible.

9.3.5 Ca TRANSPORT ACROSS INTRACELLULAR MEMBRANES

As mentioned above, the long-term maintenance of the Ca gradient between cells and medium is the result of the action of the plasma membrane transport systems. However, the fluxes in the plasma membrane account for a minor fraction of the total Ca involved in the functional cycle of cells. The Ca handled by the plasma membrane is essential as a trigger of important intracellular events, but it is now clear that the largest portion of the Ca needed for cell activity derives from intracellular stores.

9.3.6 THE ENDO(SARCO)PLASMIC RETICULUM

Most of the work on this membrane system has been performed on sarcoplasmic reticulum, essentially because of the easier availability of the system and of its key enzyme, the Ca ATPase, with respect to endoplasmic reticulum. The latter organelle, however, has recently come to the forefront, thanks to the discovery that its Ca pool is sensitive to inositol-tris-phosphate. The involvement of the latter messenger in the release of Ca from sarcoplasmic reticulum is still unclear in heart and skeletal muscle, but appears to be probable in smooth muscles (Somlyo *et al.* 1985).

The endo(sarco)plasmic reticulum is the structure responsible for the fine regulation of Ca in the cytosol. In muscles it controls the availability of Ca to the myofibrils, and it thus controls the contraction/relaxation cycle. It contains an ATPase of the same type of that of the plasma membrane, which has high affinity for Ca (K_m below 0.5 μM) and which is present in very large amounts in the membranes of sarcoplasmic reticulum. As a result, the total Ca-transporting capacity of the organelle is very high, particularly in fast skeletal muscles where it may reach 70 nmol per mg of membrane protein per sec. The ATPase has been purified by MacLennan (1970) as a single polypeptide of M_r about 100 kDa, and characterized extensively thanks to work performed in several Laboratories. It forms an aspartyl-phosphate, is inhibited by vanadate, and can be reconstituted into liposomes, where it transports Ca with a 2:1 stoichiometry to the hydrolyzed ATP. An important recent development has been the determination of the primary structure of the enzyme (MacLennan *et al.* 1985), which differs somewhat in heart and fast skeletal muscles. Also of interest is the finding that the ATPase in heart, smooth, and slow (but not fast) skeletal muscles is modulated by an acidic proteolipid termed phospholamban (Tada *et al.* 1975). This proteolipid, which is a pentamer of five identical subunits of M_r about 6 kDa, is phosphorylated by two kinases, one cAMP, one calmodulin-dependent. Once phosphorylated, phospholamban activates the ATPase-linked transport of Ca, thus transmitting to sarcoplasmic reticulum hormonal messages from the plasma membrane.

The release of Ca from heart sarcoplasmic reticulum is now the subject of very intensive investigations, particularly so in view of the great interest in the role of inositol tris phosphate in endoplasmic reticulum and in sarcoplasmic reticulum of smooth muscles. The favoured mechanism for the Ca release phenomenon in heart is the Ca-induced Ca-release (Fabiato & Fabiato 1975), in which massive liberation of Ca from the vesicles of sarcoplasmic reticulum is induced by introducing Ca into the medium at concentrations below the threshold concentration (0.1 μM). Very little is known, however on the 'Ca channel' that mediates the release phenomenon. Recent work (Meissner & Hendersen 1987) has indicated that the channel is activated by Ca, adenine nucleotides, and caffeine, and inhibited by ruthenium red, Mg, protons, and calmodulin.

9.3.7 MITOCHONDRIA

Mitochondria have long been considered as important in the regulation of cytosolic and intramitochondrial Ca (see Carafoli 1982, for a review). Recent developments, particularly the demonstration that they handle Ca with low affinity (Crompton *et al.* 1976) and the finding that they contain much less Ca *in situ* than previously assumed (Somlyo *et al.* 1979), have led to a re-evaluation of their importance as cytosolic Ca regulators, leaving as their main Ca-related task the regulation of matrix Ca. This, however, is a task of great importance, owing to the existence in the matrix of three dehydrogenases which are precisely controlled by Ca (Fig. 3). Mitochondria

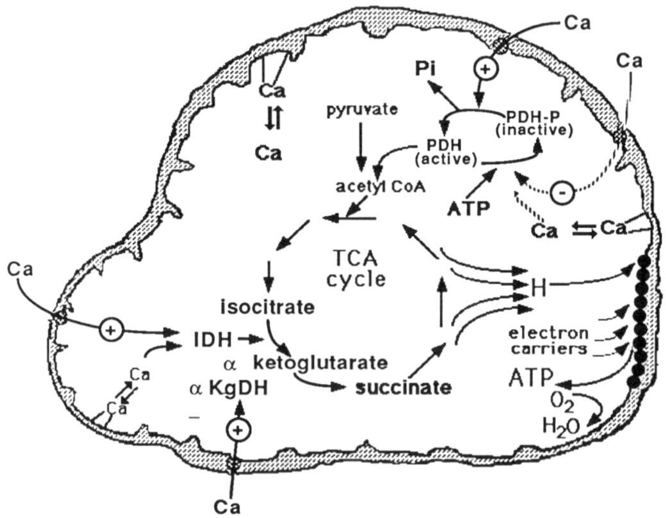

Fig. 3.—The regulation of the matrix enzmes by Ca. The information offered in the figure is taken from the work of Denton *et al.* (1972, 1978) and McCormack & Denton (1979). PDH = pyruvic acid dehydrogenase; IDH = NAD-linked isocitric acid dehydrogenase; α Kg-DH = α-ketoglutaric acid dehydrogenase.

accumulate Ca by means of a electrophoretic route which is driven by the electrical component of the proton-motive force across the inner membrane and is inhibited by ruthenium red. As mentioned, the route interacts with Ca with low affinity (K_m is 1–10 μM) and accumulates it at an optimal rate of up to 10 nmoles per mg of protein per sec. *In vivo*, however, owing to the sub-optimal concentration of Ca, and to the presence of Mg which also inhibits the route, the rate is likely to be but a fraction of the optimal. Interestingly, mitochondria also accumulate inorganic phosphate to precipitate Ca inside the matrix. This results in the damping of the changes in ionic Ca in the latter compartment, limiting the disturbance to the Ca-modulated dehydrogenases present there by newly accumulated Ca.

Since the Ca uptake process is electrophoretic, and since the transmembrane electrical potential is unlikely to fluctuate, the release of Ca does not occur through the reversal of the uptake route. It occurs through an electroneutral Na/Ca exchanger (Carafoli *et al.* 1974), which is particularly active in heart and other excitable tissues. (Crompton *et al.* 1978), and which releases Ca at a rate of about 0.2–0.3 nmol per mg of mitochondrial protein per sec. The route is insensitive to ruthenium red but is blocked by some of the agents that inhibit the plasma membrane Ca channel, e.g., the benzothiazepine diltiazem (Vaghy *et al.* 1982). Taken together, the energy-driven uptake route and the Na/Ca exchanger constitute an energy-dissipating Ca cycle (Carafoli *et al.* 1979), Fig. 4. Given the low activity of the mitochondrial Ca transport system *in vivo*, the level of energy dissipation by the cycle is minimal.

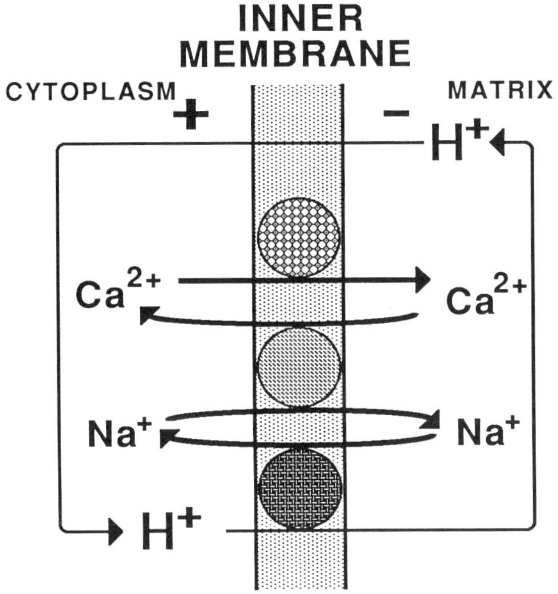

Fig. 4.—The mitochondrial Ca cycle

The role of mitochondria in the regulation of cytosolic Ca under physiological conditions is thus probably minor. However, injuring conditions may alter the permeabiliy properties of the plasma membrane, permitting the penetration of excess Ca in the cytosol. If this happens, the mitochondrial uptake system becomes activated and stores in the matrix large amounts of precipitated Ca-phosphate: the occurrence of Ca-phosphate deposits in mitochondria of injured cells, including heart cells, is indeed a common observation (see Carafoli 1982, for a review). Once the injuring condition has disappeared, mitochondria will slowly release the stored Ca, at a rate compatible with the exporting capacity of the plasma membrane systems. It is evident, then, that mitochondria play a decisive defence role against cytosolic Ca overload.

9.3.8 CONCLUSIONS

The control of cell Ca is essentially a phenomenon of reversible protein complexation. Soluble proteins contribute to Ca-buffering but are more important in the transmission of Ca signal to targets. Membrane-intrinsic proteins play the main role in the buffering of cell Ca. They may control Ca very precisely, with high affinity (ATPases) or with lower affinity (channels, exchangers, the electrophoretic uniporter of mitochondria). At a higher level of integration, the endo(sarco)plasmic reticulum is responsible for the fine, high-affinity regulation, whereas the mitochondrial Ca transporting systems have the role of controlling intramitochondrial Ca. The mitochondrial system, however, also defends the cytosol against pathological Ca increases.

REFERENCES

Babu, Y. S., Sack, J. S., Greenhough, T. J., Bugg, C. E., Means, A. R., & Cook, W. J. (1985). Three-dimensional structure of calmodulin, *Nature* **315,** 37–40.

Blaustein, M. P. & Nelson, M. T. (1982). Sodium-calcium exchange: its role in the regulation of cell calcium. In: *Membrane transport of calcium* (ed Carafoli, E.), Academic Press, London, p. 217–236.

Carafoli, E. (1989). The calcium cycle of mitochondria, *FEBS Lett.* **104,** 1–5.

Carafoli, E. (1982a). The transport of calcium across the inner membrane of mitochondria. In: *Membrane transport of calcium* (ed Carafoli, E.), Academic Press, London, p. 109–140.

Carafoli, E. (1982b). Membrane transport and the regulation of the cell calcium levels. In: *Pathophysiology of shock, anoxia, and ischemia* (eds Cowley, R. A. & Trump, B. F.), Williams and Wilkins, p. 95–112.

Carafoli, E. (1987). Intracellular calcium homeostatsis, *Ann. Rev. Biochem.* **56,** 395–433.

Carafoli, E., Tiozzo, G., Lugli, F., Crovetti, F., & Kratzing, C. (1974). The release of calcium from heart mitochondria by sodium, *J. Molec. Cell. Cardiol.* **6,** 361–371.

Caroni, P. & Carafoli, E. (1981). Regulation of Ca^{2+}-pumping ATPase of heart sarcolemma by a phosphorylation-dephosphorylation process, *J. Biol. Chem.* **256,** 9371–9373.

Caroni, P. & Carafoli, E. (1983). The regulation of the Na^{+}/Ca^{2+} exchanger of heart sarcolemma, *Eur. J. Biochem.* **132,** 451–460.

Crompton, M., Sigel, E., Salzmann, M., & Carafoli, E. (1976). A kinetic study of the energy-linked influx of Ca^{2+} into heart mitochondria, *Eur. J. Biochem.* **69,** 429–434.

Crompton, M., Moser, R., Lüdi, H., & Carafoli, E. (1978). The interrelations between the transport of sodium and calcium in mitochondria of various mammalian tissues, *Eur. J. Biochem.* **82,** 25–31.

Denton, R. M., Randle, P. J., & Martin, B. R. (1972). Stimulation by calcium ions of pyruvate dehydrogenase phosphate phosphatase, *Biochem. J.* **128,** 161–163.

Denton, R. M., Richards, D. A., & Chin, J. G. (1978). Calcium ions and the regulation of NAD^{+}-linked isocitrate dehydrogenase from the mitochondria of rat heart and other tissues, *Biochem. J.* **176,** 899–906.

Fabiato, A. & Fabiato, F. (1975). Contractions induced by a calcium from the sarcoplasmic reticulum of single skinned cardiac cells, *J. Physiol.* **249,** 457–495.

Fleckenstein, A. (1983). *Calcium antagonism in heart and smooth muscle*, John Wiley, New York.

Grand, R. J. A., Perry, S. V., & Weeks, R. A. (1979). Troponin-C like proteins (calmodulin) from mammalian smooth muscle and other tissues, *Biochem. J.* **177,** 521–529.

Herzberg, O. & James, M. N. G. (1985). Structure of the calcium regulatory muscle protein troponin-C at 2.8 A resolution, *Nature* **313,** 665–669.

Kretsinger, R. H. & Nockolds, C. E. (1973). Carp muscle calcium-binding protein. *J. Biol. Chem.* **248,** 3313–3326.

Kretsinger, R. H. & Nelson, D. J. (1977). Calcium in biological systems, *Coord. Chem. Rev.* **18,** 29–34.

MacLennan, D. H. (1970). Purification and properties of an adenosine triphosphate from sarcoplasmic reticulum, *J. Biol. Chem.* **245,** 4508–4518.

MacLennan, D. H., Brandl, C. J., Korczak, B., & Green, N. M. (1985). Amino-acid sequence of a $Ca^{2+} + Mg^{2+}$-independent ATPase from rabbit muscle sarcoplasmic reticulum, deduced from its complementary DNA sequence, *Nature* **316,** 696–700.

McCormack, J. G. & Denton, R. M. (1979). The effects of calcium ions and adenine nucleotides on the activity of pig heart 2-oxoglutarate dehydrogenase complex, *Biochem. J.* **180,** 533–544.

Meissner, G. & Henderson, J. S. (1987). Rapid calcium release from sarcoplasmic reticulum vesicles is dependent on calcium and is modulated by Mg^{2+}, adenine nucleotide, and calmodulin, *J. Biol. Chem.* **262,** 3065–3072.

Niggli, V., Adunyah, E. S., Penniston, J. T., & Carafoli, E. (1981). Purified ($Ca^{2+} - Mg^{2+}$)-ATPase of the erythrocyte membrane; reconstitution and effect of calmodulin and phospholipids, *J. Biol. Chem.* **256,** 395–407.

Nilius, B., Hess, P., Lansmann, J. B., & Tsien, R. W. (1985). A novel type of cardiac calcium channel in ventricular cells, *Nature* **316,** 443–446.

Reeves, J. P. & Sutko, J. L. (1979). Sodium-calcium exchage in cardiac membrane vesicles, *Proc. Natl. Acad. Sci. USA* **76,** 590–594.

Reuter, H. (1984). Ion channels in cardiac cell membranes, *Ann. Rev. Physiol.* **46,** 473–484.

Reuter, H., Stevens, C. F., Tsien, R. W., & Yellen, G. (1982). Properties of single calcium channels in cardiac cell culture, *Nature* **297,** 501–504.

Schatzmann, H. (1982). The calcium pump of erythrocytes and other animal cells. In: *Membrane transport of calcium* (ed Carafoli, E.), Academic Press, London, p. 41.

Somlyo, A. P., Somlyo, A. V., & Shuman, H. (1979). Electron probe analysis of vascular smooth muscle, Composition of mitochondria, nuclei, and cytoplasm, *J. Biol. Chem.* **81,** 316–335.

Somlyo, A. V., Bond, M., Somlyo, A. P., & Scarpa, A. (1985). Inositol tris phosphate-induced calcium release and contraction in vascular smooth muscle, *Proc. Natl. Acad. Sci. USA* **82,** 5231–5235.

Szebenyi, D. M. E., Obendorf, S. K., & Moffat, K. (1981). Structure of vitamin D-dependent calcium binding protein from bovine intestine, *Nature* **294,** 327–332.

Tada, M., Kirchberger, M. A., & Katz, A. M. (1975). Phosphorylation of 22.000-Dalton component of the cardiac sarcoplasmic reticulum by adenosine 3″:5″-monophosphate-dependent protein kinase, *J. Biol. Chem.* **250,** 2640–2647.

Tanabe, T., Takeshima, H., Mikami, A., Flockerz, V., Takahashi, H., Kangaura, K., Kojima, M., Matsuo, H., Hirose, T., & Numa, S. (1987). Primary structure of the receptor for calcium channel blockers from skeletal muscle, *Nature* **328,** 313–318.

Vaghy, P. L., Johnson, J. D., Matlib, M. A., Wang, T., & Schwarz, A. (1982). Selective inhibition of Na^+-induced Ca^{2+} release from heart mitochondria by diltiazem and certain other Ca^{2+} antagonist drugs, *J. Biol. Chem.* **257,** 6000–6002.

9.4 Biochemical properties of adrenergic receptors: possible involvement in cardiovascular diseases

Susanna Cotecchia†

Many hormones and drugs initiate their actions on target cells by binding to specific cell surface receptors located in the plasma membrane. Among these are the catecholamines, adrenaline, and noradrenaline, and a large number of synthetic agonist and antagonist drugs which occupy a significant place in the current practice of medicine.

This paper describes some recent findings concerning the biochemical nature of the adrenergic receptors, their mechanisms of activation and coupling to effectors, and recent discoveries about the ways in which their function is regulated. This information provides the framework for attempts to understand their role in physiological and pathological conditions.

9.4.1 CLASSIFICATION OF ADRENERGIC RECEPTORS AND EFFECTORS

Adrenergic receptors were initially classified by Ahlquist into two major types, termed α and β, based on their pharmacological specificites for binding agonists and antagonists (Fig. 1) (Ahlquist 1948). Subsequently, two subtypes of each termed α_1 and α_2 and β_1 and β_2 adrenergic receptors were also defined, based on nuances of pharmacological specificity as well as different functional correlates. The effector mechanisms of these different adrenergic receptor subtypes appear to represent paradigms for each of the known transmembrane signalling pathways which are utilized by hormones and drugs which bind to plasma membrane receptors. Both β_1 and β_2-adrenergic receptors activate the plasma membrane enzyme adenylate cyclase, leading to the generation of cAMP, activation of cAMP-dependent protein kinase, and the phosphorylation of crucial cellular substrates which lead to physiological effects. As shown in Fig. 1, the receptors are coupled to the catalytic moiety of the adenylate cyclase by a special heterotrimeric protein known as the stimulatory guanine nucleotide regulatory protein, generally abbreviated as N_s or G_s (Casey & Gilman 1987).

By contrast, α_2-adrenergic receptors were to mediate effects of catecholamines to inhibit the enzyme adenylate cyclase. Such mechanisms are found, for example, in the human platelet, on presynaptic nerve terminals, and on vascular smooth muscle.

† Box 3821, Duke University Medical Center, Durham, North Carolina 27710, USA

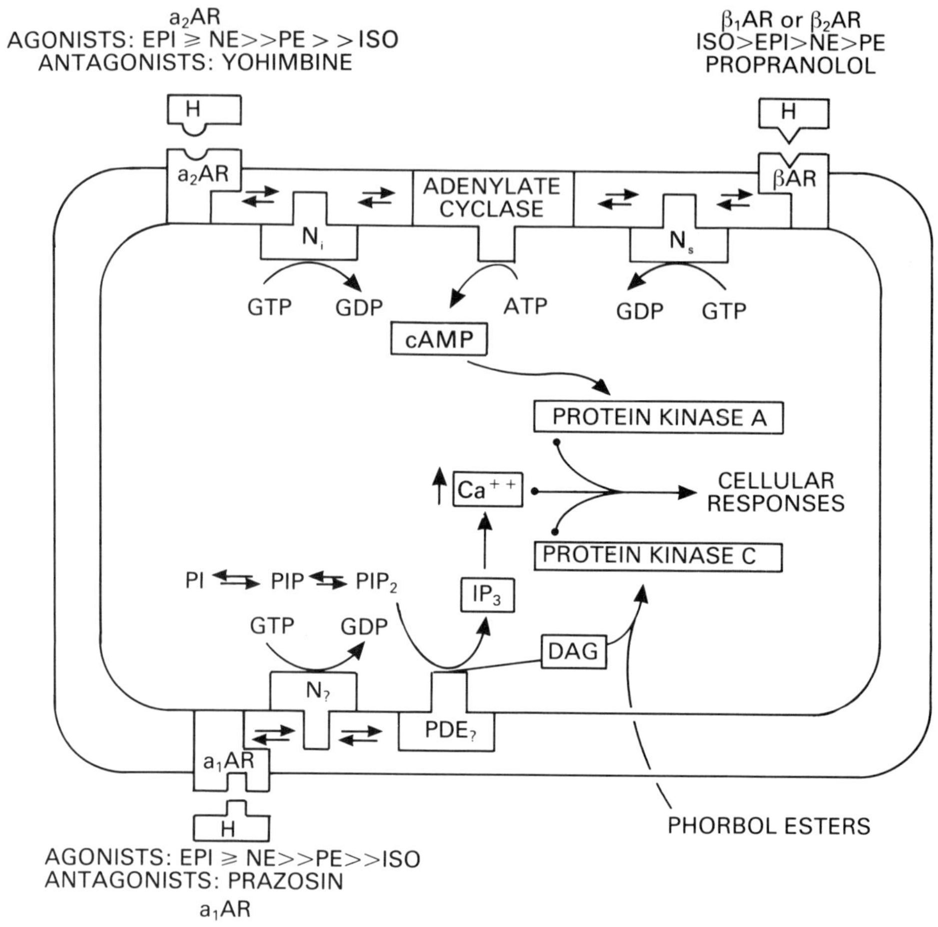

Fig. 1.—Adrenergic receptors and transmembrane signalling systems. AR, Adrenergic receptor; N_s, stimulatory guanine nucleotide regulatory protein; N_i, inhibitory guanine nucleotide regulatory protein; ISO, isoproterenol; EPI, epinephrine; NE, norepinephrine; PE, phenylephrine; H, hormone; DAG, diacylglycerol; IP_3, inositol 1,4,5-trisphosphatase; PDE, phosphodiesterase; PI, phosphatidylinositol; PIP, phosphatidylinositol 4-phosphate; PIP_2, phosphatidylinositol 4,5-bisphosphate.

α_2-Adrenergic receptors are coupled to the inhibition of adenylate cyclase via a class of guanine nucleotide regulatory proteins distinct from stimulatory receptors, and are generally abbreviated N_i or G_i for inhibitory guanine nucleotide regulatory protein (Casey & Gilman 1987).

Finally, the α_1-adrenergic receptors are coupled to processes which lead to changes in phosphatidylinositol turnover and subsequently to the release of two distinct candidate second messengers. These are diacylglycerol and inositol trisphosphate, both of which are formed from the hydrolysis of phosphatidylinositol bisphosphate (PIP_2) by phospholipase C (Berridge & Irvine 1984). Diacylglycerol activates protein kinase C, which may be involved in regulating cell growth and differentiation. Inositol trisphosphate mobilizes intracellular Ca^{2+} stores leading to a variety of responses such as smooth muscle contraction. For many hormones mediating their effects through this signalling pathway the synergistic action of these two second messengers appears important in eliciting maximal biological effects.

Recent evidence suggests that a guanine nucleotide regulatory protein may be involved in coupling agonist occupancy of such receptors to the stimulation of phospholipase C.

9.4.2 THE BIOCHEMICAL NATURE OF THE ADRENERGIC RECEPTORS

The adrenergic receptors, as most plasma membrane receptors, are present in extremely low concentrations. Purification of these receptors to homogeneity requires solubilization with detergent, followed by as much as 100 000-fold purification of the receptor protein.

Two techniques have proved invaluable in the characterization and purification of the adrenergic receptors, i.e., affinity and photoaffinity labelling and affinity chromatography. With the technique of affinity and photoaffinity labelling an analog of a high-affinity agonist or antagonist is derivatized with a reactive or photoactivatable group. By such procedures, receptor binding subunits can be visualized even in whole cells or crude membrane preparations. With the second technique, affinity chromatography, a drug or a hormone is covalently immobilized to a solid support such as Sepharose beads. Solubilized receptor preparations are then passed over the support, and the receptor is specifically absorbed. After various washing steps to remove nonspecifically absorbed proteins, the receptor binding activity can be specifically eluted by the inclusion of competing agonists or antagonits. Coupling of this procedure with chromatography of receptor preparations on immobilized lectin gels and molecular sieve high-performance liquid chromatography has proved useful in the purification of the various adrenergic receptor subtypes. The adrenergic receptors purified to homogeneity from different mammalian tissues have been identified as distinct glycoproteins of 64 000 molecular weight in the case of β_2, 64 000 molecular weight for α_2, and 80 000 molecular weight or α_1 receptor (Benovic *et al.* 1984, Regan *et al.* 1986, Lomasney *et al.* 1986).

To further understand the molecular structure of the adrenergic receptors and how this determines their function and regulatory properties, the cloning of their cDNAs and genes has been undertaken. The genes encoding for the mammalian β_2, α_2, and β_1 adrenergic receptors have been coned, and the deduced amino acid sequence of these receptor proteins is now known (Dixon *et al.* 1986, Kobilka *et al.* 1987, Frielle *et al.* 1987).

The availability of this structural information opens the way to detailed biochemical studies based on synthetic peptides, antibodies, and site-directed mutagenesis, all of which should combine to elucidate the detailed molecular architecture of the relevant functional domains of the β-adrenergic receptor.

9.4.3 MECHANISMS OF REGULATION OF RECEPTOR FUNCTION

A common property of the adrenergic receptors is the dynamic regulation of their functional response. Since receptors are the first step in the response of a target cell to a hormone or drug, they represent a crucial point in the cellular functional regulation.

Two distinct mechanisms of regulation can be envisated. First, the number of receptors present in the plasma membrane of a target cell can be modulated. For the adrenergic receptors, a wide variety of agonists, antagonists, and hormones can increase or decrease the number of cell surface adrenergic receptors. These effects probably involve altered rates of synthesis or degradation of the plasma membrane receptors. A second mechanism for regulation of receptor function is the modulation of the activating function of a receptor (i.e. the ability of a receptor to elicit activation of an effector system) by covalent modification. Recent studies suggest that the function of the adrenergic receptors is indeed regulated by phosphorylation/dephosphorylation reactions.

One of the most investigated examples of receptor regulation is densitization. Desensitization refers to the attenuation of responsiveness to a hormone or drug despite the continued presence of that drug. Such desensitization reactions markedly diminish the therapeutic efficacy and duration of adrenergic catecholamines and many other pharmacological agents.

Pharmacologists have distinguished two major categories of desensitization. 'Homologous' desensitization refers to a situation where, after stimulation of a system by one specific agonist, sensitivity is lost only to stimulation by that agonist, while responsiveness to other diverse types of agonists remains normal. In 'heterologous' desensitization stimulation by one agonist leads to decreased responsiveness to a whole series of structurally unrelated agonists working through distinct receptors, and sometimes even to stimulants which bypass normal receptor mechanisms.

Table 1—Pattern of adrenergic receptor desensitization

Agonist specific	No	Yes
Time course	Slow	Fast
Receptor sequestration	No	Yes
Receptor phoshorylation	Yes	Yes

As shown in Table 1, both types of desensitization have been observed in the adrenergic system in experimental conditions (Sibley & Lefkowitz 1985). The biochemical mechanisms underlying the homologous desensitization involve both the sequestration of the receptors from the cellular surface and the phosphorylation of the receptor protein. cAMP-dependent kinase and a new kinase termed β adrenergic receptor kinase βARK) (Benovic *et al.* 1987) seem to be involved in the heterologous and homologous β-adrenergic receptor desensitization respectively. Protein kinase C seems to play a role in both heterologous and homologous desensitization of α_1 adrenergic receptors (Leeb-Lundberg *et al.* 1986).

9.4.4 CLINICAL IMPLICATONS OF RECEPTOR REGULATION

Clinical examples of desensitization to catecholamines abound, including the rapid loss of the bronchodilating effects of β-adrenergic agonists administered to patients with asthma; the transient effect of vasconstrictor α-adrenergic amines administered to patients with hypotension; the waning inotropic effect of β-agonists administered to patients with congestive heart failures; the attenuated response to α-adrenergic constrictor amines used topically as nasal decongestants; and the decreased responsiveness to catecholamines of patients with pheochromocytomas, such that normal resting pulse and blood pressure values may be found at times when circulating catecholamine levels are well above normal.

A wide spectrum of diseases might also involve disordered adrenergic receptor function, as shown in Table 2 (Lefkowitz 1979). The recent understanding of the biochemical and molecular basis of the adrenergic receptor function might provide a framework for trying to modify these receptor regulatory phenomena for therapeutic purposes. Although these research endeavours are still in the early stages they represent a good example of direct application of biochemical advances to problems of therapeutics and medicine.

Table 2—Factors regulating adrenergic receptor binding sites*

Regulatory agent or condition	Effect on receptors
Beta-adrenergic receptors	
Beta-adrenergic catecholamines	Decrease the number
Propranolol	Increase the number
Denervation (6-hydroxydopamine, guanethidine, surgical)	Increase the number
Hyperthyroidism	Increase the number
Hypothyroidism	Decrease the number
Cortisone	Decrease the number
Malignant transformation	Increase the number
Spontaneously hypertensive rat	Decrease the number
Alcohol withdrawal	Increase the number
Alpha-adrenergic receptors	
Alpha-adrenergic catecholamines	Decrease the number
Denervation	Increase the number
Hyperthyroidism	Decrease the number, affinity
Estrogen	Increase the number
Thrombocytosis	Decrease the number

* From Lefkowitz, R. J. (1979). *Ann. Intern. Med.* **91,** 450.

REFERENCES

Ahlquist, R. (1948). A study of the adrenotropic receptors. *Am. J. Physiol.* **153,** 586–600.

Benovic, J. L., Shorr, R. G. L., Caron, M. G., & Lefkowitz, R. J. (1984). The mammalian β_2-adrenergic receptor: Purification and characterization. *Biochem.* **23,** 4510.

Benovic, J. L., Strasser, R. H., Caron, M. G., & Lefkowitz, R. J. (1986). β-Adrenergic receptor kinase: Identification of a novel protein kinase that phosphorylates the agonist occupied form of the receptor. *Proc. Natl. Acad. Sci. USA* **83,** 2797–2801.

Berridge, M. J. & Irvine, R. F. (1984). Inositol triphosphate, a novel second messenger in cellular signal transduction. *Nature* **312,** 315–321.

Casey, P. J. & Gilman, A. G. (1987). G Protein involvement in receptor-effector coupling. *J. Biol. Chem.* **263,** 2577–2580.

Dixon, R. A. F., Kobilka, B. K., Strader, D. J., Benovic, J. L., Dohlman, H. G., Frielle, T., Bolanowsi, M. A., Bennett, C. D., Rands, E., Diehl, R. E., Mumford, R. A., Slater, E. E., Sigal, I. S., Caron, M. G., Lefkowitz, R. J., & Strader, C. D. (1986). Cloning of the gene and cDNA for mammalian β-adrenergic receptor and homology with rhodopsin. *Nature* **321,** 75–79.

Frielle, T., Collins, S., Daniel, K., Caron, M. G., Lefkowitz, R. J., & Kobilka, B. K. (1987). Cloning of the cDNA for the human β_1-adrenergic receptor. *Proc. Natl. Acad. Sci. USA* **84,** 7920–7924.

Kobilka, B. K., Matsui, H., Kobilka, T. S., Yang-Feng, T. L., Francke, U., Caron, M. G., Lefkowitz, R. J., & Regan, J. W. (1987). Cloning, sequencing and expression of the gene encoding for the human platelet α_2-adrenergic receptor. *Science* **238,** 650–656.

Leeb-Lundberg, L. M. F., Cotecchia, S., DeBlasi, A., Caron, M. G., & Lefkowitz, R. J. (1987). Regulation of adrenergic receptor function by phosphorylation. *J. Biol. Chem.* **262,** 3098–3105.

Lefkowitz, R. J. (1979). Direct binding studies of adrenergic receptors: biochemical, physiologic and clinical implications. *Ann. Intern. Med.* **91,** 450–458.

Lomasney, J. W., Leeb-Lundberg, F. L. M., Cotecchia, S., Regan, J. W., DeBernardis, J. F., Caron, M. G., & Lefkowitz, R. J. (1986). Mammalian α_1-adrenergic receptor: purification and characterizaton of the native receptor ligand binding subunit. *J. Biol. Chem.* **261,** 7710–7716.

Regan, J. W., Nakata, H., DeMarinis, R., Caron, M. G., & Lefkowitz, R. J. (1986). Purification and characterization of the human platelet α_2-adrenergic receptor. *J. Biol. Chem.* **261,** 3894–3900.

Sibley, D. R. & Lefkowitz, R. J. (1985). Molecular mechanisms of receptor desensitization using the β-adrenergic receptor-coupled adenylate cyclase system as a model. *Nature* **317,** 124–129.

9.5 Myocardial ischaemia: diagnostic approaches and therapeutic perspective

Sabino Iliceto & Paolo Rizzon†

Diagnostic techniques commonly used for the detection of coronary artery disease are based on the conjunction of a stress capable of inducing myocardial ischaemia and a procedure capable of detecting indirect signs of ischaemia itself.

In the last few years new, safe and effective stresses have been developed and considerable improvement in the potential of diagnostic technique has also been achieved.

In the same period important progress has also been made in the therapy of acute myocardia ischaemic events.

9.5.1 INTRODUCTION

Diagnostic approaches aimed at the recognition of acute myocardial ischaemia are based on the detection of electrical, functional, perfusional, or metabolic abnormalities induced by the ischaemic event. These abnormalities can be detected by various kinds of cardiac techniques (imaging or non-imaging ones), though, in the majority of instances, they are not present at rest because of the absence of myocardial ischaemia in resting conditions. Consequently, stresses capable of safely inducing reversible myocardial ischaemia often have to be used in conjunction with one of the various diagnostic techniques. Diagnostic accuracy of these techniques is determined by their ability to detect myocardial ischaemia and by the efficacy of the stress used to induce it. The ideal test would: (a) have a 100% sensitivity and specificity; (b) be safe, non-invasive, and easily repeatable; and (c) be relatively inexpensive. Such a test does not exist, and, probably, will never exist. Currently used diagnostic approaches are, in fact, far from being ideal.

9.5.2 DIAGNOSTIC TECHNIQUES

In the last decade, for the diagnosis of coronary artery disease the old, yet still useful, electrocardiogram has been aided by sophisticated cardiac imaging techniques which can evaluate left ventricular wall motion (radionuclide ventriculography and two-dimensional echo-cardiography) and myocardial perfusion (thallium scintigraphy). The information which can be obtained by studying myocardial perfusion and function enables a more sensitive and specific diagnosis. This greater diagnostic potentiality can easily be explained by the changes which take place over the course of time in the alterations induced by acute ischaemia. Experimental and clinical studies (Tennant

† Division of Cardiology, University of Bari, Bari, Italy

& Wiggers 1935, Theroux *et al.* 1974, Battler *et al.* 1980, Scheurer & Brachfeld 1966) have clearly demonstrated how, during an acute ischaemic episode, electrocardiographic alterations are the last to appear, while mechanical, and even more so perfusion alterations, appear much earlier on. This means that alterations in wall motion and perfusion may be observed even when there are no electrical ones (in cases where the ischaemia is not serious enough to alter the electrocardiogram). Consequently, techniques which are able to monitor these alterations over the course of time have a better diagnostic potential.

Among the existing cardiac imaging techniques, echocardiography is undoubtedly the one which has undergone the most intense development over the last few years.

9.5.3 TWO-DIMENSIONAL ECHOCARDIOGRAPHY AND DOPPLER

This diagnostic tool is based on the use of ultrasound beams which, emitted from a transducer placed on the chest surface, pass inside the thorax, exploring the cardiac structures (two-dimensional echocardiography) and the direction and velocity of blood flows in various areas (Doppler) in detail.

The diagnostic potential of two-dimensional echocardiography used in conjunction with Doppler has opened up seemingly unlimited diagnostic and physiopathological perspectives to the world of ultrasounds.

Even if it is extremely useful (Maurer & Nanda 1981, Wann *et al.* 1979, Morganroth *et al.* 1981, Visser *et al.* 1983, Iliceto *et al.* 1986), this method has not been used much in the diagnosis of coronary artery disease owing to some methodological problems (hyperventilation, excessive chest wall motion, and chest muscle contractions) which occur when echocardiography is done during physical exercise aimed at inducing ischaemia with its consequent alterations in wall motion or myocardial thickening.

The limits of exercise echocardiography have been largely overcome by a stress test which has recently been developed in our laboratory (Iliceto *et al.* 1984, 1985a,b, Papa *et al.* 1985): two-dimensional echocardiography during transesophageal atrial pacing (see 9.5.4.2).

9.5.4 STRESSES USED TO INDUCE MYOCARDIAL ISCHAEMIA

To assess latent coronary insufficiency, there are several types of stress which can provoke, by means of an increase in oxygen consumption, myocardial ischaemia and consequently perfusion and overall and/or regional functional deficits of the left ventricle.

9.5.4.1 Physical exercise

Physical exercise is the most physiological form of stress. The haemodynamic alterations brought on by this sort of stress are: an increased cardiac output, vasodilatation with an augmented blood flow to the skeletal muscles; and increased arterial pressure, heart rate, and myocardial oxygen consumption. Currently, physical exercise is generally done by using either a bicycle ergometer (in the supine or upright positions) or a treadmill. The haemodynamic variables behave differently, depending on the manner chosen to carry out the test. The treadmill enables one to reach a higher level of stress than the bicycle ergometer, and, therefore, some authors consider it to be the most efficient technique for inducing myocardial ischaemia (Ford *et al.* 1983),

9.5.4.2 Atrial pacing

Unlike physical exercise, this sort of stress leads to a reduction in the cardiac volumes without significant changes in arterial pressure; in most cases, therefore, double product values equal to those obtained with physical exercise are not reached. This sort of stress can induce clinical and instrumental signs of myocardial ischaemia in patients with coronary artery disease.

Until recently, this technique, used in conjunction with various forms of imaging, was done invasively by placing a transvenous pacing catheter in the right atrium. Some studies done by Chapman *et al.* (1984) and by our group (Iliceto *et al.* 1984, 1985a,b, 1986, Papa *et al.* 1985) have evaluated the feasibility of the transesophageal approach for rapid atrial stimulation. Taking advantage of the fact that the left atrium is anatomically next to the distal oesophagus, we have made atrial pacing much less invasive: a specially designed pacing catheter is introduced 30–35 cm down into the oesophagus, and then transesophageal atrial pacing is carried out during a two-dimensional echocardiographic exam. Done in this way, the examination quality is as good as that obtained during resting conditions: neither the hyperventilation nor the chest wall motion which limit the execution of the echocardiographic examination during physical exercise occur. This new diagnostic test has shown good sensitivity and specificity in displaying echocardiographic signs of ischaemia (wall motion abnormalities); indeed, in a group of 81 patients, we found a sensitivity of 91% and a specificity of 88% (Iliceto *et al.* 1985a).

9.5.4.3 Cold pressor test

This type of stress, described for the first time by Hines & Brown (1936), is based on the alpha-adrenergic stimulation caused by putting one's hand in water and ice; in this manner one generates a reflex, starting at the skin receptors, which leads to a widespread vasconstriction even in the parts of the body not directly touching the cold. The reflex induces an increase in the heart rate and the arterial pressure which may then, in subjects with coronary artery disease, give rise to ischaemia because of the increased myocardial request for oxygen. Moreover, as Mudge *et al.* (1970) have demonstrated, in coronary patients the cold pressor test reduces the coronary flow because of an augmented coronary resistance.

9.5.4.4 Dypiridamole

Dypiridamole is a vasoactive substance which, by means of a complex and not yet fully understood mechanism, can induce myocardial ischaemia in the presence of critical stenoses. The mechanisms responsible for this myocardial ischaemia appear to be:

(1) a drop in the perfusion pressure downstream of fixed and severe stenoses, following on an increase in the coronary flow;

(2) the phenomenon of 'blood stealing' which leads to a rechannelling of blood flow towards areas supplied by healthy coronaries or by ones with haemodynamically not significant stenoses with a consequent insufficient supply to areas with critical stenoses.

9.5.5 MYOCARDIAL ISCHAEMIA: THERAPEUTICAL PERSPECTIVES

Enormous progress has been made over the last few years in the therapy of acute myocardial ischaemia. Though traditional nitrates are still used, there are now new generations of B-blockers and calcium antagonists. These drugs are particularly useful in treating exercise-induced ischaemia and vasospastic angina, respectively. New drugs belonging to these two groups are being studied by researchers working on basic and clinical projects.

The fact that in both the first phases of acute myocardial infarction and during the phases of the extreme instability of angina, intracoronary thrombotic processes can play a decisive role, has led to great interest in the clinical evaluation of substances which are able to inhibit coagulating processes or even to exert a thrombolitic effect on recently formed thrombi.

9.5.6 CONCLUSIONS

The rapid and continuous evolution of technologies and pharmacological research is changing the clinical approach to myocardial ischaemia. Today, a more reliable and earlier identification of coronary patients is possible as is, consequently, a quicker and more appropriate medical treatment. The modern cardiac imaging diagnostic techniques are important not only for identifying the patient with coronary artery disease but also for evaluating the effects of the therapy used in each particular case.

REFERENCES

Battler, A., Froelin, V. F., Gallagher, K. P., Kemper, W. S., & Ross, J., Jr. (1980). Dissociation between regional myocardial dysfunction and ECG changes during ischaemia in the conscious dog. *Circulation* **62,** 735–44.

Chapman, P. D., Doyle, T. P., Troup, P. J., Gross, C. M., & Wann, L. S. (1984). Stress echocardiography with transesophageal atrial pacing: preliminary report of a new method for detection of ischaemia wall motion abnormalities. *Circulation* **70,** 445–50.

Ford, D., Maddahi, J., Berman, D., Rozanski, A., & Swan, H. J. C. (1983). Differing ability of treadmill and upright bicycle exercise testing to induce clinical cardiac ischaemia in patients with coronary artery disease (abstr). *J. Am. Coll. Cardiol.* **1,** 650.

Hines, E. A. & Brown, G. E. (1936). The cold pressor test for measuring the reactibility of the blood pressure: data concerning 571 normal and hypertensive subjects. *Am. Heart J.* **11,** 1–4.

Iliceto, S., Sorino, M., D'Ambrosio, G., Papa, A., Favale, S., & Rizzon, P. (1984). Detection of coronary artery disease by two-dimensional echocardiography during transesophageal atrial pacing: sensitivity and specificity (abstr). *Circulation* **70,** II–185.

Iliceto, S., Sorino, M., D'Ambrosio, G., Papa, A., Favale, S., Biasco, G., & Rizzon, P. (1985a). Detection of coronary artery disease by two-dimensional echocardiography and transesophageal atrial pacing. *J. Am. Coll. Cardiol.* **5,** 1188–97.

Iliceto, S., Sorino, M., D'Ambrosio, G., Papa, A., Amico, A., & Rizzon, P. (1985b). Wall motion abnormalities induced by atrial pacing in patients with suspected coronary artery disease. Analysis of 176 cases studied by 2D Echo during transesophageal atrial pacing (abstr). *Eur. Heart J.* **6,** 124.

Iliceto, S., D'Ambrosio, G., Sorino, M., Papa, A., Amico, A., Ricci, A., & Rizzon, P. (1986). Comparison of post exercise and transesophageal atrial pacing two-dimensional echocardiography for detection of coronary artery disease: feasibility, specificity and sensitivity. *Am. J. Cardiol.* **57,** 547–53.

Maurer, G. & Nanda, N. C. (1981). Two-dimensional echocardiographic evaluation of exercise-induced left and right ventricular asynergy: correlation with thallium scanning. *Am. J. Cardiol.* **48,** 720–7.

Morganroth, J., Chen, C. C., David, D., Sawin, H. S., Naito, M., Parrotto, C., & Meixell, L. (1981). Exercise cross-sectional echocardiographic diagnosis of coronary artery disease. *Am. J. Cardiol.* **47,** 20–6.

Mudge, G. H., Goldberg, S., Gunther, S., Mann, T., & Grossman, W. (1979). Comparison of metabolic and vasoconstrictor stimuli on coronary vascular resistance in man. *Circulation* **59,** 544–50.

Papa, A., Iliceto, S., D'Ambrosio, G., Sorino, M., Graziadei, R., & Rizzon, P. (1985). Value of wall motion abnormalities during atrial pacing in the prediction of the extent of coronary artery disease (abstr). *Eur. Heart J.* **6,** 14.

Scheurer, J. & Brachfeld, N. (1966). Coronary insufficiency: relations between hemodynamic, electrical and biochemical parameters. *Circ. Res.* **18,** 178–86.

Tennant, R. & Wiggers, C. (1935). The effect of coronary occlusion on myocardial contraction. *Am. J. Physiol.* **112,** 351–8.

Theroux, P., Franklin, D., Ross, J., & Kemper, W. S. (1974). Regional myocardial function during acute coronary occlusion and its modification by pharmacologic agents in the dog. *Circ. Res.* **35,** 896–902.

Visser, C. A., Van der Wieken, R. L., Kan, G., Lie KI, Busemann-Sokele, E., Meltzer, R. S., & Durrer, D. (1983). Comparison of two-dimensional echocardiography with radionuclide angiography during dynamic exercise for the detection of coronary artery disease. *Am. Heart J.* **106,** 528–34.

Wann, L. S., Faris, J. V., Childress, R. H., Dillon, J. C., Weyman, A. E, & Feigenbaum, H. (1979). Exercise cross-sectional echocardiography in ischaemic heart disease. *Circulation* **60,** 1300–8.

Part 10

Diagnostic probes

10.1 Molecular diagnostic probes in human malignant brain tumours: a preliminary report

Massimo A. Gerosa†, Daniela Talarico‡, Caterina Fognani‡, Elena Raimodi‡, Luigi De Carli‡, Marco Colombatti§, Giuseppe Tridente§, & Giuliano Della Valle‡

(1) Expression of a panel of oncogenes was investigated by northern blot hybridization in 5 human glioblastoma cell lines.
(2) N-*ras* oncogene expression was significantly higher in all 5 cell lines than in long-term cultures of 'normal' glial cells. Abnormal expression of Epidermal-Growth-Factor-receptor (EGF-r) gene was detected in 4/5 cases, and was closely correlated with the increase in copy number of chromosome 7.
(3) Analysis of EGF-r and N-*ras* overexpression was then extended to fresh brain tumour and non-neoplastic brain tissue biopsies.
(4) Overexpression of N-*ras* protooncogene and EGF-r gene was confirmed in 5/5 glioblastomas, but not in relatively benign well-differentiated gliomas (fibrillary astrocytoma, ependymoma), or in non-neoplastic brain tissue specimens.
(5) Overexpression of these two oncogenes might play a key role in the uncontrolled proliferation of highly malignant brain tumours.

10.1.1 INTRODUCTION

Transcriptional activation of cellular oncogenes has been demonstrated in several human malignant solid tumours (Varmus 1984) and cell lines (Eva *et al.* 1982). In the case of neuro-ectodermal malignancies, particularly brain tumours, a key role in neoplastic progression has been attributed to abnormal expression of the epidermal growth factor receptor (EGF-r)-gene. High EGF-r levels have been observed in human brain tumours, and EGF-r gene amplification or overexpression have frequently been found in glioblastomas (Libermann *et al.* 1984, 1985, Talarico in press).

Human *ras* oncogenes code for a plasma membrane protein (p21) which shows an intrinsic guanosine triphosphatase activity (Levinson 1986). Enhanced expression of *ras* genes, resulting from gene amplification, has been observed in various tumours (Schwab *et al.* 1985), and high p21 levels have been related to local aggressiveness in colon carcinoma (Thor *et al.* 1984).

† Dept. of Neurosurgery, University of Verona, ‡ Dept. of Genetics, University of Pavia, and § Dept. of Immunology, University of Verona, Italy

Recent experimental evidence indicates that *ras* proteins may play a role in the EGF-r system (Kamata 1984, Wakelam *et al.* 1986). We therefore analysed a series of human malignant brain tumour cell lines and surgical biopsies to investigate the possibility that increased EGF-r gene expression might be related to *ras* gene overexpression.

10.1.2 MATERIALS AND METHODS

10.1.2.1 Cell lines

Five human glioblastoma-multiforme-derived primary cell lines (Hu70, Hu104, Hu112, Hu195, and Hu197) had been established from surgical specimens as previously described (Rosenblum *et al.* 1983). Monolayer cultures were grown in Ham's F12 supplemented with 20% fetal calf serum (Flow Laboratories), incubated in a 5% CO_2 humidified atmosphere and split 1:2–1:4 when confluent. The main techniques and markers for phenotypic characterization—routinely performed every 5–7 culture passages—have already been reported (Gerosa *et al.* 1986). Long-term cultures of non-neoplastic brain (Hu175) served as controls.

10.1.2.2 Surgical specimens

Analysis of EGF-r and N-*ras* gene expression was extended to human primary brain tumours. Primary brain tumours and control brain tissue samples were obtained, either by endocranial biopsy or during major neurosurgery, from untreated patients. Surgical specimens included: (a) highly malignant, undifferentiated gliomas (glioblastoma multiforme, 5 cases, Hu233, Hu235, Hu237, Hu242-A, and Hu243); (b) relatively benign, well-differentiated gliomas (fibrillary astrocytoma, 1 case, Hu244; ependymoma, 1 case, Hu231); (c) peritumoural brain tissue sample (Hu242-B, 1 case); and (d) 'normal' brain (vascular surgery, 1 case, Hu245). All specimens were frozen immediately after excision and stored in liquid nitrogen.

10.1.2.3 Nucleic acid analysis

Culture dishes were washed twice with PBS. Cells were scraped and collected by centrifugation. Frozen tissue samples were pulverized in liquid nitrogen and processed for nucleic acid purification. DNA was extracted by standard procedures (SDS lysis, proteinase K treatment, phenol-chloroform extraction, RNAase digestion, ethanol precipitation).

Ten μg of purified DNA from each sample were digested with *Eco*RI restriction enzyme, fractionated on 0.8% agarose slab gels, treated with 0.2 M HCl, denatured, and transferred to Amersham's Hybond-N nylon membranes (AHNM) according to the manufacturer's specifications.

RNA was isolated from cells and frozen tissues by the guanidine thiocyanate/CsCl method described by Chirgwin *et al.* (1979). Dot blot RNA analysis of serially diluted samples (10 μg to 1.25 μg) was performed as described by White & Bancroft (1982); samples were dotted onto AHNM under slow vacuum suction.

For northern blot analysis, 20 μg samples of total RNA were denatured in 50%

formamide, 2.2 M formaldehyde, and 1 × gel running buffer (20 mM MOPS pH 7.0, 5 mM sodium acetate, 1 mM EDTA pH 8.0) for 10 min at 65°C.

RNAs were fractionated on 1% agarose gels containing 2.2 M formaldehyde and 1 × gel running buffer and subsequently transferred in 20 × SSC to AHNM. Filters were hybridized with ^{32}P nick-translated DNA probes (2×10^8 cpm/μg DNA) for 20 h at 42°C in 50% formamide, 5 × SSC, 1 × Denhardt's solution, 20 mM sodium phosphate buffer pH 7.0, 0.1% SDS, 10% sodium dextran sulfate, and 100 μg/ml denatured salmon sperm DNA. Membranes were washed under high stringency conditions to avoid cross-hybridization with related species, and exposed at −70°C using Kodak X-Omat SO-282 films for varying lengths of time.

DNA probes specific for EGF-r, N-*ras*, Ha-*ras*, Ki-*ras*, c-*myc*, N-*myc*, *mos*, *neu*, *ros*, *sic*, *src*, and β-actin sequences were used. The following fragments were used for the hybridization reported in Table 1 and Fig. 1: a 1.8 kb *Eco*RI fragment of human EGF-r c-DNA from the plasmid 64-1; a 1.5 kb *Eco*RI N-*ras* fragment from N-*ras* plasmid (Oncor); a 2.9 kb c-Ha-*ras* *Sac*I fragment from T24-C3; a 1.0 kb *Eco*RI v-Ki-*ras* fragment from pHiHi3; and a 0.6 kb *Bam*HI-*Eco*RI β-actin fragment from pHFBA-3′ UT.

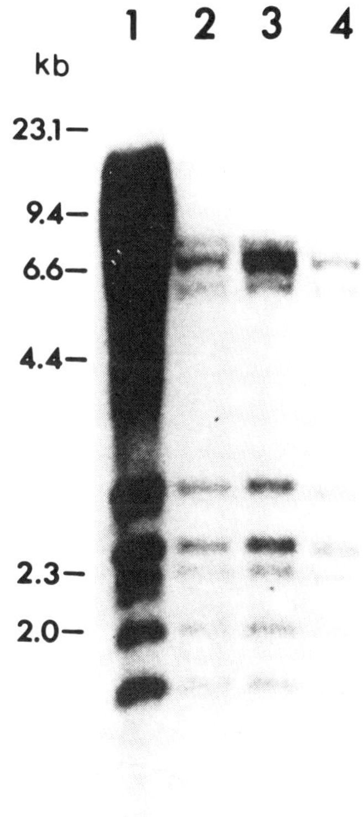

Fig. 1.—Southern blot analysis of EGF-receptor sequences in human brain tumors and 'normal' brain tissue sample.
10 μg samples of DNA from glioblastomas Hu243 (lane 1), Hu242-A (lane 2), and Hu233 (lane 3), and from non-neoplastic brain Hu245 (lane 4) were digested with *EcoRI* restriction enzyme. Hydribization was performed with a radiolabelled EGF-receptor 1.8 kb *Eco*RI fragment. Numbers on the left indicate sizes of Hind III DNA fragments.

Table 1—Oncogene expression in human glioblastoma-derived cell lines

Probes	Cell lines					
	Hu70	Hu104	Hu112	Hu195	Hu197	Hu175*
EGF-r	+++	+++	+	+++	+++	+
c-myc	+++	+++	++	++	+++	++
Ha-ras	+	+	+	+	+	+
Ki-ras	+	+	+	+	+	+
N-ras	+++	+++	+++	+++	+++	+
ros	0	++	0	0	0	0
sis	0	+	0	0	0	0

Dot blot analysis of serially diluted samples (10 μg to 1.25 μg) dotted onto Amersham's Hybond-N nylon membranes and hybridized with oncogene-specific probes. The amount of transcripts was estimated by comparison of the intensity of the hybridization signals: 0 = no expression detected; + to +++ = low to high level expression. No specific transcripts for N-myc, mos, src, or neu genes were detected in any of the cell lines analysed.
* Hu 175 = 'Normal' glial cell line (see text).

10.1.3 RESULTS

10.1.3.1 Cell lines

Table 1 gives the results for oncogene expression (amount of transcripts in total RNA) as estimated by dot blot analysis of serially diluted samples. As we previously reported (Talarico *et al.* in press), EGF-r overexpression was found in cell lines Hu70, Hu104, Hu195, and Hu197, all of which showed increased number of chromosome 7, where the EGF-r gene has been mapped. A significant increase in N-*ras* expression was displayed by all five glioblastoma cell lines, while c-Ha-*ras* c-Ki-*ras* m-RNAs were present to a comparable extent in both tumour and 'normal' glial cells. High-level expression of c-*myc* oncogene was observed in both tumour and 'normal' cells; c-*ros* and c-*sis* transcripts were present only in the Hu104 cell line. No expression of c-*mos*, c-*src*, N-*myc* or *neu* was detected.

Southern blot analysis failed to reveal any increase in N-*ras* copy number, thus indicating that augmented N-*ras* expression in the glioblastoma cell lines was not the result of gene amplification.

10.1.3.2 Primary tumours

Northern blot hybridization showed increased levels of the 1.5 and 5.8 kb EGF-r specific transcripts in all 5 glioblastomas. Densitometric quantification of the signals on the autoradiographic film revealed that the amount of EGF-r specific m-RNA in these tumours was 4 to 50 fold higher than in controls. In Hu244 (astrocytoma) and in Hu231 (ependymoma) EGF-r gene expression was only slightly increased (about 2-fold).

Southern blot analysis showed that the EGF-r gene was amplified 40 to 60-fold in Hu243 and 3 to 5-fold in Hu233 (Fig. 1).

High levels of the 5.5 kb and 2.2 kb N-*ras* specific transcripts, 5 to 15 times higher than in 'normal' brain tissues, were detected in the 5 glioblastomas, whereas in Hu244 and Hu231 N-*ras* expression was not significantly increased as compared to control tissues. No significant differences in Ha-*ras* and Ki-*ras* expression were detected.

10.1.4 DISCUSSION

Multiple oncogenes were transcriptionally active in all glioblastomas examined. The importance of activation of multiple oncogenes in malignancy is suggested by data showing that more than one oncogene is needed to transform normal primary embryo fibroblasts into tumourigenic cells (Land *et al.* 1983). Although non-neoplastic host cells, and particularly vascular or stromal glial elements, were present in most of the surgical tumour samples, these cells are unlikely to be responsible for the high levels of oncogene-specific transcripts observed. Indeed, the same oncogenes were expressed at low levels in 'normal' brain tissue and in non-neoplastic glial cells in culture, and overexpressed only in the glioblastoma cell lines. If oncogene overexpression is of pathogenetic significance in brain tumours, then this differential transcriptional levels are consistent with a quantitative model.

EGF-r gene overexpression was consistently observed in our glioblastoma series (5/5 in biopsies, 4/5 in cell lines) compared to 'normal' brain tissue and non-neoplastic glial cells. High EGF-r levels have been reported in several human tumours and tumour-derived cell lines, mainly of neuro-ectodermal origin. Enhanced EGF-r activity has been found in malignant glioma homogenates (Libermann *et al.* 1984, 1985), and in cell cultures (Harsch *et al.* 1985), but not in normal adult brain (Libermann *et al.* 1984, 1985). An amplified, overexpressed, rearranged EGF receptor has been identified in a human astrocytoma cell line (Filmus *et al.* 1985), and a high-affinity EGF receptor in a malignant glioma cell line (Westphal *et al.* in press).

In glioblastomas, enhanced EGF-r expression has been related either to amplification of the specific gene (Libermann *et al.* 1985) or to increased copy number of chromosome 7 (Talarico *et al.* in press). EGF-r gene amplification seems to be more common in primary tumours than in glioblastoma-derived cell lines (Filmus *et al.* 1985); our southern blot analysis showed DNA amplification in 2/5 surgical biopsies.

As previously reported (Talarico *et al.* in press), 4/5 glioblastoma cell lines displayed an increased number of chromosome 7. In 3 cases (Hu104, Hu195, and Hu197), the increase in gene copy number was higher than expected from the number of chromosome 7 identified, thus suggesting the occurrence of either subliminal gene amplification events or translocations of part of the short arm of chromosome 7 to unclassified marker chromosomes (Talarico *et al.* in press). Furthermore, the increase in EGF-r expression was greater both in glioblastoma tumours and cell lines than expected from the augmented gene dosage, indicating that a loss of control of transcriptional activity of the gene also occurred.

N-*ras* oncogene overexpression was found in all glioblastoma cell lines and primary tumours. The gene loci of several oncogenes have been found to lie at or very close to, the breakpoints of chromosomal rearrangements (Yunis 1983). N-*ras* oncogene has been mapped on the short arm of chromosome 1 (1p12-p21) (Davis *et al.* 1983). Structural abnormalities of the latter have been shown in various neuro-ectodermal tumours: deletions distal to 1p32 and 1p22 are associated with neuroblastomas and malignant melanomas respectively (Garret 1986); 2/4 of our N-*ras* positive glioblastoma cell lines showed minor terminal deletions (1p33-pter and 1p35-ter): however, these were not very close to the mapped gene.

The normal location of certain oncogenes has been shown to be neighbouring to genes that code for cell growth factors or their receptors (Gordon 1985): on the short arm of chromosome 1, the N-*ras* oncogene is a neighbour to the gene for the nerve growth factor (1p21-pter) (Gordon 1985). This apparent 'neighbourliness' might be coincidental, or might indicate an early evolutionary relationship.

Finally, recent experimental evidence suggests that EGF-r and *ras* proteins, which reside in the same cellular compartment, may interact directly or indirectly in response to mitogenic stimulation, namely: (i) addition of EGF to membranes isolated from c-Ha-*ras*-transformed rat cells enhances the guanine nucleotide binding activity of $p21^{ras}$ (Kamata & Feramisco 1984); and (ii) the growth promoting effect of EGF is greatly enhanced in NIH 3T3 cells which express high levels of N-*ras* protein (Wakelam *et al.* 1986). As EGF is present in human cerebrospinal fluid in concentrations comparable to those in plasma (Guroff 1983), such a mechanism might be of relevance in glial tumour cell proliferation.

Overexpression of these two proto-oncogenes might entail a putatively predictive role in human malignant brain tumours.

ACKNOWLEDGEMENTS

We wish to thank J. Haley for the gift of plasmid 64-1, E. Scolnick for plasmid pHiHi3, and S. Pulciani for T24-C3. Our thanks also go to M. Negri for his expert technical assistance and to A. Steele for his help with the English text.

This work was supported by grants from the Italian Ministry of Education (MPI), the Ass. Ital. Ric. Cancro, the CNR (Progetto Finalizzato Oncologia), and the Regione Veneto.

REFERENCES

Chirgwin, J. M., Przybyla, A. E., MacDonald, R. J., & Rutter, W. J. (1979) Isolation of biologically active ribonucleic acid from sources enriched in ribonuclease. *Biochemistry* **18,** 5294–5299

Davis, M., Malcom, A. H., & Marshall, C. J. (1983) Localization of the human N-*ras* oncogene to chromosome Icen-p21 by *in situ* hybridization. *EMBO J.* **2,** 2281–2283

Eva, A., Robbins, K. C., Andersen, P. R., Srinivasan, A., Tronick, S. R., Reddy, E. P., Ellmore, N. W., Galen, A. T., Lautenberger, J. A., Papas, T. S., Westin, E. H., Wong-Staal, F., Gallo, R. C., & Aaronson, S. A. (1982) Cellular genes analogous to retroviral *onc* genes are transcribed in human tumour cells. *Nature* **295,** 116–119

Filmus, J., Pollack, M. N., Cairncross, J. G., & Buick, R. N. (1985) Amplified, overexpressed and rearranged epidermal growth factor receptor gene in a human astrocytoma cell line. *Biochem. Biophys. Res. Comm.* **131,** 207–215

Garret, C. T. (1986) Oncogenes. *Clin. Chim. Acta* **156,** 1–40.

Gerosa M. A., Rosenblum, M. L., & Tridente, G. (1986) *Brain tumors: biopathology and therapy.* Pergamon Press, Oxford

Gordon, H. (1985) Oncogenes. *Mayo Clin. Proc.* **60,** 697–713

Guroff, G. (1983) *Growth and maturation factors.* Vol. I, Wiley, New York

Harsch, G. R., Rosenblum, M. L., & Williams, L. T. (1985) Oncogene related growth factors in human brain tumor cell lines. *Proc. Am. Ass. Neurol. Surg.* **53,** 264–265

Kamata, T. & Feramisco, J. M. (1984) Epidermal growth factor stimulates guanine nucleotide binding activity and phosphorylation of *ras* oncogene proteins. *Nature* **310,** 147–149

Land, H., Parada, L. F., & Weinberg, R. A. (1983) Tumorigenic conversion of primary embryo fibroblasts requires at least two cooperating oncogenes. *Nature* **304,** 596–602

Levinson, A. D. (1986) Normal and activated *ras* oncogenes and their encoded products. *Trends Genet* **2,** 81–85

Libermann, T. A., Razon, N., Bartal, A. D., Yarden, Y., Schlessinger, J., & Soreq, H. (1984) Expression of epidermal growth factor receptors in human brain tumors. *Cancer Res.* **44,** 753–760

Libermann, T. A., Nusbaum, H. R., Razon, N., Kris, R., Lax, I., Soreq, H., Whittle, N., Waterfield, M. D., Ullrich, A., & Schlessinger, J. (1985) Amplification, enhanced expression and possible rearragement of EGF receptor gene in primary human tumors of glial origin. *Nature* **313,** 144–147

Rosenblum, M. L., Gerosa, M. A., Wilson, C. B., Barger, G. R., Pertuiset, B. F., De Tribolet, N., & Dougherty, D. V. (1983) Stem cell studies of human malignant brain tumors. *J. Neurosurg.* **58,** 170–176

Schwab, M., Alitalo, K., Varmus, H. E., Bishop, J. M., & George, D. (1983) A cellular oncogene (c-Ki-*ras*) is amplified, overexpressed, and located within karyotypic abnormalities in mouse adrenocortical tumor cells. *Nature* **303,** 497–501

Varmus, H. E. (1984) The molecular genetics of cellular oncogenes. *Ann. Rev. Biochem.* **18,** 553–612

Talarico, D., Raimondi, E., Fognani, C., Gerosa, M. A., Gregotti, S., Della Valle, G., & De Carli, L. Increased number of chromosome 7 is related to overexpression of EGF receptor gene in human glioblastomas. *Cytotechnology* in press

Thor, A., Horan Hand, P., Wunderlich, D., Caruso, A., Muraro, R., & Schlom, J. (1984) Monoclonal antibodies define differential *ras* expression in malignant and benign colonic diseases. *Nature* **311,** 562–565

Wakelam, M. J. O., Davies, S. A., Huslay, M. D., McKay, I., Marshall, C. J., & Hall, A. (1986) Normal p21-N-*ras* couples bombesin and other growth factor receptors to inositol phosphate production. *Nature* **323,** 173–176

Westphal, M., Harsch, G. R., & Rosenblum, M. L. Epidermal growth factor receptors in the human glioblastoma cell line SF268 differ from those in epidermoid carcinoma cell line A431. *Biochem. Biophys. Res. Comm.* in press

White, B. A. & Bancroft, F. C. (1982) Cytoplasmic dot hybridization. *J. Biol. Chem.* **257,** 8569–8572

Yunis, J. J. (1983) The chromosomal basis of human neoplasia. *Science* **221,** 227–236

10.2 Oncogenes as diagnostic and prognostic tools in human haematologic neoplasms

M. Introna & J. Golay†

Studies of the expression, mutation or rearrangements of oncogenes in human hematological neoplasms has so far provided evidence for the role of only two oncogenes, N. ras and the rearranged bcr-abl oncogenes as potential prognostic or diagnostic tools in these human neoplasms. Further studies of these and other oncogenes are therefore of great clinical interest.

10.2.1 INTRODUCTION

Oncogenes have raised great interest in recent years (Kahn & Graf 1986), even though their direct and causative role in neoplasia can be proved only in the few cases of acute transforming retroviruses and in selected experimental models (Weiss-Teich-Varmus Coffin 1985). Nevertheless, extensive research efforts have been carried out to explore their possible involvement in human cancer. This paper will review the advances in the use of oncogenes as diagnostic or prognostic tools in human haematologic neoplasms with a particular interest in their potential usefulness in clinical research.

10.2.2 REVIEW

Before discussing the role of oncogenes on diagnosis and prognosis, it is necessary to provide general information on the basic research on oncogenes in haematologic neoplasms. Table 1 lists all the transforming retroviruses which can lead to several different haematologic tumours in various animal species and their related v-onc genes (Graf & Stehelin 1982). Only eight oncogenes (erbA, erbB, myb, ets, myc, raf, abl, and rel) have been so far identified which play, at least in these models, a direct transforming role in haematopoietic cells (Graf & Stehelin 1982). It should be stressed, however, that the specific contribution of each of these oncogenes in the transformation event and their mechanism of action in many cases is still far from being fully understood (Weiss-Teich-Varmus Coffin 1985).

Many other RNA viruses exist which do not carry an oncogene in their genome but are able to transform cells of the haematopoietic system. The neoplastic action

† European Molecular Biology Laboratory, Postfach 10.2209, Meyerhofstraße 1, 6900 Heidelberg, W. Germany

Table 1—Oncogenes directly involved in experimental models of haematologic neoplasms

Virus	Disease	Oncogene	Animal species
AEV	erythroleukaemia	erbB + erbA	chicken
AMV	myeloid leukaemia	myb	chicken
E26	mixed erythroid + myeloid leukaemia	myb + ets	chicken
MC29	myelocytomatosis	myc	chicken
OK10	myelocytomatosis	myc	chicken
MH2	myelocytomatosis	myc + raf	chicken
Ab MLV	pre-B lymphoma	abl	mouse
REV-T	pre-B leukaemia	rel	turkey

of such non-defective retroviruses has been related to their ability to integrate into the genome of the host cell through several distinct mechanisms (Hayward *et al.* 1981). The normal cellular genes involved in these insertional or recombinational events and which have been identified in experimental models of leukaemia and lymphomas are shown in Table 2. In a few cases these genes are indeed proto-oncogenes (the normal cellular counterparts of the viral oncogenes), but in most other cases the oncogenicity of the cellular genes involved remains an open question, even when these genes have been characterized and sequenced.

Table 2—Cellular regions of integration in retroviruses induced haematologic neoplasms

	Oncogenes	Non-oncogenes	
c-erbB	erythroleukaemia	fis-1	lymphoma and leukaemia
c-myb	leukaemia	fim-1	leukaemia
c-myc	lymphoma	fim-2	leukaemia
c-fms	leukaemia	mlvi-1	thymoma
c-mos	plasmacytoma	mlvi-2	thymoma
		mlvi-3	thymoma
		mis-1	thymoma
		pim-1	lymphoma
		dsi-1	thymoma
		pvt-1	lymphoma

A third line of evidence that points to the potential role of the known oncogenes as transforming genes in human leukaemias, comes from several studies of disease-specific chromosomal translocations in which the breaking point regions have been cloned and sequenced (Croce 1987). In several cases these lesions occur in the proximities of proto-oncogenes (Table 3), while in other examples normal cellular genes have been sequenced at the breaking points, but we still lack information on their putative role as oncogenes (Table 3).

10.2.3 DISCUSSION

The findings summarized above represent the background information that has led to many clinically oriented studies performed in man, aimed at detecting abnormalities

Table 3—Cellular regions involved in chromosomal translocations or deletions in haematologic neoplasms

Oncogenes			Non-oncogenes		
c-myc	t(8,14)	Burkitt lymphoma and T leukaemia	bcl-1	t (11,14)	B cell lymphoma and leukaemia
	t (2,8)	Burkitt lymphoma	bcl-2	t (14,18)	follicular lymphoma acute leukaemia
	t (8,22)	Burkitt lymphoma			
c-ets-1	t (9,11)	acute leukaemia	pim-1	t (6,9)	myeloid leukaemia
	t (4,11)	acute leukaemia			
			bcr	t (9,22)	chronic myelogenous leukaemia
c-ets-2	t (8,21)	acute leukaemia			
p53	t (15,17)	acute leukaemia			
c-erb-A	t (15,17)	acute leukaemia			
c-abl	t (9,22)	chronic myelogenous leukaemia			
c-fms	del 5q	acute leukaemia			

in the structure or expression of proto-oncogenes in leukemias and lymphomas with potential usefulness for diagnosis and/or prognosis. Apart from episodic reports of gene amplification (Dalla Favera *et al.* 1982), attention has been generally focused on the expression levels of proto-oncogenes in RNA extracts of neoplastic cells (Preisler *et al.* 1987, Mavilio *et al.* 1986, Rosson & Tereba 1983, Blick *et al.* 1984). As shown in Table 4, few oncogenes have been studied so far. Interestingly, no attention has been given to some oncogenes, for example erbA and erbB, which are clearly responsible for haematologic tumours in experimental models (Table 1).

Table 4—Expression of proto-oncogenes in haematopoietic neoplasms

Proto-oncogenes	Detectable in	Not detectable in
c-myb	T-ALL AML CML	B-CLL B-ALL
c-myc	some CML some AML some ALL	
c-fos	AML (M4–M5 FAB)	all the others
c-sis		always negative
c-src		always negative
c-erbB		always negative
c-k-ras	some T-ALL	
p53	some AML some ALL	

Furthermore, these studies on the expression of proto-oncogenes are, in general, largely inconclusive. Among the many possible reasons, the complete lack of understanding of the exact functional role of the proto-oncogenes in normal haematopoietic cells plays a crucial role. Expression of several proto-oncogenes can be induced in various cell types following entry into the cell-cycle (Kelly *et al.* 1983) or differentiation (Gonda & Metcalf 1984). In addition, evidence has been produced more recently showing induction of c-fos expression in mature macrophages (Introna

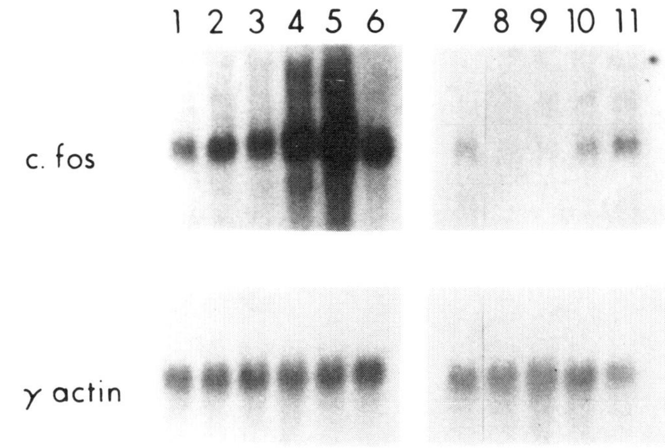

Fig. 1.—Expression of c-fos and y-actin by macrophages after incubation with LPS. Murine peritoneal macrophages were incubated with medium alone for 1 h (lane 1) or were treated with 20 ng/ml LPS for 2 min (lane 2), 5 min (lane 3), 15 min (lane 4), 30 min (lane 5), 60 min (lane 6), 2 h (lane 7), 8 h (lane 8), 12 h (lane 9), and 24 h (lane 10). Control populations were also cultivated for 24 h in medium without endotoxin (lane 11). From Introna *et al.* (1986)

et al. 1986, 1978a,b) and granulocytes (Colotta *et al.* 1987) following functional activation of these cells. As shown in Fig. 1, low doses of lipopolysaccharide (LPS) can induce a dramatic increase in c-fos transcription in terminally differentiated murine macrophages in the complete absence of detectable proliferation (Introna *et al.* 1986). Therefore, although altered levels of expression of several proto-oncogenes can be found in crude RNA extracts of transformed leukocytes (Table 4), it is unclear if they simply reflect the contribution of different subpopulations of cells in different moments of their cell-cycle or their stage of differentiation or even their functional status. For these reasons they do not usually provide more diagnostic information than the classical methods of classification of leukaemias.

Only very recently have reports appeared which provide positive data on the use of oncogenes as diagnostic or prognostic tools in human leukaemias (Table 5). Hirai *et al.* (1987) extracted DNA from the bone marrow of 8 myelodysplastic syndrome (MDS) patients and transfected in the murine 3T3 cell line. Only three patients could be scored positive for transformation in this assay, and the 'activated' responsible oncogene has been identified as an N-ras which had undergone a point mutation at codon 13 in all the cases. Interestingly, all 3 patients showed an aggressive disease developing a full AML within one year of diagnosis. In this study, the presence

Table 5—Studies in which the use of oncogenes as diagnostic or prognostic tools has been shown in human haematologic neoplasms

H. Hirai *et al.* (1987) *Nature* **327** 3/8 patients with MDS carry point mutations at codon 13 of N-ras and develop AML in one year from diagnosis
C. M. Morris *et al.* (1986) *Nature* **320** T. S. Ganbsan *et al.* (1986) *Blood* **68** The presence of a bcr-abl transcript may help in diagnosis of Ph-negative CML patients.

of an activated oncogene seems therefore to correlate with a more malignant biology of the disease within an apparently homogeneous group of patients.

A number of reports points to the role of a recombinational event between the two genes bcr and abl (only the latter being a 'bona fide' proto-oncogene) in the pathogenesis of CML (Shtivelman *et al.* 1985). As already known, the vast majority of these recombinations occur as a consequence of a massive translocation of portions of chromosomes which leads usually to the formation of the 'Philadelphia chromosome'. Nevertheless, as pointed out in recent reports (Ganesan *et al.* 1986, Morris *et al.* 1986), this recombination between bcr and abl can also be detected in a few cases of Philadelphia-negative patients, and may absolutely correlate with true CML. This implies that (a) more limited lesions at the DNA level can give rise to the same phenotype, and (b) the abnormal transcripts generated by translocation of abl to the bcr locus may have a causative role in the pathogenesis of the disease. Obviously the use of 'bcr' or 'abl' probes should be helpful in the diagnosis of Philadelphia-negative leukaemias.

In conclusion, the impressive amount on the biology of oncogenes and proto-oncogenes has not yet been proved to be of direct usefulness for diagnosis or prognosis in human haematologic neoplasms, but this may reflect the fact that this area of research is still in its early days. Recent results suggest that clinical investigations with a solid research background should be extended and encouraged.

REFERENCES

Blick, M. *et al.* (1984) Oncogene expression in human leukemia. *Blood* **64,** 1234–1239

Colotta, F. *et al.* (1987) Expression of c-fos proto-oncogene in normal human peripheral blood granulocytes. *J. Exp. Med.* **165,** 1224–1229

Croce, C. M. (1987) Role of chromosome translocations in human neoplasia. *Cell* **49,** 155–156

Dalla Favera, R. *et al.* (1982) Onc gene amplification in promyelocytic leukaemia cell line HL-60 and primary leukaemia cells of the same patient. *Nature* **299,** 61–63

Ganesan, T. S. *et al.* (1986) Rearrangement of the bcr gene in Ph-negative chronic myeloid leukemia. *Blood* **68,** 4–960

Gonda, T. J. & Metcalf, D. (1984) Expression of myb, myc and fos proto-oncogenes during the differentiation of a murine myeloid leukemia. *Nature* **310,** 249–251

Graf, T. & Stehelin, D. (1982) Avian leukemia viruses. Oncogenes and genome structure. *Biochem. Biophys. Acta* **651,** 245–271

Hayward, W. *et al.* (1981) Activation of a cellular onc gene by promoter insertion in ALV-induced lymphoid leukemia. *Nature* **290,** 475–480

Hirai, H. *et al.* (1987) A point mutation at codon 13 of the N-ras oncogene in myelodysplastic syndrome. *Nature* **327,** 430–434

Introna, M. *et al.* (1986) Treatment of murine peritoneal macrophages with tacterial LPS alterns expression of c-fos and c-myc oncogenes. *J. Immunol.* **137,** 2711–2715

Introna, M. *et al.* (1987a) Homologous and heterologous desensitisation of proto-oncogene c-fos expression in murine peritoneal macrophages. *J. Cell Physiol.* **131,** 36–42

Introna, M. *et al.* (1987b) The effect of LPS on expression of the 'early' competence genes JE and KC in murine peritoneal macrophages. *J. Immunol.* **138,** 3891–3896

Kahn, P. & Graf, T. (eds) (1986) *Oncogenes and growth control*, Springer-Verlag

Kelly, K. *et al.* (1983) Cell-specific regulation of the c-myc gene by lumphocytes mitogenes and PDGF. *Cell* **35,** 603–610

Mavilio, F. *et al.* (1986) Expression of cellular oncogenes in primary cells from human acute leukemias. *PNAS* **83,** 4394–4398

Morris, C. M. *et al.* (1986) Genomic diversity correlates with clinical variation in Ph-negative chronic myeloid leukaemia. *Nature* **320,** 281–283

Preisler, H. D. *et al.* (1987) Expression of the protooncogenes c-myc, c-fos and c-fms in AML at diagnosis and at remission. *Cancer Research* **47,** 874–880

Rosson, D. & Tereba, A. (1983) Transcription of hematopoietic-associated oncogenes in childhood leukemia. *Cancer Research* **43,** 3912–3918.

Shtivelman *et al.* (1985) Fused transcript of abl and bcr genes in chronic myelogenous leukaemia. *Nature* **315,** 550–554

Weiss-Teich-Varmus Coffin, C. S. H. (eds) (1985) *RNA tumor viruses: molecular biology of tumour viruses*

10.3 Membrane diagnostic probes: situation and perspectives

Roland Glaser†

It is well known that many diseases affect membrane properties. Therefore the measurement of membrane parameters can be used for diagnostic purposes.

The following kinds of membrane diagnostic probes can be used:

—Measurements of the directly affected cells.
—Measurements on easily obtainable cells reflecting a disfunction of other parts of the body.
—Utilisation of body cells for tests of the individual drug sensitivity.

Particular membrane properties which can be measured by routine methods are listed in a table. These methods are applicable partly for single cells partly for cell suspensions, and partly for tissues.

In general the real degree of application of these methods for routine diagnosis is unsatisfactory as yet. The reasons for this are various. The rapid development of highly-automated methods and the progress in membranology, will obviously (and hopefully) change this in future.

10.3.1 INTRODUCTION

There is no doubt that membrane investigations are very important for medical research. Nearly all diseases somehow effect membrane properties. This concerns processes of virus–cell interaction as well as nervous, muscular, metabolic, or other disorders finally leading to abnormalities in membrane properties. In general, one has to differentiate between the following fields of medical membrane research:

- Basic investigations of causes and consequences of membraneous dysfunctions.
- Research and tests of the influence of drugs on membrane properties for therapeutic reasons.
- Development of new diagnostic techniques using measurements of membrane properties.

The separation of the basic membrane research, mentioned in the first point of this list, from the fields of application in the following two, at first glance seems to be very artificial and even impossible: no pharmaceutical development seems to be

† Humboldt-Univ., Sektion Biologie, Bereich Biologie, Berlin—DDR

reasonable without a profound knowledge of the basic manner of its molecular action. The same may be said of diagnostic probes: no simple correlation between a definite membrane parameter and the occurrence of a special disease should be sufficient for introducing a new diagnostic probe.

These statements seem to be rather trivial. The reality, however, teaches us the opposite: most drugs are used in therapy without sufficient knowledge of the molecular mechanisms of its action. As an example for diagnostic probes: erythrocyte sedimentation rate is used daily throughout the world as a quick check for inflammationary processes in the body. Obviously, this parameter reflects the increased aggregation affinity of blood cells (Oka 1985). The causal chain between the inflammation processes and the agglutination, however, is still unknown.

This contradiction between the demands of basic science and the really existing (and doubtless sometimes necessary) pragmatism of the clinical application is the source of a number of diagnostic and therapeutic failures. A typical and in some respect even alarming example is the cancer tests using electrophoretic-motility of blood cells. These tests are based exclusively on certain correlations between the occurrence of cancer in the body and the change of surface charges of blood cells after a definite preparation. After an initial enthusiasm 10 years ago, leading to the development of corresponding equipment, serious objections have been raised concerning the reliability of this test (Mross 1985). Consequently, the simple correlation between the occurrence of a definite disease and a particular membrane parameter is in no case sufficient for introducing a new reliable diagnostic probe.

In general, one has to differentiate between two kinds of membrane diagnostic probes: firstly, the direct checking of the pathologically affected cell (for example: the erythrocyte in cases of haemolytic anaemia, the muscle cell in myotonia, etc.), and secondly, the use of any other simply obtainable cell (such as a blood cell) as a representative of the tissue cells of a diseased organ. In this second case one supposes that either the dysfunction in a definite organ is accompanied by an abnormality of membranes of all body cells (as for example in cases of hereditary abnormalities of transport proteins, or changes in lipid metabolism), or that toxic compounds in the blood plasma as a result of the disease cause an overall effect on each body cell simultaneously.

Membrane dysfunctions are mostly reflected even by abnormalities in definite cytoplasmic properties. For example, a measured change in the K^+/Na^+-relation in the cell can be taken as caused by transport abnormalities of the membrane. Therefore, knowing the physiological mechanisms of the observed cell, even non-direct membrane probes may lead to information about membrane dysfunctions.

In some cases, the measured effect can be ambiguous: changes in the electrical membrane potential, for example, can be the result either of permeability changes in the membrane or of modified cellular ionic composition. The same holds for haemorheological parameters, for haemolytic resistance, and many others. To avoid misinterpretation, one needs, of course, a good knowledge of the causal connections of these parameters; and, in some cases, a combination of the results obtained by different methods is necessary.

What is the real situation in the application of membrane probes in medicine today? It is impossible to review all the papers touching on this problem. Only a few examples can be discussed here. Generally, immunological as well as haematological tests, as special fields of membraneous and cellular probes, will be excluded.

10.3.2 PROBES AND THEIR APPLICATIONS

It is almost impossible to arrange this report according to the systematics of diseases. It seems to be better to check different parameters and methods in membrane research, and to discuss their significance for diagnostic purpose (see Table 1).

The rapid progress of analytical techniques in recent years enables the quick and detailed chemical analyses of the composition of membrane constituents in small samples. In contrast to transport measurements which requires more or less undisturbed living cells, this analysis can be performed even on biopsy samples of the relevant tissue. It is not possible to list and discuss all these methods here. Basically, these analyses concentrate on protein separation, on checking alterations in enzymes, and, in this respect, also transport proteins, as well as in analyses of membrane lipids and there fatty acid composition. In recent years, especially, receptor analyses has become an interesting and important field. The following findings are mentioned only as examples: alteration in transport protein in brush-border membrane diseases (Crane *et al.* 1987), changes in arachidonic acid content in haemolytic uraemia (Powell *et al.* 1987), modification of fatty acid composition after *Plasmodium* infection (Beaumelle & Vial 1986), and many others. In most cases, however, these probes did not become part of a diagnosis procedure, but they rather were of purely scientific interest or, at most, they became part of a probe for differential diagnosis.

A large number of papers indicate that, in many cases, blood cells, especially erythrocytes, reflect abnormalities in the transport properties of those tissue cells which are directly affected by the disease. This can be illustrated, for example, by patients with myotonia (Bryant 1987, Appel & Roses 1987), where abnormalities in the Cl^- conductance and the stoichiometry of the cationic exchange could be found in the red blood cells. Measurement of the ion transport can indicate the effect of the dialysis of uraemic patients (Corry *et al.* 1986). Even the effect of the Li^+-therapy has been followed by checking erythrocytes (Sen *et al.* 1987). An increasing number of papers deal with transport anomalies in erythrocytes from patients with hypertension (Haddy 1983). In no case, however, have these observations led to the introduction of a clinically applied diagnostic method. The reason for this seems to be on the one hand a lack of the basic knowledge of the mechanisms underlying the effects, and on the other hand the fact that the measurement of transport parameters, and even the determination of the ionic composition of the cells, are too time-consuming for routine laboratory diagnostics. It seems to be possible, however, that in the future this situation might be changed by the introduction of new fluorescence methods (for example, for the measurement of Ca^{++}-concentration) or NMR-measurements of sodium and potassium content of isolated cells or even of tissue cells *in vivo*.

The rapid development of the haemorheology in recent years has led not only to new insights into the processes of blood circulation, but has given rise to several new analytic methods (see Table 1). The question is now: what mechanical parameters of the cell really are reflected by a particular method? (Schmidt-Schönbein & Teitel 1987). This makes possible a profound valuation of the measured haemodynamic parameters, although even in this case the reasons for the measured abnormalities in the mechanical parameters of the cells are not fully clarified. But even in spite of the development of many new methods and a large number of observed haemorheological abnormalities caused by various diseases, these probes have been used only

Table 1—Membrane probes and their applications

Parameters: Methods	Application for: Single cells	Cells in suspension	Tissue
Mechanical properties:			
Viscosimetry		+	
Rigidometry	+	+	
Filtrometry		+	
Optical shape determination	+	+	
Transport properties:			
Tracer methods	+	+	+
Cytolytic resistance	+	+	
Ionic content analysis	+	+	+
Chemical membrane composition		+	+
Electrical properties:			
Cell electrophoresces	+		
Microelectrode techniques	+		+
Fluorescence labelling	+	+	+
Electrorotation	+		
Impedance measurement		+	+

hesitantly in routine diagnosis. In the future, however, the rapidly growing knowledge about membrane mechanisms, and the highly developed level of techniques in this field, combined with a large degree of automatization and computerization, will certainly speed up this process.

The electrical methods listed in Table 1 allow measurement of surface potential (cell electrophoresces), transmembrane potential (microelectrode techniques, fluorescence labelling), and passive electric properties (electrorotation, impedance measurements) such as membrane conductance, membrane capacitance, and cytoplasmatic conductivity of cells. It seems that surface potential and surface charge can be applied as diagnostic indicators only in combination with immunological probes, using charged antibodies for the detection of specific receptors. The microelectrode technique, especially the patch-clamp technique, is obviously too awkward for use in diagnostic techniques in everyday use, even despite its great significance in membrane research in general. The introduction of fluorescent dyes for measurement of transmembrane potential of cells in suspension, however, could probably become a useful method for diagnostic probes. This sort of measurement can also be realized with a large degree of automation.

A new method involves the measurement of the spin of single cells in measuring chambers between four electrodes driven by an electrical field, rotating with frequencies between some kHz and some MHz. Because of its dependence on membrane resistance, membrane capacity, and internal conductivity of the cell, resonance effect occur at definite field frequencies, leading to a more or less fast rotation of the observed cell. This 'electrorotation' of cells reflects modifications of transport properties and membrane resealing, and in this respect it is a quick and sensitive test for cell vitality (Glaser & Fuhr 1986, 1987). The activation kinetics of a single platelet can be measured, as well as the sensitivity of the process to the influence of various drugs (Egger *et al.* 1986). It is also possible to check the activation of single lymphocytes (Ziervogel *et al.* 1986). The capacity of this method has not yet been fully exploited, and even the techniques itself needs much more development before it can be introduced into routine measurement. We are hopeful, however, that it will become a useful test in the future.

10.3.3 CONCLUSION

A large number of diseases are accompanied by a specific pattern of membrane alterations. Up to now, these alterations have been measured, but the results were obtained almost exclusively to further the understanding of the basic mechanics of the disease. The reason for the hesitant introduction of these probes into clinical practice are two-fold:

- The methods are too expensive and time-consuming for practical use.
- The causal chain between the parameter and the pathological process is not fully recognized.

This situation will obviously change. The rapid development of highly-automated methods on the one hand and our increasing knowledge of normal and pathological membrane processes on the other, will surely accelerate the introduction of particular membrane probes into diagnostic practice, at least as a part of differential diagnosis as well as for aetiological reasons. Additionally, cellular *in vitro* tests could be increasingly introduced into clinical practice. They would help to determine the correct drug application; and they could be used as a viability test of cells provided for transfusion or transplantation, and for checking the success of a therapeutic treatment. In any case, one has to be careful about the introduction of diagnostic probes on the sole basis of simple correlation between a definite parameter and a disease.

REFERENCES

Appel, St. H. & Roses, A. D. (1987). Membrane biochemical studies in myotonic muscular dystrophy. In: Bolis *et al.* (1987), 183–195

Beaumelle, B. D. & Vial, H. J. (1986). Modification of the fatty acid composition of individual phospholipide and neutral lipids after infection of the simian erythrocyte by *Plasmodium knowlesi*. *Biochim. Biophys. Acta* **877,** 262–270

Bolis, L., Hoffman, J. F., & Leaf, A. (eds) (1987). *Membranes and disease*, Raven Press, New York

Bryant, S. H. (1976). Altered membrane properties in myotonia. In: Bolis *et al.* (1987), 197–206

Corry, D. B., Tuck, M. L., Brickman, A. S., Yanagawa, N., & Lee, D. B. N. (1986). Sodium transport in red blood cells from dialyzed uremic patients. *Kidney International* **29,** 1197–1202

Crane, R. K., Menard, D., Preiser, H., & Cerda, J. (1987). The molecular basis of brush-border membrane disease: In: Bolis *et al.* (1987) 229–241

Egger, M., Donath, E., Ziemer, S., & Glaser, R. (1986). Electrorotation—a new method for investigating membrane events during thrombocyte activation. Influence of drugs and osmotic pressure. *Biochim. Biophys. Acta* **861,** 122–130

Glaser, R. & Fuhr, G. (1986). Electrorotation of single cells—a new method for assessment of membrane properties. In: *Electrical double layers in biology* (Blank, M. ed), Plenum Press, New York, 227–241

Glaser, R. & Fuhr, G. (1987). Electrorotation—the spin of cells in rotating high frequency electric fields. In: Blank, M. & Findl, E. *Mechanistic approaches to interaction of electric and electromechanic fields with living systems.* Plenum Press, New York

Haddy, F. J. (1983). Abnormalities of membrane transport in hypertension. *Hypertension Suppl.* **5,** 66–72

Mross, K. B. (1985). Cancer diagnosis and other applications using the electrophoretic mobility test during the last years (1974–1984)—A critical review. In: Schutt & Klinkmann (1985), 871–893

Oka, S. (1985). A physical theory of erythrocyte sedimentation. *Biorheology* **22,** 315–321

Powell, H. R., Groves, V., McCredie, D. A., Yong, A., & Pitt, J. (1987). Low red cell arachidonic acid in hemolytic uremic syndrome. *Clinical Nephreology* **27,** 8–10

Schmidt-Schönbein, H. & Teibel, P. (1987). *In vitro* assessment of 'covertly abnormal' blood rheology; critical appraisal of presently available microrheological methodology. *Clinical Hemorheology* **7** 203–238

Sen, A. K., Murthy, R., Stancer, H. C., Awad, A. G., Godse, D. D., & Grof, P. (1987). The mechanisms of action of lithium ion in affective disorders: A new hypothesis. In: Bolis *et al.* (1987), 109–122

Ziervogel, H., Glaser, R., Schadow, D., & Heymann, S. T. p1986). Electrorotation of lymphocytes—the influence of membrane events and nucleus. *Bioscience Reports* **6,** 873–982

10.4 Clinical, ultrasonographic, and hystopathological findings in cerebral atherosclerosis

C. Sabbà†, D. Pugliese†, G. Caruso‡, V. Zupo†, A. Odero§, & O. Albano†

Echo–Doppler examination is commonly considered to be a reliable non-invasive method to quantify the extent of the atherosclerotic lesions. In the ultrasonographic study of the carotid we consider topographic, quantitative, qualitative, and haemodynamic aspects of the lesions. Our protocol includes the post mortem echographic examination of the isolated carotids and the serial hystologic examination of the vessel.

In our experience, Echo–Doppler seems to offer the highest reliability in assessing the topography, the quantitative features, and the haemodynamic relevance of the process.

On the other hand, the relationship between the ultrasonographic patterns and the hystopathological findings is not undisputed, and its clinical meaning remains partly unknown.

10.4.1 INTRODUCTION

The atherosclerosis of the common and internal carotid arteires in their extracranial segments is a relevant factor in the pathogenesis of cerebral ischaemic attacks. Arteriography has been, and still is, considered by most clinicians to be the major pre-operative diagnostic tool. However, most of the cases that the clinician has to deal with are represented by patients with weakness, dizziness, or confusion, diagnostic dilemmas in which the suspicion of transient ischaemic attack is very weak. At the same time, in these cases the clinician is required to evaluate the possibility of preventing a stroke by sending the patient to the vascular surgeon. Obviously, angiographic examination cannot be proposed for all these cases. For all these reasons, non-invasive investigations of carotid axes has been developed in recent years. The present study describes our protocol of study of the carotid arteries, including post mortem comparison between ultrasonographic and hystopathological findings, and discusses the relations between ultrasonograhic, hystopathological, and clinical aspects of the lesions.

† Istituto di Clinica Medica I, Università di Bari, Italy
‡ Cattedra di Patologia Cardiovascolare, Università di Bari, Italy
§ Cattedra di Chirurgia Vascolare, Università di Bari, Italy

10.4.2 METHODS

We used a Duplex scanner, with a 10 MHz high-resolution probe (Biosound 2000).

In the ultrasonographic study of the carotid we considered topographic, morphologic, quantitative, qualitative, and haemodynamic aspects of the lesions (Table 1).

Table 1—Aspects of atherosclerotic lesions

Topography	Level: Common (superior/medium/inferior portion) Bifurcation Internal (distance from bifurcation) Medial/lateral wall
Morphology and extension	Longitudinal and transversal diameter Regular/irregular/ulcerated surface Number of lesions
Ultrasonic patterns	Soft (hypo-echoic) Mixed (hypo/hyper-echoic) Hard (hyper-echoic) With/without acoustic shadowing
Haemodynamics	Laminar flow Low/high grade stenosis Occlusion

Besides the Echo–Doppler examination of the carotid we performed in all cases, a standard CW Doppler examination of the subclavian, vertebral, and ophthalmic arteries (Albano & Palasciano 1982).

Furthermore, our protocol include the post mortem echographic examination of the isolated carotids. After resection, carotids were immersed in isotonic saline and were observed under the best conditions for high quality imaging. Finally, macroscopic and serial hystolic examination of the vessel were performed.

10.4.3 CLINICAL AND ULTRASONOGRAPHIC FEATURES OF PATIENTS

From January 1984 to September 1987 we performed 452 ultrasonographic examinations of carotid axes (mean age 62 ± 13 years, range 26–84, Male: 291, Female: 161). In 160 cases a TIA was suspected; in 43 cases patients had had a major ischaemia episode; in the other cases, the examination had been requested as a screening test in patients having one or more vascular risk factors and/or previous diagnosis of atherosclerosis of lower limbs. We used an arbitrary score for the association of risk factors, giving the value of one to each of them (e.g.: smoke + hypertension = 2). The diagnosis of atherosclerosis of lower limbs was made in most cases by clinical and CW–Doppler examination, and in 53 cases it was confirmed by angiography. In 330 patients we found one or more lesions of the vessel wall; all these cases were considered pathological. Among these lesions 265 did not determine alterations of the blood flow, 43 provoked a stenosis, and in 22 cases the internal carotid was occluded. In 14 cases we diagnosed subclavian steal syndrome. Among pathological examinations the number of lesions was significantly correlated with the age ($p < 0.05$), and the presence of one or more risk factors ($p < 0.005$). The presence of haemodynamically significant stenosis was significantly higher in symptomatic than in asymptomatic patients ($p < 0.05$), without any difference among those who had major and transitory neurologic symptoms. Internal carotid occlusion was more frequent in symptomatic patients ($p < 0.05$) than in asymptomatic and in patients with stroke compared with those with TIA, although in this case the difference was less significant ($p < 0.07$). Patients with symptomatic subclavian steal syndrome had a higher incidence of carotid lesions than asymptomatic patients ($p < 0.05$). Lesions of the carotid were significantly more frequent (76%) in patients with atherosclerosis of the lower limbs than in those without ($p < 0.01$). The finding of more than one lesion on one side was very often (68% of cases) associated with lesions on the other side.

Since August 1987 we have examined 16 carotids from 8 consecutive autopsies (Male: 6, Female: 2; mean age 72 ± 5 years) by post mortem echography. The comparison with macroscopic and hystologic examination gave the following results. There was a very strong correlation between US and macroscopic findings concerning the level ($r = 0.91$, $p < 0.001$) and the longitudinal diameter ($r = 0.86$, $p < 0.005$) of the lesions. The echographic examination was also very accurate in differentiating lesions with regular surface, while it was not so accurate as to differentiate irregular from ulcerated lesions. Echography was unable to detect 30% of non-stenosing lesions situated more than 2.5 cm from carotid bifurcation.

A statistical analysis of microscopic findings is not possible, because of the small number of lesions examined. Mixed echographic patterns represented 78% of lesions. Hystologically, this pattern corresponded both to uncomplicated lesions (40% of observations, fibrous tissue/foam cells) and complicated lesions (60% of observations haemorrhage/thrombosis/calcium). Among homogeneous patterns, 65% were described as hyperechoic. In these cases the lesions were more often fibrous plaques, but in 25% of cases lesions were considered to be complicated by hystology. Hypoechoic homogeneous pattern was observed in only two cases, corresponding to small non-complicated plaques, rich in lipids. The correlation between acoustic shadowing and the presence of calcium in complicated lesions was confirmed in all cases. The association of three signs (mixed pattern with acoustic shadowing, irregular/ulcerated surface, longitudinal diameter > 2 cm) corresponded in all cases to the hystological finding of complicated lesions.

10.4.4 CONCLUSIONS

Many authors (Harrison & Marshall 1982, Julian *et al.* 1963, Moore *et al.* 1978, Powers *et al.* 1987, Ziegler *et al.* 1973) have reported the correlation between the extension and severity of atherosclerotic lesions and the occurrence of clinical events, but the predictive value of carotid lesions is still very unclear. In our opinion, this could be due to two main factors. First, we cannot evaluate in all patients with suspected neurologic ischaemic symptoms of the intracranial and extracranial extent of vascular lesions. Second, we do not know the hystopathological equivalent of the lesions that we are able to diagnose. We have essentially two methods for evaluating the extent of atherosclerosis in cerebral vessels: ultrasounds (echographic and Doppler examinations) and angiographic techniques.

Echo–Doppler examination is commonly considered to be a reliable non-invasive method of identifying atherosclerotic lesions. This conviction is based on the fact that previous observations have shown good correlations between individual atherosclerotic lesions identified by B-mode ultrasonography and by angiography. We do not believe that the meaning of this correlation should be over-estimated, since the focus of the angiographic assessment is the arterial lumen, while that of B-mode is the arterial wall. Furthermore, we believe that high-resolution US devices are more sensitive than angiography in detecting small lesions (i.e. less than 2 mm), and many reports indicate that even for extensive lesions echography is more accurate than venous digital subtraction angiography. For these reasons we do not consider angiography as the reference method for evaluating the reliability of Echo–Doppler, and we believe that contrastographic examination should be performed only in very selected cases of symptomatic patients who are proposed for surgery.

On the other hand, the possibility of investigating the intracranial vascular system is the undeniable advantage of the contrastographic techniques.

In our experience, Echo–Doppler seems to offer the highest reliability in assessing the topography, the quantitative features, and the haemodynamic relevance of the process. This study shows that the severity of atherosclerotic disease is correlated with the presence, but not with the severity, of neurological symptoms, except perhaps for the association between haemodynamic occlusion and stroke. It also confirms our previous observation on the higher frequency of symptomatic subclavian steal syndrome in patients with concomitant carotid lesions (Sabbà *et al.* 1983). Furthermore, it confirms the importance of ultrasonographic screening examination in middle-aged subjects, with one or more risk factors (Crouse *et al.* 1986, Landi *et al.* 1987, Mannarino *et al.* 1986).

On the other hand, the relationship between the ultrasonographic patterns and the hystopathological findings is not universally accepted, and its clinical meaning remains partly unknown. The isolated US findings do not seem clearly correlated with the symptoms or with the hystopathological findings, as previously described by other authors (Spagnoli *et al.* 1985). However, the association between three US signs (i.e. mixed pattern, irregular-ulcerated surface, longitudinal diameter >2 cm) is highly correlated with the findings of complicated lesions by hystology. Whether this could be considered as a predictive sign for the occurrence of neurologic ischaemic symptoms is obviously not deducible from a retrospective study such as the present one. Thus, if the final results of this study confirm the high predictivity of the association of echographic signs in the diagnosis of complicated atheroma, the predictivity of non-invasive investigation for the occurrence of ischaemic cerebrovascular episodes will deserve a prospective study.

REFERENCES

Albano, O. & Palasciano, G. (eds) (1982). Atlante di ecografia clinica. *Masson-Italia*, **82,** 112.

Crouse, J. R., Harpold, G. H., Kahl, F. R., Toole, J. F., & McKinney, W. M. (1986). Evaluation of a scoring system for extracranial carotid atherosclerosis extent with B-mode ultrasound. *Stroke* **17** No 2, 270–275.

Harrison, M. J. G. & Marshall, J. (1982). Prognostic significance of severity of carotid atheroma in early manifestations of cerebrovascular disease. *Stroke* **13,** 567–579.

Julian, O. C., Dye, W. S., Javid , H., & Hunter, J. A. (1963). Ulcerative lesions of the carotid artery bifurcation. *Arch. Surg.* **86,** 803–809.

Landi, G., Guidotti, M., & Valsecchi, F. (1987). Influence of age on carotid atheroma in patients with reversible ischemic attacks. *Stroke* **18** No. 1, 43–45.

Mannarino, E., Susta, A., Tazza, D., Pistola, L., & Senin, U. (1986). Arteriosclerotic carotid lesions in hyperlipoproteinemia. *Angiography* Nov. 1986, 797–800.

Moore, W. S., Boren, C., Malone, J. M. *et al.* (1978). Natural history of nonstenotic asymptomatic ulcerative lesions of the carotid artery. *Arch. Surg.* **113,** 1352–1358.

Powers, W. G., Press, G. A., Grubb, R. L., Gado, M., & Raichle, M. E. (1987). The effect of hemodynamically significant carotid artery disease on the hemodynamic status of the cerebral circulation. *Ann. Int. Med.* **106,** 27–35.

Sabbà, C., Pugliese, D., Morizio, R., Carbone, P., Buonamico, P., Altamura, P., Portincasa, P., & Albano, O. (1983). La sindrome da furto della succlavia. *Minerva Angiol., Atti 5 Congr. Naz. Soc. It. Patol. Vasc.* 269–271.

Spagnoli, L. G., Zanette, E., Faraglia, V., Mauriello, A., & Buttinelli, C. (1985). Validazione istopatologica dei reperti ecotomografici di placche carotidee. *Gior. Arterioscl.* **2,** 95–108.

Ziegler, D. K. & Hassanein, R. S. (1973). Prognosis in patients with transient ischaemic attacks. *Stroke* **4,** 666–673.

10.5 A method proposed for the preparation of plasma membranes from myocytes of human gall bladders

P. Portincasa†, G. M. Murphy†, R. H. Dowling†, G. Palasciano‡, & O. Albano‡

Gall bladder (GB) emptying is slower and less complete in gallstone patients whether assessed by scintigraphic techniques or by ultrasound. One possible hypothesis is that cholelithiasis is associated with an altered cholecystokinin (CCK) receptor interaction at the level of smooth muscle membranes in the GB (impaired 'end-organ' response).

The isolation of plasma membranes (PMs) from target organs provides receptor-enriched fractions suitable for morphological, enzymatic, and radioligand characterization.

The authors employed and compared three methods for the isolation of PMs (Percoll density gradient, differential centrifugation along, and discontinuous sucrose density gradient) from human GBs in 34 patients with gallstones. Morphological (electron microscopy) and enzymatic characterization (specific marker: 5′-nucleotidase) indicated that the second two methods provided the best PM recovery.

The authors suggest that these PM fractions are suitable for further studies, including radioligand assays for specific CCK receptors in humans GBs.

10.5.1 INTRODUCTION

Little is known about myocyte membranes and hormone interaction in the animal and human gall bladders (GB). Moreover, impaired GB motor-function is frequent in gallstone patients, as shown by several studies where GB emptying is slower and less complete than normal whether assessed by scintigraphic methods or by ultrasound (Forgacs *et al.* 1984, Krishnamurthy *et al.* 1983, Thompson *et al.* 1982, Zhu *et al.* 1985). One possible explanation for these findings is that cholelithiasis is associated with an altered cholecystokinin (CCK) receptor interaction at the level of myocyte membranes in the GB wall. Plasma membranes (PMs) are obtained by physical separations from the extracellular environment (Evans 1978), and several authors used different separation techniques to obtain purified fractions from a variety of tissues and cellular preparations (De Duve 1971, Takeuki & Terayama 1965, Neville 1976, Peter *et al.* 1972, Carroll & Sereda 1968). In the present paper we describe methods developed for the isolation of human GB muscle membranes which are suitable for morphological, enzymatic, and receptor binding studies.

† Gastroenterology Unit, Dept. of Medicine, UMDS, Guy's Hospital, London SE1 9RT, UK
‡ Istituto di Clinica Medica I, University of Bari, Policlinico, 70124 Bari, Italy

10.5.2 MATERIALS AND METHODS

Bovine Serum Albumin (BSA), MES, bacitracin and SBTI (Soybean Tripsin Inhibitor), were purchased from SIGMA Chemicals. Percoll and density marker beads were purchased from Pharmacia Fine Chemicals.

10.5.21 Biochemical assays

Protein was determined by the method of Lowry (1951) using BSA as standard. The marker enzyme 5′-nucleotidase (EC 3.1.3.5) was measured in the membrane fractions, using the method described by Matlib *et al.* (1979).

10.5.2.2 Tissue handling

Human gall bladders, obtained from patients undergoing elective cholecystectomy, were placed immediately on ice. The pathologist kept a body-fundus strip plus the neck for histological examination; the remaining samples were rinsed free of bile and washed with saline at 4°C. The serosa was dissected off from the underlying muscle, and discarded: the mucosal surface was also removed (as much as possible) by scraping with a blade. The weight of the 'pure' muscle preparation ranged from 3 to 6 g for each GB. The specimens were either used individually or pooled (see Table 1). The tissue was blotted dry on filter paper, weighed, and minced in a 10% w/v solution (50 mM TRIS pH 7.4, 8% sucrose + 1 mg/ml SBTI + 0.25 mg/ml bacitracin and 1 mM EDTA). The homogenate obtained with an Ultra-Turrax homogenizer (30 s, allowing some cooling between the bursts) was filtered first through two and then through four layers of cheesecloth. The pools were collected.

10.5.2.3 Percoll gradient preparation

An iso-osmotic solution was obtained by adding 9 parts (v/v) of Percoll to 1 part (v/v) of 2.5 M sucrose to yield a final density of 1.05 g/ml. The homogenate was first spun at 25 000 × *g*, 20 min, the pellets (2–3 ml) layered on the top of the Percoll solution (in 38.5 ml polycarbonate Beckman tubes) and spun at 50 000 × *g*, 25 min in a 70 Ti fixed angle rotor on a L-8M BecKman ultracentrifuge). A broad band was collected (density ranging from 1.039 to 1.049 g/ml as assessed in preliminary experiments using different times of centrifugation and colour-coded marker beads to monitor the gradient shape) (Pertoft & Laurent 1977, Pertoft *et al.* 1978, Laurent *et al.* 1980, Jenkins *et al.* 1979).

10.5.24 Differential centrifugation

The homogenate was spun at 1500 × *g*, 15 min, the supernatant collected (Post Nuclear Supernatant) and spun at 10 000 × *g*, 15 min. Again, the supernatant remaining was spun at 25 000 × *g*, 30 min (Pellets = PM1) and the last supernatant spun at 200 000 × *g*, 60 min (Pellets = PM2). The fractions PM1, PM2 were collected.

10.5.25 Discontinuous sucrose density gradient

The method developed by Steigerwalt *et al.* (1984) for bovine GBs was used and modified (Ahmad *et al.* 1987). The homogenate was first spun at 40 000 × *g*, 25 min, the pellets were then resuspended a in few ml of buffer, homogenized again, and layered onto the top of a discontinuous sucrose gradient (14%, 25%, 35%, 40%, 48% w/v). Membranes were spun at 100 000 × *g*, 65 min using the swinging bucket SW1 rotor of a Beckman L-8M ultracentrifuge. The fractions formed at each sucrose interface (F0 at 8–14%, F1 at 14–25%, F2 at 25–35%, F3 at 35–40%, F4 at 40–48%, and debris at the bottom of the tube) were collected, washed, and suspended in 1 ml of binding buffer (MES pH 6.5 + EGTA 1 mM + SBTI 0.2 mg/ml + BAC 0.25 mg/ml but without BSA). The fractions were stored at −70°C before analysis.

10.5.2.6 Morphological characterization (EM)

Membrane fractions were fixed in glutaraldehyde, dehydrated in ethanol, and impregnated with medium-TAAB epoxy-resin polymerized. Thin sections (70–100 nm) werecut, stained with saturated uranyl-acetate and lead citrate, and examined with an Hitachi-HU-12-TM transmission electron microscope. Photomicrographs of randomly selected areas were taken at various magnifications.

10.5.3 RESULTS (see Table 1)

As described in the *Materials and methods* section myocytic plasma GBs were collected from 34 patients. Isolation of membranes was achieved with Percoll density gradient in 15 GBs (5 pools of 1 to 4 GBs). Differential centrifugation was used in 4 GBs (2 pools of 3 and 1 GB each). 15 GBs were studied, using discontinuous sucrose density gradient (6 pools from 1 to 4 GBs each). Females represented the majority of the

Table 1—Clinical, biochemical, and morphological features of the GBs and PM fractions studied as described in the *Material and methods* and *Results* sections

	Percoll density gradient	Differential centrifugation	Discontinuous sucrose density gradient
GBs (n)	15	4	15
pools	5	2	5
GBs/pool			
min–max	1–4	1–3	1–4
M:F	6:9	0:4	2:13
Age years			
(mean ± SD)	52 ± 17	61 ± 19	51 ± 18
(range)	(25–80)	(44–88)	(23–80)
Stones:			
single	5	—	2
multiple	10	4	13
Fractions isolated	1 band	PM1, PM2	F0–F4 + debris
EM (morphology)	+ (vesicles)	+ + + (vesicles)	+ + (vesicles)
5′-NT enrichment			
(folds; means)	1.7 ($n = 5$)	3.6 ($n = 4$)	F0 = 1.5 ($n = 1$) F1 = 4 ($n = 6$) F2 = 3 ($n = 6$) F3 = 1.6 ($n = 6$)

patients undergoing cholectystectomy were woman who were, on average, younger (13 yr) than the men (48 ± 18 SD vs 63 ± 10 SD yr). All the cholecystectomy specimens contained gall stones which ranged in number from 1–200. The size of each stone varied from 2–3 mm to 25 mm in diameter. All the stones were classified as 'mixed type' at the gross examination.

10.5.3.1 Histology

All the GB specimens (routine H-E sections) showed inflammation with fibrosis extending into, and disrupting, a mildly hypertrophic muscle layer. The final histopathological diagnosis was of a chronic calculous cholecystitis and in a few cases, areas of 'acute on chronic' cholecystitis were found.

10.5.3.2 Electron microscopy

Percoll density gradient ultracentrifugation yielded a very broad band which was contaminated with other cellular subfraction. PMs were present mainly as vesicles which were spread throughout the fields. After differential centrifugation, vesicles were present in both PM1 and PM2 fractions. Larger (0.35 ± 0.09 SD μm) and smaller (0.18 ± 0.04 μm) vesicles were found in PM1 whereas a uniform population of smaller vesicles (0.13 ± 0.03 μm) was found in PM2 (Fig. 1). All the other fractions (homogenate, and 1000 × g and 10 000 × g) pellets were contaminated with lysosomes and mitochondria. EM, performed on the sucrose discontinuous density gradient, showed vesicles in F0 (identified in only preparation), F1, F2, F3 fractions (mixed population of bigger and smaller vesicles ranging from 0.11 to 0.70 μm) with very few mitochondria.

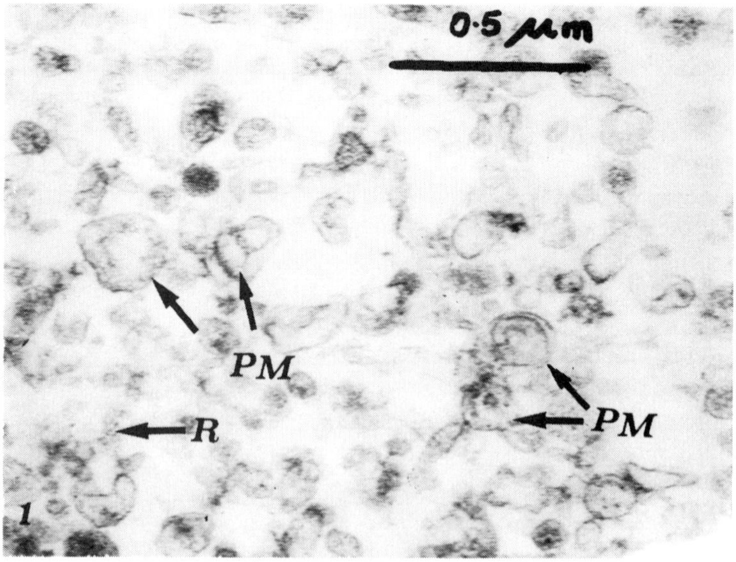

Fig. 1.—High-power electron micrograph of the fraction PM2 obtained after differential centrifugation as described in the *Material and methods* section. Note the presence of several vesicles (PM). Small amounts of ribosomes (R) are present in this fraction.

10.5.3.3 5′-nucleotidase (5′-NT) assay

The lowest degree of 5′-NT enrichment was seen in the band obtained with Percoll (1.67 ± 0.4 folds SEM) compared with the original homogenate. In 2 out of 5 preparations there was no enrichment with 5′-NT. After differential centrifugation, there was a better 5′-NT enrichment in both the PM1 and PM2 fractions (3.67 ± 0.53 SEM fold, $p < 0.02$) Table 1). Finally, with discontinuous sucrose density gradient, enzymatic enrichment was variable in the various fractions. Several experiments on each of them confirmed a max of 4, 3, and 1.6 fold enrichment for F1, F2, and F3 respectively (Table 2). There was no enrichment in the $40\,000 \times g$ supernatant and very low activity in the debris. Fractions F1 and F2 contained 40–91% of total enzymatic activity among the sucrose step fractions.

Table 2—5′-nucleotidase-specific activity in various fractions collected after sucrose discontinuous density gradient as described in detail in the *Material and methods* section. Specific activity expressed as μmol Pi/hr/mg protein (Matlib *et al.* 1979)

Fraction	5′-nucleotidase	No. of experiments
Homogenate	7.1 ± 1.2	7
F0	10.4	1
F1	28.0 ± 9.4	6
F2	21.1 ± 9.0	6
F3	11.0 ± 2.4	6
F4	8.6 ± 6.0	6
debris	4.62 ± 0.8	5

10.5.4 DISCUSSION

The first step in induced GB contraction is ligand binding of hormones and other endogenous substances as shown by human and animal models to specific membrane receptors. CCK is the most important stimulus (Amer 1972, Amer & McKinney 1972, Lin 1975, Yau *et al.* 1973) with the target area in the muscle layer of the organ. Although an impaired 'end organ' response has been found in GBs from gallstone patients (Fisher *et al.* 1982, Forgacs *et al.* 1984, Zhu *et al.* 1985, Pomeranz & Shaffer 1985) and in several animal models (Doty *et al.* 1983; Pellegrini *et al.* 1986, Fridhlander *et al.* 1983) we still do not know whether the altered motility antedates, or results from, the development of gallstones.

The isolation of PMs from target tissues is, therefore, an important way to provide receptor-enriched fractions suitable for further radioligand studies using a variety of hormones and endogenous/exogenous substances. Similar studies have been carried out using pancreas (Innis & Snyder 1980, Miller *et al.* 1981, Pearson & Miller 1986), gastric smooth muscle cells (Miller 1984, Pearson & Miller 1986), or GBs from animals (Steigerwalt *et al.* 1984, Singh *et al.* 1986, Shaw *et al.* 1986): from bovine/rabbit, dog, and rabbit or man (gallstone patients) (Portincasa *et al.* 1986, Upp *et al.* 1987). We evaluated the techniques currently available to isolate smooth muscle PMs, trying to overcome some of the peculiar problems when working with human samples. In our experience, the GB serosa was easily dissected from the underlying layers in all cases. Even when specimens were inflammed and thickened, a layer of fibrous, or sometimes fatty, tissue provided a natural plane of cleavage from which the external layer could be peeled off. On the other hand, preliminary histologial studies showed that irregularly oriented smooth muscle bundles (200–1000 μM) were often deeply intertwined with fibrous tissue and frequently extended into the superficial folds, thus making mucosal dissection almost impossible. Scraping of the mucosal surface with a blade guaranteed a 'purer' muscle preparation whilst preserving the muscle layer intact. Effective fragmentation of the muscle preparation was ensured by using the Ultra-Turrax (or Polytron) homogenizer, owing to the hardness of the fibrous tissue of the GB wall. Indeed, the EM carried out in some of the homogenates did not show intact cells or nuclei, a prerequisite for a better isolation of PM fractions.

The activity of the enzyme 5′-NT was considered to be the best PM marker (Kidwai *et al.* 1976, Matlib *et al.* 1979, Ahmad *et al.* 1987, Kwan *et al.* 1982, Miller 1984). The low enrichment shown in the bands after Percoll procedures might be the result of small PM vesicles production during homogenization which reduces the amount of vesicles spun down at $25\,000 \times g$ (with high 5′-NT activity left in the supernatant). Indirect support for this hypothesis was obtained from differential centrifugation when low enzymatic activity was shown in the $1500 \times g$ and $10\,000 \times g$ pellets with most of the activity in the PM1 ($25\,000 \times g$) and PM2 ($200\,000 \times g$) fractions as confirmed by EM. It must be pointed out, however, that 5′-NT activity was still detected in the $200\,000 \times g$ supernatant, resulting either from the presence of very small and few vesicles or from a 'soluble' enzymatic activity (hypothesis supported by Kidwai *et al.* 1971 and Portincasa, unpublished observations).

The data on discontinuous sucrose density gradient showed a consistent enrichment in the lightest fractions (F0, F1, F2, F3). The enzymatic assay give reproducible results. Moreover, preliminary experimental data with radioligand assay carried out in our lab, confirm that reversible and saturable CCK-OP binding can be shown in these fractions, allowing an estimation of the hormone-binding capacity and affinity for specific receptors.

The lack of enough membrane preparations in the pools studied represented a serious problem in our study. We believe that the amount of muscle in normal GBs is about 8–10% of the total wall as assessed by morphometric studies of strips from the body-fundus (Portincasa *et al.* 1987) with a tendency to increase during chronic cholecystitis (without massive fibrosis). Despite this and the dissection, muscle mass can represent a minor part of the whole tissue (20 to 40%). This problem induced us to pool the specimens in order to increase the amount of smooth muscle membranes available for morphological and enzymatic studies and for subsequent radioligand assay.

However, a more extensive study involving several enzymatic markers (e.g. for mitochondria and endoplasmic reticulum), complete EM and radioligand assay will need more samples in each pool, and we cannot exclude, at this stage, the need for both differential centrifugation and sucrose density gradient, in order to obtain more enriched PM fractions.

10.5.5 CONCLUSIONS

Our study shows that isolation of smooth muscle PMs from human GBs is feasible, the most reliable techniques being differential centrifugation and/or discontinuous sucrose density gradient. However, the small amount of smooth muscle mass in the wall is still a limit to a full study in each GB. On the other hand, the PM fractions we purified are suitable for morphological, enzymatic, and binding studies to be applied to normal and inflamed tissues.

ACKNOWLEDGEMENTS

We are indebted to Dr Malcom Higgins, Dept. of Biochemistry, Guy's Hospital, to Dr Edwin E. Daniel and Dr Sultan Ahmad, McMaster University, Hamilton, Canada for helpful scientific discussions, to the Staff of the EM Unit, Guy's Hospital for technical assistance, to the Dept. of Surgery, Guy's Hospital for continuing longstanding cooperation, and to Ms Anna D'amico for secretarial assistance.

REFERENCES

Ahmad, S., Berezin, I., Vincent, J. P., Daniel, E. E. (1987). Neurotensin receptors in canine intestinal smooth muscle: preparation of plasma membranes and characterization of (Tyr3-125I)-labeled neurotensin binding. *Biochim. Biophys. Acta* **896,** 224–238.

Amer, M. S. (1972). Studies with cholecystokinin *in vivo*. III. Mechanism of the effect on the isolated rabbit gallbladder strips. *J. Pharmacol. Exp. Ther.* **183,** 527–34.

Amer, M. S. & McKinney, G. R. (1972). Studies with cholecystokinin *in vivo*. IV. Effects of cholecystokinin and related peptides on phosphodiesterase. *J. Pharmacol. Exp. Ther.* **183,** 535–48.

Carroll, P. M. & Sereda, D. D. (1968). Cell membrane of uterine smooth muscle. *Nature* **217,** 666–7.

Daniel, E. E., Grover, A. K., & Kwan, C. Y. (1982). Isolation and properties of plasma membrane from smooth muscle. *Fed. Proc.* **41,** 2898–2904.

De Duve, C. (1971). Tissue fractionation. Past and present. *J. Cell Biol.* **50,** 20D–55D.

Doty, J. E., Pitt, H. A., Kuchenbecher, S. L., & DenBesten, S. A. (1983). Impaired gallbladder emptying before gallstone formation in the prairie dog. *Gastroenterology* **85,** 168–174.

Evans, H. (1978). Preparation and characterisation of mammalian plasma membranes. In: *Laboratory techniques in biochemistry and molecular biology* (eds Work, T. S. & Work, E.). North Holland Publ. Comp. New York, Oxford.

Fisher, R. S., Rock, E., & Malmud, L. S. (1985). Cholinergic effects on gallbladder emptying in man. *Gastroenterology* **89,** 716–22.

Forgacs, I. C., Murphy, G. M., & Dowling, R. H. (1984). Influence of gallstones and UDCA on gallbladder emptying. *Gastroenterology* **87,** 299–307.

Fridhlander, T. M., Davison, J. S., & Shaffer, E. A. (1983). Defective gallbladder contactility in the ground squirrel and prairie dog during the early stages of cholesterol gallstone formation. *Gastroenterology* **85,** 830–836.

Innis, R. B. & Snyder, S. H. (1980). Distinct cholecystokinin receptors in brain and pancreas. *Proc. Natl. Acad. Sci. USA* **77,** 6917–21.

Jenkins, W. J., Clarkson, E., Milsom, J., & Sherlock, S. (1979). A simple analytical subcellular fractionation of liver biopsies with Percoll. *Clin. Sci.* **57,** 29P.

Kaminsky, D. L., Deshpande, Y., Thomas, L., Qualy, J., & Blank, W. (1985). Effect of oral ibuprofen on formation of prostaglandins E and F by human gallbladder muscle and mucusa. *Dig. Dis. Sci.* **30**(10), 933–940.

Kidwai, A. M., Radcliffe, M. A., & Daniel, E. E. (1977). Studies on smooth muscle plasma membrane. Isolation and characterization of plasma membranes from rat myometrium. *Biochim. Biophys. Acta* **233,** 538–549.

Krishnamurthy, G. I., Bobba, V. R., McConnell, D, Turner, F., Mesgazadeh, M., & Kingston, E. (1983). Quantitative biliary dynamics: introduction of a new noninvasive scintigraphic technique. *J. Nucl. Med.* **24,** 217–223.

Kwan, C. Y., Sakai, Y., Grover, A. K., & Lee, R. M. K. W. (1982). Isolation and characterization of plasma membrane fraction with gastric fundus smooth muscle of the rat. *Mol. Physiol.* **2,** 107–120.

Laurent, T. C., Ogston, A. G., & Pertoft, H. (1980). Physical chemical characterization of Percoll. II. Size and interaction of colloidal particles. *J. Colloid Interface Sci.* **76,** 133–141.

Laurent, T. C. & Pertoft, H. (1980). Physical chemical characterization of Percoll. III. Sodium binding. *J. Colloid Interface Sci.* **76,** 142–145.

Laurent, T. C., Pertoft, H., & Nordli, O. (1980). Physical chemical characterization of Percoll. I. Particle weight of the colloid. *J. Colloid Interface Sci.* **76,** 124–132.

Lennon, F., Feeley, T. M., Clanachan, A. S., & Scott, G. N. (1984). Effect of histamine receptor stimulation on diseased gallbladder and cystic duct. *Gastroenterology* **87,** 257–62.

Lin, T. M. (1975). Actions of gastrointestinal hormones and related peptides on the motor function of the biliary tract. *Gastroenterology* **69,** 1006–1022.

Lowry, O., Rosenbrough, N., Farr, A. L., & Randall, R. J. (1951). Protein measurement with folin reagent. *J. Biol. Chem.* **193,** 265–275.

Matlib, M. A., Crankshaw, J., Garfield, R. E., Kwan, C. Y., Branda, L. A., & Daniel, E. E. (1979). Characterization of membrane fractions and isolation of purified plasma membranes from rat myometrium. *J. Biol. Chem.* **254,** 1834–1839.

Miller, L. J., Reilly, W. M., Rosenzweig, S. A., & Jamieson, J. D. (1981). Preparation and characterization of a probe for the CCK-8 receptor N-alfa(125I-desamino-tyrosil)CCK-8 and its interactions with pancreatic acini. *J. Biol. Chem.* **193,** 265–275.

Miller, L. J. (1984). Characterization of cholecystokinin receptors on human gastric smooth muscle tumors. *Am. J. Physiol.* **247,** G402–G410.

Neville, D. M. Jr. (1976). The preparation of cell surface membrane enriched fractions. In: *Biochemical analysis of membranes* (Maddy, A. H. ed), London, Chapman and Hall, J. Wiley & Sons, Inc., NY. pp. 27–54.

Pearson, R. K. & Miller, L. J. (1986). A novel CCK binding protein in pancreatic membranes identified by affinity labelling with short receptors probes. *Gastroenterology* **90**(II), 1581. (abstract)

Pearson, R. K. & Miller, L. J. (1986). Structural analysis of the CCK receptor on human gastric smooth muscle tumor. *Gastroenterology* **90**(II), 1581. (abstract)

Pellegrini, C. A., Ryan, T., Broderick, W., & Way, L. W. (1986). Gallbladder filling and emptying during cholesterol gallstone formation in the prairie dog. A cholescintigraphic study. *Gastroenterology* **90,** 143–149.

Pertoft, H. & Laurent, T. C. (1977). Isopycnic separation of cells and cell organelles by centrifugation in modified colloidal silica gradients. In: *Methods of cell separation*, Vol. I (Catsimpoolas, N., ed). Plenum, Press NY, pp. 25–65.

Pertoft, H., Laurent, T. C., & Laas, T. (1978). Density gradients prepared from colloidal silica particles coated by PVP (Percoll). *Anal. Biochem.* **88,** 271–82.

Peter, T. J., Muller, M., & De Duve, C. (1972). Lysosomas of the arterial wall. Isolation and subcellular fractionation of cells from normal rabbit aorta. *J. Exp. Med.* **136,** 1117–1139.

Pomeranz, I. S. & Shaffer, E. A. (1985). Abnormal gallbladder emptying in a subgroup of patients with gallstones. *Gastroenterology* **88,** 787–791.

Portincasa, P., Howard, A., Murphy, G. M., & Dowling, R. H. (1986a). Cholecystokinin receptor binding by human gallbladder myocyte membranes. *Gut* **27,** A1261.

Portincasa, P., Howard, A., Murphy, G. M., & Dowling, R. H. (1986b). Cholecystokinin (CCK) receptors on human gallbladder myocyte membranes. *Reg. Peptides* **15,** 188.

Portincasa, P., Mittra, P., Maghsoudldoo, M., Murphy, G. M., & Dowling, R. H. (1987). An integrated study of gallbladder (GB) motorfunction in gallstone patients. *Gut* **28,** A1395.

Scatchard, G. (1949). Attraction of proteins for small molecules and ions. *Ann. NY Acad. Sci.* **46,** 660–672.

Shaw, M. J., Hadac, E. M., Pearson, R. K., Power, S. P., & Miller, J. (1986). Functional and biochemical characterization of gallbladder muscular CCK receptors. *Gastroenterology* **90**(5)II, 1636.

Shepherd, A. N., Gallacher, C., Ross, P. E., & Bouchier, I. A. D. (1986). Effect of cholecystokinin on epithelial cell proliferation in the guinea pig gallbladder and on human gallbladder tissue culture. *Gastroenterology* **90**(5), 1767.

Singh, P., Rae-Venter, B., Towsend, C. M. Jr., Khalil, T., & Thompson, J. C. (1985). Gastrin receptors in normal and malignant gastrointestinal mucosa: age-associated changes. *Am. J. Physiol.* **249,** G761–G769.

Singh, P., Singh, H., Towsend, C. M., Lardjiani, A., Lluis, F., Gomez, G., & Thompson, J. C. (1986). Binding kinetics of CCK receptor on gallbladder and pancreas are similar in humans, rabbit and dogs. *Gastroenterology* **90**(5)II, 1630.

Singletary, B. K., Van Thiel, D. H., & Eagon, P. K. (1986). Estrogen and progesteron receptors in human gallbladder. *Hepatology* **6**(4), 574–78.

Steigerwalt, R. W., Goldfine, I. D., & Williams, J. A. (1984). Characterization of cholecystokinin receptors on bovine gallbladder membranes. *Am. J. Physiology* **247,** G709–G714.

Takeuki, M. & Terayama, M. (1965). Preparation and chemic of composition of rat liver cell membranes. *Exp. Cell. Res.* **40,** 32–44.

Thompson, J. C., Fried, G. M., Odgen, D. N., Fagan, C. G., Inove, K., Wiener, I., & Watson, L. C. (1982). Correlation between release of cholecystokinin and contractions of the gallbladder in patients with gallstones. *Ann. Surg.* **145,** 670–5.

Upp, J. R., Nealon, W. H., Singh, P., Fagan, C. J., Jonas, A. S., Greeley, G. H., & Thompson, J. C. (1987). Correlation of cholecystokinin receptors with gallbladder contractility in patients with gallstones. *Ann. Surg.* **205**(6), 641–648.

Yau, W. M., Makhlouf, G. M., Edwards, L. E., & Farrar, J. T. (1973). Mode of action of cholecystokinin and related peptides on gallbladder muscle. *Gastroenterology* **65,** 451–456.

Zhu, X. G., Greeley, G. H., Newman, J., Wiener, I., Fagan, J. C., & Thompson, J. C. (1985). Correlations of *in vivo* measurements of contractility of the gallbladder with *in vitro* ultrasonographic findings in patients with gallstones. *Surg. Gynaecol. Obs.* **161,** 470–2.

10.6 Is an integrated study of gall bladders from normal and gallstone patients possible?

G. Palasciano, P. Portincasa, G. Baldassarre, V. Palmieri, E. Altomare, G. Vendemiale, & O. Albano†

Gallstone disease is a frequent condition in western countries.

Gallbladder (GB) motor-dysfunction is common in gallstone patients maybe because of an altered cholecystokinin receptor interaction at the level of the hormone target area (smooth muscle cells).

A possible way to answer whether the observed dysfunction is primitive or secondary (e.g. chronic cholecystitis) is an integrated study of the GB considering tensiometric properties of GB strips, histological score to assess chronic inflammation, measurement of muscle mass (morphometry), and cholecystokinin (CCK) radioligand assay.

In the present paper the authors describe the techniques which are being adopted.

10.6.1 Introduction

Gallstone disease is a frequent condition in western countries (Ingelfinger 1968, Friedman *et al.* 1966, GREPCO 1984, Barbara *et al.* 1984) with 70 to 80% of gallstones mainly composed of cholesterol.

In recent years more data have been given about the pathogenesis of the disease, and different approaches have been employed in order to study gallbladder (GB) motor-function which is frequently impaired in gallstone subjects.

The present paper describes an integrated *in vivo* study of the GB we are currently adopting to relate tensiometric properties of GB strips to the degree of inflammation, to the morphometry of GB wall, and to radioligand assay of cholecystokinin hormone (CCK).

10.6.2 MATERIALS AND METHODS

Fresh gall bladders (GBs) were collected from patients either undergoing elective cholecystectomy or organ transplant donors and immediately placed in Tyrode solution (37°C,) pH 7.4, pregassed with O_2 (95%) + CO_2 (5%).

The specimen was examined by a pathologist, and strips from both the neck and the body-fundus were kept for histological examination (routine H-E sections).

† Istituto di Clinica Medica I, University of Bari, Policlinico, 70124 Bari, Italy

10.6.2.1 Tensiometric studies

The remaining sample was placed on a dissecting plate where two to four longitudinal strips were dissected from the body-fundus (1.2 cm length × 0.2 cm width). The strips were suspended in a 10 ml organ-bath (Aimer Ltd U.K.) whose solution was prewarmed and continuously gassed. Contractile activity was recorded isometrically on a force displacement transducer (Grass FT03C, Quincy, Mass. USA) and displayed on a chart recorder. A resting tension of 0.5–0.7 g was initially applied, as suggested by several authors (Amer 1972, Behar & Biancani 1980, Doty *et al.* 1983) to guarantee the most reproducible response to stimuli.

Cumulative or single dose-response curves were subsequently constructed with various agonists either alone (e.g. cholecystokinin octapeptide: CCK-OP; acetylcholine: ACH; histamine) or with antagonists (e.g. proglumide, atropine, H1 and H2 blockers) (Fig. 1).

Finally, each strip was washed several times and fixed in formaline for histological studies and quantitative morphometry.

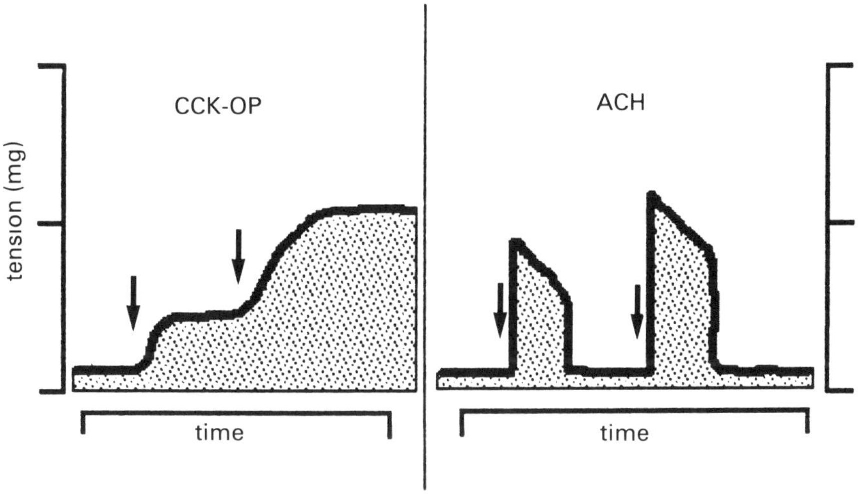

Fig. 1.—Tensiometric study: the schematic example shows the typical dose-response curves for increasing doses of CCK-OP and ACH respectively in human GB strips.

On the left: when CCK is added to the organ-bath, the tension increases slowly, reaching a plateau in 10–15 min, after which the next dose is added without washing the strip (cumulative increasing doses).

On the right: when ACH is added, the tension increases quickly, reaches the peak within seconds, and falls to the basal line in 1–2 min. The next dose is added after the tissue has been washed (single increasing or random doses).

10.6.2.2 Histological studies

The strips were stained with H-E and the degree of inflammation in the GB wall was assessed by a pathologist (unaware of all the previous studies), considering six parameters scored 0 to 3: fibrosis, Rokitansky–Aschoff sinuses, oedema, inflammatory infiltrate, cholesterolosis, necrosis (Kaminsky *et al.* 1985, Nahrwold *et al.* 1976, Portincasa *et al.* 1987). Myohypertrophy was separately assessed with quantitative morphometry.

10.6.2.3 Morphometry

Each strip used for tensiometric studies and already fixed in formalin, was embedded in paraffin and H-E stained; five consecutive transversal sections were cut and placed on the same slide. A personal computer (PC) coupled to a light microscope (2.5 ×) and a digitizer were used to assess the following parameters (means of five measurements per strip): thickness of the wall and muscle layer, cross-sectional area (CSA), muscle area, and percentage of muscle within the CSA (M%) (Fig. 2). Data relative to the tensiometry (tension developed as mg) can be subsequently normalized to the CSA and M% (kg/cm^2 (Herlihy & Murphy 1973, Ryan 1984, 1985).

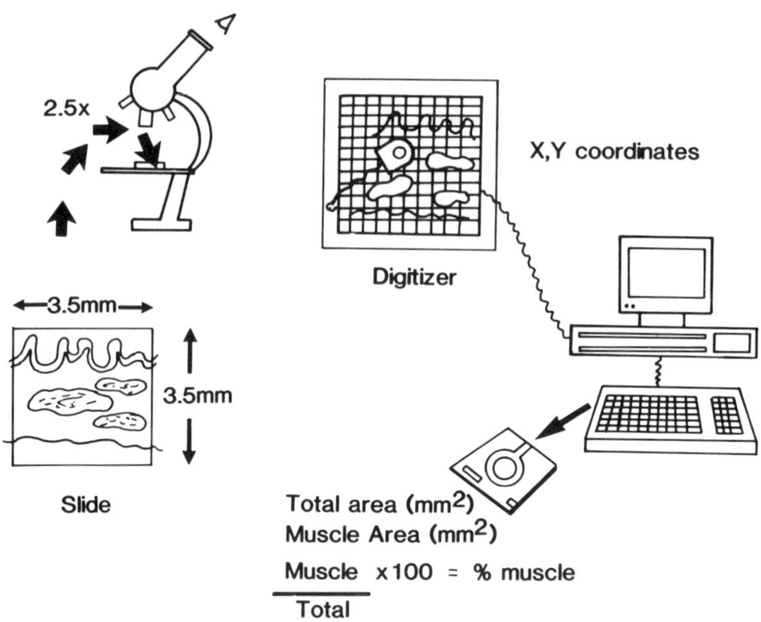

Fig. 2.—Method employed for morphometric studies of GB wall and strips: Routine H-E sections are evaluated under a light microscope. Standard fields of 3.5 × 3.5 mm are selected and different parameters are measured with a digitizer. Data are recorded and processed on a PC.

10.6.2.4 Radioligand assay

(a) Isolation of plasmamembranes

The remaining part of the GB, which was not used for tensiometric studies was immediately placed in ice. The serosa was dissected, the mucosa scraped with a blade to provide a 'pure' muscle preparation which was subsequently finely minced in a 10% w/v solution containing TRIS pH 7.4, EDTA, soybean trypsin inhibitor and bacitracin (Steigerwalt *et al.* 1984, Portincasa *et al.* in press). An ultra-Turrax homogenizer provided the final homogenate (30 s bursting time allowing some cooling between the bursts) which was collected.

The isolation of plasmamembranes (PMs) was obtained using differential centrifugation and eventually sucrose discontinuous density gradient as reported by several authors (Steigerwalt *et al.* 1984, Grover *et al.* 1980, Kidwai *et al.* 1971, Ahmad *et al.* 1987, Portincasa *et al.* in press).

Various fractions were subsequently collected and assayed for enzymatic markers (e.g. 5′-nucleotidase), morphological characterization, (electron microscopy) and radioligand assay.

(b) Binding studies
Experiments were performed in a final volume of 1 ml to which PMs (diluted to a final protein concentration of 0.1–0.2 mg/ml), radiolabelled hormone (3H-CCK-OP, 0.6–0.8 pM) and buffer (MES pH 6.5) were added. Incubation was carried out at 37°C for 90 min (Steigerwalt *et al.* 1984, Portincasa *et al.* 1986, Singh *et al.* 1986, Shaw *et al.* 1987). Non-specific binding (radiolabelled hormone which was not displaced by the addition of 'cold' hormone) was determined in a separate set of tubes to which a large excess of unlabelled CCK was added (1 μM).

The separation of bound from free hormone was obtained by filtration of the samples under reduced pressure, using a Millipore sampling manifold (mod. 1225) with nitrocellulose filters (0.45 μm pore size) on which bound hormone plus receptors were trapped. Radioactivity remaining on the filters was subsequently counted in a beta counter. Total, non-specific and specific binding were thereafter calculated and information on specific CCK-OP receptors binding capacity/affinity, association, and dissociation were derived.

10.6.3 DISCUSSION

Several animal models (Pellegrini *et al.* 1986, Fridhlander *et al.* 1983, Doty *et al.* 1983) and human studies (Table 1) have been developed to give an explanation for the reduced GB contraction seen in either all or a subgroup of patients with gallstones. Whether or not the deficit is primary or secondary to chronic cholecystitis and/or supersaturated bile (or to other factors) is still under investigation. More recently (Upp *et al.* 1987) a decrease in CCK-receptor number has been proposed as an early event in the pathogenesis of gallstone formation in some patients, by Forgacs *et al.* (1984).

Table 1—Methods employed for the study of human GB motility

in vivo:		
	Biliary output	Mok *et al.* (1980)
	Indocyanine green	van Berge Heunegouwen & Hoffmann (1978)
	Cholecystograms	Silva (1949)
	Ultrasound	Thompson *et al.* (1982), Forgacs *et al.* (1984), Upp *et al.* (1987)
	Radionuclide scanning	Fisher *et al.* (1982), Palisciano *et al.* (1983) Forgacs *et al.* (1984), Pomeranz & Shaffer (1985)
in vitro:		
	Tensiometry	Zhu *et al.* (1985), Portincasa *et al.* (1987)
	Radioligand assay	Portincasa *et al.* (1986), Upp *et al.* (1987)
	Histology	Lennon *et al.* (1984), Portincasa *et al.* (1987), Upp *et al.* (1987)

Few studies have related GB mechanics to quantitative histology of GB muscle mass, degree of inflammation of GB wall and CCK receptors (Zhu *et al.* 1985, Lennon *et al.* 1986, Portincasa *et al.* 1987, Upp *et al.* 1987); the importance of this relationship is that GB smooth muscle cells and their specific receptors represent the target area for CCK (Lin 1975, Amer *et al.* 1972, Yau *et al.* 1973). Moreover, myo-hypertrophy, -atrophy and muscle fragmentation are frequently found in inflammed GBs from gallstone patients.

The described protocol provides a detailed study of these factors in order to obtain information on muscle strength and receptor sensitivity (tensiometry), degree of inflammation and muscle mass (histology, morphometry), CCK receptor-binding affinity and capacity (radioligand study). Furthermore, newly adopted techniques (e.g. ultrasound or radionuclide scanning) can be associated to the above-mentioned methods to obtain a complete *in vitro* and *in vivo* study of the GB contractile properties in gallstone patients undergoing cholecystectomy.

In conclusion, it can be said that the described integrated studies (tensiometry, histological score, morphometry and radioligand assay) should provide new information on the role of smooth muscle and specific receptors (e.g. CCK, ACH) during different stages of gallstone disease.

ACKNOWLEDGEMENT

This chapter is based on work carried out by Dr Portincasa during the tenure of a research fellowship in the Gastroenterology Unit, Guy's Hospital, London, which was supervised by Dr G. M. Murphy and Professor R. H. Dowling.

REFERENCES

Ahmad, S., Berezin, I., Vincent, J. P., & Daniel, E. E. (1987). Neurotensin receptors in canine intestinal smooth muscle: preparation of plasma membranes and characterization of (Tyr3-125I)-labeled neurotensin binding. *Biochim. Biophys. Acta* **896,** 224–238.

Amer, M. S. (1972). Studies with cholecystokinin *in vivo*. III. Mechanism of the effect on the isolated rabbit gallbladder strips. *J. Pharmacol. Exp. Ther.* **183,** 527–534.

Barbara, L., Festi, D., Morselli-Labate, A. M., Roda, E., Rusticali, A. G., Sama, C., Sapio, C., & Taroni, F. (1984). The Sirmione study: familial frequency of gallstone disease. *Hepatology* **4,** 318–325.

Behar, J. & Biancani, P. (1980). Effect of cholecystokinin and the octapeptide of cholecystokinin on the feline sphincter of Oddi and gallbladder. Mechanism of action. *J. Clin. Invest.* **66,** 1231–1239.

Daniel, E. E., Grover, A. K., & Kwan, C. Y. (1982). Isolation and properties of plasma membrane from smooth muscle. *Fed. Proc.* **41,** 2898–2904.

Doty, J. E., Pitt, H. A., Kuchenbecher, S. L., & DenBesten, S. A. (1983). Impaired gallbladder emptying before gallstone formation in the prairie dog. *Gastroenterology* **85,** 168–174.

Fisher, R. S., Stelzer, F., Rock, E., & Malmud, L. S. (1982). Abnormal gallbladder emptying in patients with gallstones. *Dig. Dis. Sci.* **27,** 1019–1024.

Forgacs, I. C., Murphy, G. M., & Dowling, R. H. (1984). Influence of gallstones and UDCA on gallbladder emptying. *Gastroenterology* **87,** 299–307.

Fridhlander, T. M., Davison, J. S., & Shaffer, E. A. (1983). Defective gallbladder contactility in the ground squirrel and prairie dog during the early stages of cholesterol gallstone formation. *Gastroenterology* **85,** 830–836.

Friedman, D. G., Kamel, W. B., & Dawber, T. R. (1966). The epidemiology of gallbladder disease. Observations in the Framingham study. *Journal of Chronic Disease* **19,** 273–282.

GREPCO (Rome Group for the Epidemiology and Prevention of Cholelithiasis) (1984). Prevalence of gallstone disease in an Italian adult female population. *JAMA* **82,** 613–624.

Herlihy, J. T. & Murphy, R. A. (1973). Length–tension relationship of smooth muscle of the hog carotid artery. *Circulation Research* **23,** 275–283.

Ingelfinger, F. J. (1968). Digestive disease as a national problem. V. Gallstones. *Gastroenterology* **5,** 102–104.

Kaminsky, D. L., Deshpande, Y., Thomas, L., Qualy, J., & Blank, W. (1985). Effect of oral ibuprofen on formation of prostaglandins E and F by human gallbladder muscle and mucosa. *Dig. Dis. Sci.* **30**, 933–940.

Kidwai, A. M., Radcliffe, M. A., & Daniel, E. E. (1977). Studies on smooth muscle plasma membrane. Isolation and characterization of plasma membranes from rat myometrium. *Biochim. Biophys. Acta* **233,** 538–549.

Lennon, F., Feeley, T. M., Clanachan, A. S., & Scott, G. N. (1984). Effect of histamine receptor stimulation on diseased gallbladder and cystic duct. *Gastroenterology* **87,** 257–262.

Lin, T. M. (1975). Actions of gastrointestinal hormones and related peptides on the motor function of the biliary tract. *Gastroenterology* **69,** 1006–1022.

Mok, H. Y. I., von Bergmann, K., & Grundy, S. M. (1980). Kinetics of the enterohepatic circulation during fasting: biliary lipid secretion and gallbladder storage. *Gastroenterology* **78,** 1023–1033.

Nahrwold, D. L., Rose, R., & Ward, S. P. (1976). Abnormality in gallbladder morphology and function in patients with cholelithiasis. *Ann. Surg.* **184,** 415–421.

Palisciano, G., Balassarre, G., Albano, O. (1983) Ultrasonography in the study of gallbladder motility. In 'Clinical Advances in Ultrasonography', G. Labo *et al.* (Ed.), Masson Italia Editori, Milano, p. 117–119.

Pomeranz, I. S. & Shaffer, E. A. (1985). Abnormal gallbladder emptying in a subgroup of patients with gallstones. *Gastroenterology* **88,** 787–791.

Portincasa, P., Howard, A., Murphy, G. M., & Dowling, R. H. (1986a). Cholecystokinin receptor binding by human gallbladder myocyte membranes. *Gut* **27,** A1261.

Portincasa, P., Howard, A., Murphy, G. M., & Dowling, R. H. (1986b). Cholecystokinin (CCK) receptors on human gallbladder myocyte membranes. *Reg. Peptides* **15,** 188.

Portincasa, P., Mitra, P., Maghsoudldoo, M., Murphy, G. M., & Dowling, R. H. (1987). An integrated study of gallbladder (GB) motorfunction in gallstone patients. *Gut* **28,** A1395.

Portincasa, P., Murphy, G. M., Dowling, R. H., Palasciano, G., & Albano, O. A Method proposed for the isolation of plasmamembranes from GB of gallstone patients. (in press)

Ryan, J. P. (1984). Effect of pregnancy on gallbladder contractility in the guinea pig. *Gastroenterology* **87,** 674–678.

Ryan, J. P. (1985). Calcium and gallbladder smooth muscle contraction in the guinea pig: effect of pregnancy. *Gastroenterology* **89,** 1279–1285.

Scatchard, G. (1949). Attraction of proteins for small molecules and ions. *Ann. NY Acad. Sci.* **46,** 660–672.

Shaw, M. J., Hadac, E. M., Pearson, R. K., Power, S. P., & Miller, J. (1986). Functional and biochemical characterization of gallbladder muscular CCK receptors. *Gastroenterology* **90**(5)II, 1636.

Silva, G. (1949). A simple method for computing the volume of the human gallbladder. *Radiology* **52,** 904–912.

Singh, P., Singh, H., Towsend, C. M., Lardjiani, A., Lluis, F., Gomez, G., & Thompson, J. C. (1986). Binding kinetics of CCK receptor on gallbladder and pancreas are similar in humans, rabbits and dogs. *Abs. Gastroenterology* **90**(5)II, 1630.

Steigerwalt, R. W., Goldfine, I. D., & Williams, J. A. (1984). Characterization of cholecystokinin receptors on bovine gallbladder membranes. *Am. J. Physiology* **247,** G709–G714.

Thompson, J. C., Fried, G. M., Odgen, D. N., Fagan, C. G., Inove, K., Wiener, I., & Watson, L. C. (1982). Correlation between release of cholecystokinin and contractions of the gallbladder in patients with gallstones. *Ann. Surg.* **145,** 670–675.

Upp, J. R., Nealon, W. H., Singh, P., Fagan, C. J., Jonas, A. S., Greeley, G. H., & Thompson, J. C. (1987). Correlation of cholecystokinin receptors with gallbladder contractility in patients with gallstones. *Ann. Surg.* **205**(6), 641–648.

van Berge Heunegouwen, G. & Hoffmann, A. F. (1978). Nocturnal gallbladder storage and emptying in gallstone patients. and healthy subjects. *Gastroenterology* **75,** 879–885.

Yau, W. M., Makhlouf, G. M., Edwards, L. E., & Farrar, J. T. (1973). Mode of action of cholecystokinin and related peptides on gallbladder muscle. *Gastroenterology* **65,** 451–456.

Zhu, X. G., Greeley, G. H., Newman, J., Wiener, I., Fagan, J. C., & Thompson, J. C. (1985). Correlations of *in vivo* measurements of contractility of the gallbladder with *in vitro* ultrasonographic findings in patients with gallstones. *Surg. Gynaecol. Obs.* **161,** 470–472.

10.7 Thyroid hormone lowers the stimulatory effect of insulin on lipogenesis in cultured rat hepatocytes

G. V. Gnoni† & M. J. H. Geelen‡

(1) The rate of lipogenesis in hepatocyte cultures from hypothyroid rats is about half that in cultures from euthyroid animals.
(2) Addition of 3,3′,5 triiodo-L-thyronine (T_3) stimulates lipogenesis in both types of cultures, and brings the rate of lipogenesis in 'hypothyroid' cultures to values similar to those of 'euthyroid' cells.
(3) Treatment of the cultures with insulin results in a dose-dependent stimulation of lipogenesis in 'euthyroid' as well as 'hypothyroid' cells in both the absence and presence of T_3.
(4) Addition of T_3, however, reduces the insulin stimulation by about 30% and 15% in 'hypothyroid' and 'euthyroid' cells, respectively.

10.7.1 INTRODUCTION

Insulin is known to influence cellular behaviour. After binding to its receptor, this hormone initiates a large variety of cellular responses. The mechanism by which insulin-binding sets off these responses is unknown. One of the earliest events following insulin-binding is enhanced phosphorylation of the insulin receptor (Kasuga *et al.* 1982).

Thyroid hormones appear to influence the phosphorylation of the insulin receptor, e.g. thyroidectomy results in a several-fold increase in insulin-dependent phosphorylation of the β-subunit moiety of the insulin receptor in adipocytes (Corrèze *et al.* 1985). Whether this increase in receptor phosphorylation triggers any change in early cellular responses following insulin addition is not yet clear.

Lipogenesis in rat hepatocytes maintained in primary culture offers a suitable and convenient experimental system to study such early effects (Geelen & Gibson 1975, Gnoni *et al.* 1985). We, therefore, decided to investigate the effects of insulin and thyroid hormone on lipogenesis in monolayer cultures of hepatocytes isolated from hypothroid and from euthyroid donor rats.

† Laboratory of Biochemistry, University of Lecce, 73100 Lecce, Italy.
‡ Laboratory of Veterinary Biochemistry, University of Utrecht, P.O. Box 80.177, 3508 TD Utrecht, The Netherlands.

10.7.2. MATERIALS AND METHODS

Radioactive chemicals were purchased from the Radiochemical Centre, Amersham, bovine serum albumin (fraction V), collagenase type I, 3,3′,5 triiodothyronine and 6-*n*-propyl-2-thiouracil were from Sigma; culture medium was from Flow; other chemicals were from Baker. Crystalline bovine insulin was kindly donated by Lilly Labs. (Indianapolis, IN, USA).

Male Wistar rats weighing 250–300 g were used throughout in this study. The animals had free access to water and were fed a stock pelleted diet. A group of rats was made hypothyroid by continuous administration of 6-*n*-propyl-2-thiouracil (0.1% in drinking (tap) water) for 3–4 weeks (Corrèze *et al.* 1982). Animals were sacrificed between 8 and 9 a.m., and hepatocytes isolated essentially according to Seglen (1976) with modifications described earlier (Geelen *et al.* 1978). Culturing of cells was exactly as described previously (Gnoni *et al.* 1985). Following a 2-h plating period fresh medium without foetal calf serum was added with or without T_3 and/or insulin as indicated. In the sixth hour of the experiment lipogenesis was measured by following the rate of [1-^{14}C] acetate (0.96 mCi/mmol) or [^{3}H]H_2O (1mCi/ml) incorporation into fatty acids. Fresh medium, with the indicated hormonal addition, was added together with labelled substrates one hour before ending the experiment. Incubations were performed in triplicate. Other procedures were as described by Gnoni *et al.* (1985).

10.7.3 RESULTS AND DISCUSSION

To vary the thyroid hormone status of the cell preparation as much as possible hepatocytes from euthyroid as well as from hypothyroid donor rats have been incubated in the absence and presence of triiodothyronine (T_3). In agreement with earlier studies (Gnoni *et al.* 1985) the hepatocyte cultures from hypothyroid animals showed a smaller rate of lipogenesis than cultures from euthyroid animals (Fig. 1). Incubation of the cells with T_3 (1.48×10^{-5} M) enhances the rate of fatty acid synthesis in the two types of cultures (Fig. 1). The stimulation due to addition of T_3 is most pronounced in 'hypothyroid' cells. As a result of the T_3-treatment, the rate of fatty acid synthesis in 'hypothyroid' cultures reaches values similar to those of 'euthyroid' cultures.

In the two types of cultures the rate of fatty acid synthesis as a function of the insulin concentration was determined. If insulin was added to the cells following the 2-h plating period and the cultures were incubated for an additional 4 h, acetate incorporation in the last hour was markedly enhanced in comparison to controls that were incubated in the absence of added insulin (Fig. 1). In 'hypothyroid' as well as in 'euthyroid' cells a marked dose-dependent stimulation of fatty acid synthesis is apparent. In percentage terms the insulin-stimulation of fatty acid synthesis is most noticeable in hepatocytes from hypothyroid rats; however, at all insulin levels the actual values are less than those observed with 'euthyroid' cells.

Increasing the concentration of insulin in combination with a constant concentration of T_3 progressively enhances the rate of fatty acid synthesis in the two cell types (Fig. 1). However, the insulin stimulation in the presence of T_3 is consistently less as compared to the situation with no added T_3. In 'euthyroid' cells the insulin stimulation drops about 15%, whereas in 'hypothyroid' cells the fall is approximately 30%.

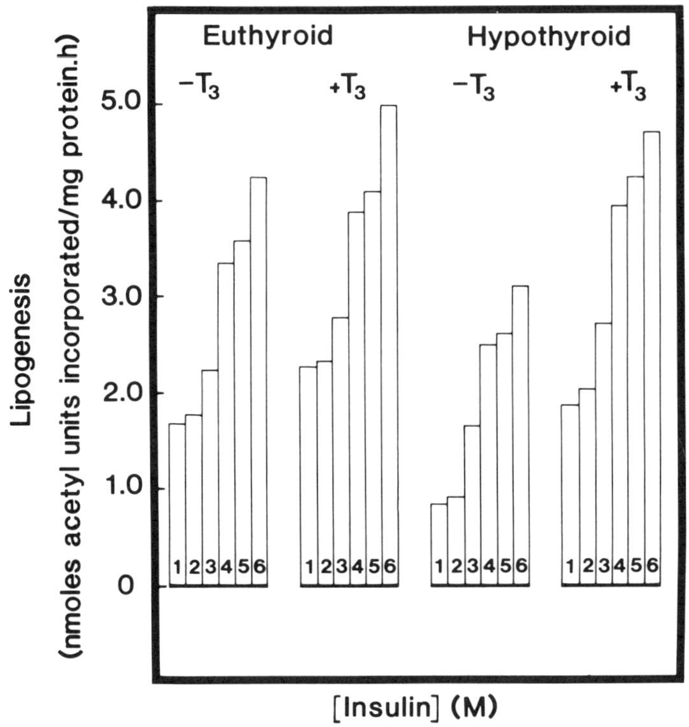

Fig. 1.—Effect of increasing concentrations of insulin on the rate of lipogenesis in hepatocyte cultures from euthyroid and hypothyroid rats, incubated in absence or presence of T_3 (1.48×10^{-5} M). Following a 2-h plating period the medium was changed and hormones added. After 3 h, fresh medium containing the appropriate additions together with labelled acetate was added. Reactions were stopped after incubation for an additional hour, and lipids extracted. Insulin was either absent (1) or present at one of the following concentrations: 2×10^{-11} M (2), 2×10^{-10} M (3), 2×10^{-9} M (4), 2×10^{-8} M (5) or 2×10^{-7} M (6). Values are expressed as the means of 3 experiments with triplicate assays for each experiment.

It could be argued that insulin and/or T_3 might affect the specific radioactivity of the intracellular [^{14}C] acetyl-CoA pool and thereby seemingly effect a stimulation of fatty acid synthesis. Therefore, studies were performed using [^{3}H]H_2O incorporation into lipids as an independent index of lipogenic activity (Jungas 1968). As shown in the experiment described in Table 1, insulin as well as T_3 increase the rate of synthesis of fatty acids, as measured by the rate of tritium incorporation.

Since the insulin response in maintenance cultures of hepatocytes is dependent on the thyroid hormone status of the cell donor, this isolated cell system should be useful in answering the question whether changes in the phosphorylation of the insulin receptor triggers changes in cellular response following addition of insulin and/or thyroid hormone.

From the results of this study, it would appear that, in maintenance cultures of isolated hepatocytes, thyroid hormones regulate the action of insulin. Whether this is the result of changes in the phosphorylation degree of the insulin receptor is under investigation.

Table 1—Effect of insulin and triiodothyronine (T_3) on fatty acid synthesis as measured by the ^3H_2O method

Addition	Fatty acid synthesis (nmoles acetyl units/mg protein per h)	
	Euthroid†	Hypothyroid†
None	2.99 ± 0.33	2.03 ± 0.27
T_3	3.62 ± 0.42	3.98 ± 0.47
Insulin	6.22 ± 0.90	5.01 ± 0.55

Cells were in contact with T_3 (1.48×10^{-5} M) or with insulin (2×10^{-8} M) for a total period of 4 h. Further details as described in Fig. 1. Values are expressed as the means $\pm$S.D. of 3 experiments. In each experiment determinations were done in triplicate.
† Thyroid state of the cell donor.

ACKNOWLEDGEMENTS

The authors wish to thank Prof. Dr S. G. van den Bergh for critically reading the manuscript. This research was supported by the Netherlands Foundation for Chemical Research (SON) with financial aid from the Netherlands Organization for the Advancement of Pure Research (ZWO). M.J.H.G. was the recipient of a travel grant from the latter organization.

REFERENCES

Corrèze, C., Berriche, S., Tamayo, L., & Nunez, J. (1982). Effect of thyroid hormones and cyclic AMP on some lipogenic enzymes of the fat cell. *Eur. J. Biochem.* **122,** 387–392.

Corrèze, C., Pierre, M., Thibout, H., & Toru-Delbauffe, D. (1985). Autophosphorylation of the insulin receptor in rat adipocytes is modulated by thyroid hormone status. *Biochem. Biophys. Res. Commun.* **126,** 1061–1068.

Geelen, M. J. H. & Gibson, D. M. (1975). Lipogenesis in maintenance cultures of rat hepatocytes. *FEBS Lett.* **58,** 334–339.

Geelen, M. J. H., Beynen, A. C., Christiansen, R. Z., Lepreau-Jose, M. J., & Gibson, D. M. (1978). Short-term effects of insulin and glucagon on lipid synthesis in isolated rat hepatocytes. *FEBS Lett.* **95,** 326–330.

Gnoni, G. V., Geelen, M. J. H., Bijleveld, C., Quagliariello, E., & van den Bergh, S. G. (1985). Short-term stimulation of lipogenesis by triiodothyronine in maintenance cultures of rat hepatocytes. *Biochem. Biophys. Res. Commun.* **128,** 525–530.

Jungas, R. L. (1968). Fatty acid synthesis in adipose tissue incubated in tritiated water. *Biochemistry* **7,** 3708–3717.

Kasuga, M., Zich, Y., Blithe, D. L., Karlsson, F. A., Harring, H. V., & Kahn, C. R. (1982). Insulin stimulation of phosphorylation of the β subunit of the insulin receptor. *J. Biol. Chem.* **257,** 9891–9894.

Seglen, P. O. (1976). Preparation of isolated rat liver cells. *Meth. Cell. Biol.* **13,** 29–83.

10.8 Isoelectric separation of prestained plasma lipoproteins: diagnostic and preparative aspects

D. Stathakos†, D. Kletsas†, G. Rekoumis‡, A. Avgerinos‡, & T. Kanaghinis‡

(1) Plasma lipoproteins prestained with tetrazolium blue can be separated by isoelectric focusing on 3.8% polyacrylamide gel-rods containing 3% carrier ampolytes, at 500 V.
(2) Low-density and high-density lipoproteins (LDL and HDL) are fractionated into their subspecies, which reach equilibrium at their isoelectric points in approx. 6 hours.
(3) Very-low-density lipoproteins (VLDL) enter the gel-matrix, but do not migrate to final focusing due to the porosity of the gel which is restrictive for these molecules.
(4) Lp-patterns obtained by this method are reproducible, and seem to be characteristic for various types of liver dysfunction.
(5) Furthermore, the fractionation of prestained lipoproteins on preparative scale by multiphasic electrofusing is discussed.

10.8.1 INTRODUCTION

During recent decades the nomenclature of plasma lipoproteins has been based mainly on operational terms, depending on the physical parameter used in each separation technique. Thus, hydrated density in ultracentrifugation determined their classification in chylomicrons, VLDL, LDL, and HDL, whereas molecular size and/or charge expressed in relative mobilities in electrophoresis suggested their classification in chylomicrons, pre-β, β, and α lipoproteins, respectively. Recently, new important parameters have been introduced, such as the specific apoprotein content in connection with the bound lipid in each subclass (Gotto *et al.* 1986), while reasonable suggestions have been made in favour of classifying lipoproteins according to their surface antigens (Coulhon *et al.* 1985).

For lipoprotein separation, composite multi-step procedures ranging from selective precipitation, chromatographic and immunochemical techniques to ultra-filtration have been added to the traditional ultracentrifugational methodology, with varying success (Busbee *et al.* 1981, McVicar *et al.* 1984, Luley *et al.* 1985). Among

† Laboratory for Enzyme Research, Biology Department, N.R.C. 'Demokritos', ‡ Research Unit, 'Evangelismos' Hospital, Athens, Greece.

Abbreviations: Lp, lipoprotein; VLDL, very-low-density lipoproteins; IDL, intermediate-density lipoproteins; LDL, low-density lipoproteins; HDL, high-density lipoproteins; PAGE, polyacrylamide gel electrophoresis; EDTA, ethylenediamine tetraecetic acid.

these, isoelectric focusing, in spite of its high resolving capacity, has been of limited efficiency in lipoprotein fractionation (Marcel & Weech 1986). In early experiments in liquid systems, aggregation and flocculation of focused lipoproteins was a major drawback, while the great disparity of their molecular size, ranging from 17.5×10^4 to $10–80 \times 10^6$ (Gotto *et al.* 1986) was practically prohibitive for focusing in gel systems. Nevertheless, isoelectric fractionation methods still offer the highest resolution in charge separation, especially for monitoring the heterogeneity of lipoprotein subfractions (Luley *et al.* 1985, Marcel & Weech 1986, Carlson *et al.* 1986). In an earlier report we described gel electrofocusing of plasma lipoproteins prestained with tetrazolium compounds (Stathakos *et al.* 1983). In more recent work, we have observed a high reproducibility of the isoelectric patterns obtained, and a consistent separation of the three major lipoprotein groups, suggesting the preparative potential of this technique. Some of these observations are reported here.

10.8.2 MATERIALS AND METHODS

Reagents

Tetrazolium blue chloride, NADH (disodium salt), phenazine methosulfate, acrylamide 4Xcryst, N,-N′-methylene bisacrylamide and N,N,N′,N′-tetramethyl ethylenediamine were purchased from Serva Feinbiochemica; Ampholine carrier ampholytes from LKB produkter AB.

Samples

Venous blood was collected with EDTA as anticoagulant after a 14 h fast. After centrifugation for the removal of chylomicrons, the plasma was stored at 2°C and processed within 4 h after collection.

Procedures

Prestaining of 1 ml of plasma was carried out by adding the following solutions: 100 μl of 5% NADH, 500 μl of 0.3% tetrazolium blue, and 20 μl of 0.1% phenazine methosulfate. The mixture was incubated for 60 min at 25°C and centrifuged for 6 min at 15 000 *g* to remove the insoluble formazan not bound to lipoproteins (Busbee *et al.* 1981).

The tetrazolium mixtures used here for prestaining are light-sensitive. Therefore, it is important to avoid exposure to direct light during staining of the plasma and electrofocusing.

Electrofocusing was performed in a vertical-gel-rod apparatus (M.R.A. Corp); 0.01 M H_3PO_4 and 0.02 M NaOH were used as anolyte (lower chamber) and catholyte (upper chamber), respectively, 3.8% polyacrylamide gels were used (if not otherwise indicated) in 100 mm-long tubes of I.D. 3 mm. Prerunning time was 30 min and the duration of the run 6 h at 500 V under constant cooling at 2°C. At the end of the run the gel was scanned (Joyce-Loebl Chromoscan) or segmented by use of a Hamilton syringe (Righetti & Drysdale 1974); the gel segments were shaken in CO_2-free water and pH was measured (Orion 801 pH meter) at 2°C.

10.8.3 RESULTS AND DISCUSSION

After pre-running, the sample is applied on the upper surface of the gel underneath an aqueous layer which separates it from the alkaline catholyte.

In the case of normal plasma, soon after the beginning of the run the bulk of prestained lipoproteins migrates readily toward the anode, while VLDL enter, very slowly, the gel matrix. At the end of the run, after 6 h at 500 V, the lipoprotein fractions have reached an apparent equilibrium as shown in Fig. 1A, and a clear-cut separation of three fractions is observed.

The farthest migrating fraction (HDL) is focused within the pH range 5.1–5.4. At higher pHs, approx. 6.1–6.8, a second fraction (LDL) focuses in a highly resolved pattern of very sharp intensely stained bands. The third fraction (VLDL) has barely

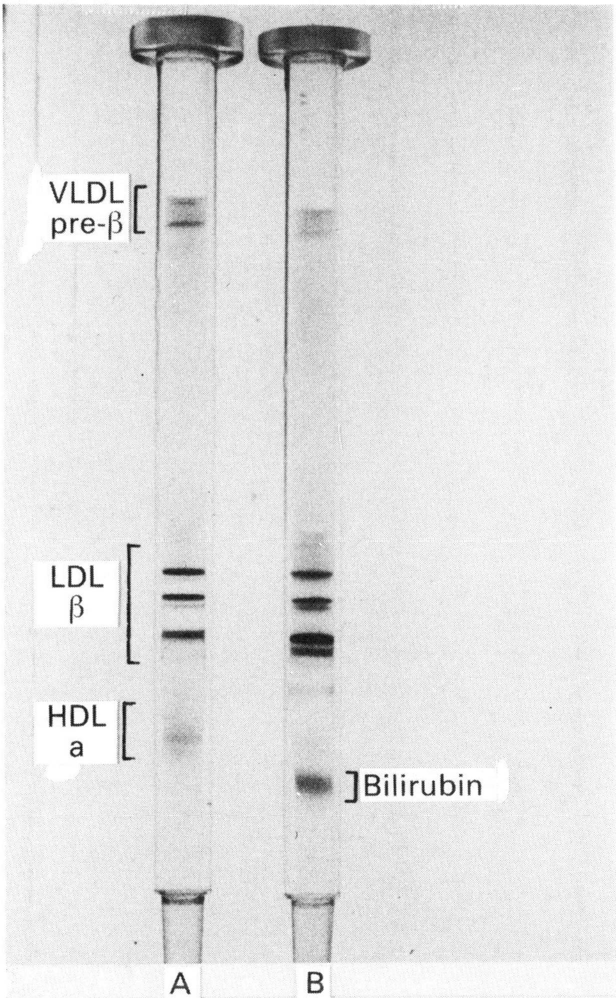

Fig. 1.—Isoelectric pattern of plasma lipoproteins, pH 3.5–10.0 (Sample: 20 μl of the tetrazolium-prestained mixture have been applied on the gel; for details see text)
A. Normal pattern.
B. Mild obstructive jaundice (see text).

penetrated the gel, albeit with the tendency to resolve into more than one subfractions. To identify the focused lipoproteins we compared them in their isoelectric distribution with the α, β, and pre-β fractions obtained by polysacrylamide gel electrophoresis according to Masket *et al.* (1973). Therefore, normal plasma prestained with tetrazolium blue was fractionated in polyacrylamide gels; the segments of the gel which contained the α, β, and pre-β lipoproteins were cut out, subsequently positioned separately on electrofocusing gel rods, and were run under the electrofocusing conditions described above. Indeed, after the normal 6-h run each fraction focused at the pH regions designated HDL, LDL, and VLDL, respectively, virtually reconstituting the initial isoelectric pattern as represented in Fig. 1A (Stathakos *et al.* 1983). Furthermore, when the lipoprotein fractions of Fig. 1 were cut out and refocused, the same Lp-profile was obtained and no deviations from the initial pIs suggestive of artifacts were observed.

Having thus established the identity of the focused fractions, we proceeded to examine how lipoprotein abnormalities would be expressed in the obtained pattern. Certainly, liver diseases are among those most extensively studied by gel electrophoresis, whereby considerable knowledge in lipoprotein phenotyping has accumulated. Thus, a generally accepted common feature of PAGE-patterns of plasma in hepatic lesion is the decrease or even deletion of α and pre-β lipoprotein bands (Taketa & Watanabe 1981). By applying our procedure to electrophoretically well-defined cases we obtained analogous changes in the Lp-pattern.

Fig. 1B represents a case of mild obstructive jaundice. The obstruction was established 20 days prior to the assay, and was due to choledocholithiasis: VLDL are reduced as compared to normal plasma (Fig. 1A), HDL are barely visible, while LDL are more dense with concomitant appearance of extra bands. A diffuse bilirubin band appears near the bottom of the gel rod.

Fig. 2 shows the electrofocusing pattern of plasma from a patient with severe long-standing obstructive jaundice due to carcinoma of the pancreas. Here, the VLDL and HDL fractions of normal plasma (cf. Fig. 2A) are deleted, while the LDL region presents a pattern resembling the one in Fig. 1B. The pattern of Fig. 2B, also observed in other similar cases, corresponds to that of obstructive jaundice with significant hepatocellular dysfunction, possibly related to the duration of the lesion. The method can also provide characteristic reproducible Lp-patterns for some types of parenchymal liver injury (e.g. cirrhosis, acute viral hepatitis), as well as recognize successive changes of the lipoprotein fractions during the course of the disease (Stathakos *et al.* 1984).

At this point some particular features of this procedure are worth considering for further development on analytical or scale-up level.

Firstly, it becomes obvious that before the method can be put to clinical use, extensive epidemiologic studies are needed to establish direct correlation between an isoelectric lipoprotein pattern as the ones presented and the clinical profile of each type of lipoprotein disorder. It must be emphasized that the Lp-subfractions are separated according to the pIs of the lipoprotein complexes, while the focused fractions are visualized by lipid staining. This presents a composite problem in trying to quantitate their isoelectric pattern by densitometry. Fig. 3 shows such a densitogram of normal plasma. Tetrazolium blue gives a uniform blue colour and a satisfactory quantitation of total lipoprotein in each peak. Efficient quantitation techniques have also been reported by Busbee *et al.* (1981) for the fractionation of neotetrazolium-prestained lipoproteins by size-exclusion chromatography. This, however, does not

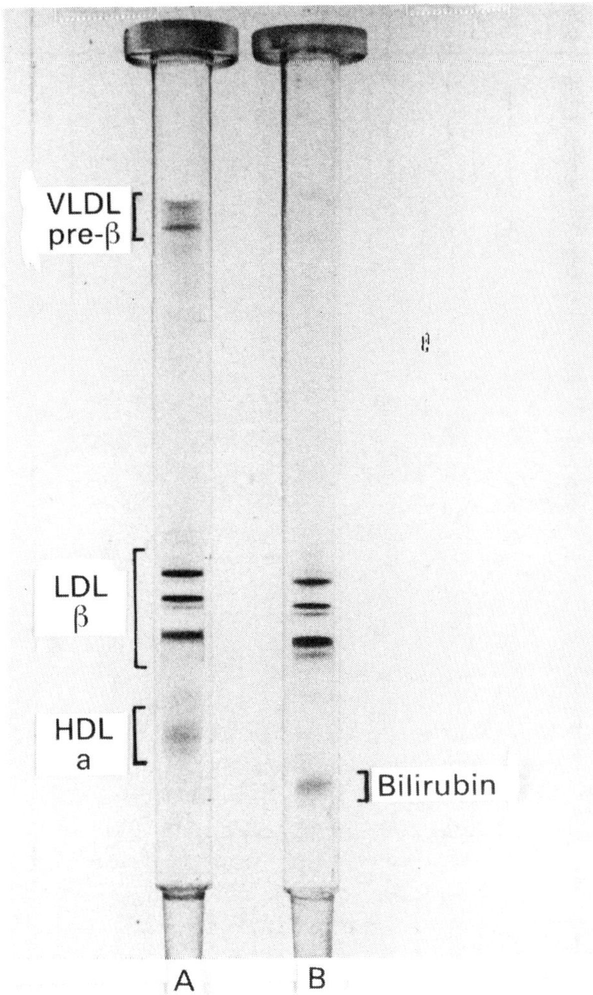

Fig. 2.—Isoelectric pattern of plasma lipoproteins, pH 3.5–10 (Sample as in Fig. 1).
A. Normal pattern.
B. Severe obstructive jaundice (see text).

always apply to isoelectric patterns of patient sera, where a change in apoprotein composition—and the pI—of a band may transpose it to a new position, while analogous changes of the lipid may affect the intensity of the colour, regardless of the lipoprotein content of the scanned fraction (Busbee *et al.* 1981). Hence, a systematic study of each subfraction in terms of lipid and apoprotein composition is needed. The latter has become quite feasible in recent years through immunological techniques (Coulhon *et al.* 1985).

Secondly, it seems reasonable to assume that this system can provide a clear one-step separation of the three major lipoprotein classes and also the isoelectric fractionation of HDL and LDL into their subspecies at reproducible isoelectric points. On the other hand, VLDL (and IDL) with particle sizes ranging from 20 to 80 nm (Gotto *et al.* 1986) are clearly unable to migrate through the gel to reach their pIs

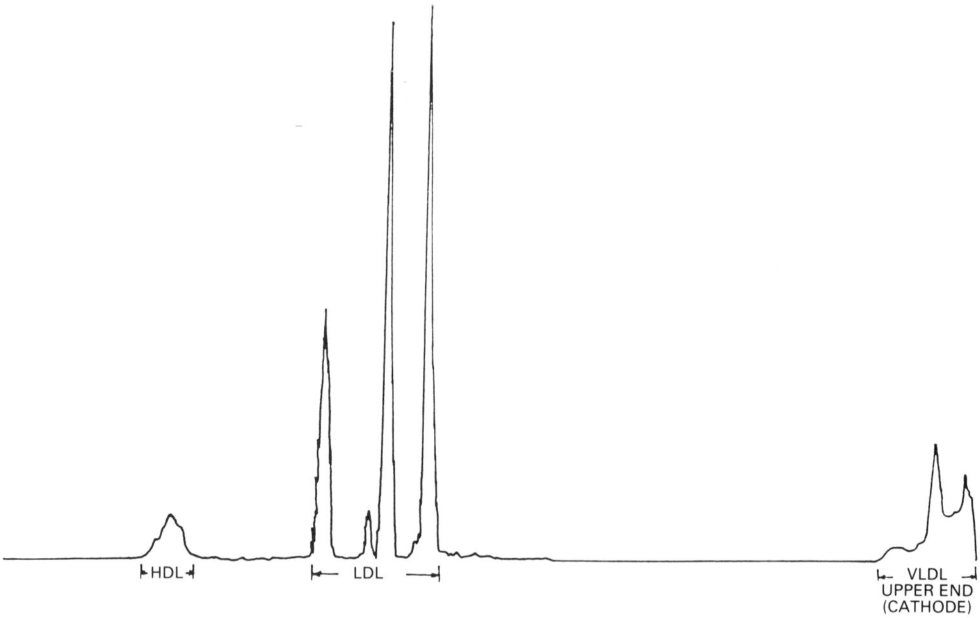

Fig. 3.—Densitogram of the pattern of normal plasma (620 nm filter; for details see text).

which can range down to about pH 5 (Stinson 1975, Marcel & Weech 1986). Moreover, their free migration to final equilibrium would result in a distribution of VLDL bands extending far into the LDL—and HDL pI patterns. It is the molecular-sieve effect of the 3.8% polyacrylamide-gel matrix which actually immobilizes VLDL while the other two Lp groups reach isoelectric equilibrium. In practical terms a higher resolution of HDL and LDL can thus be achieved by expanded-scale electrofocusing, e.g. in a pH gradient 5–8 instead of 3.5–10, while the VLDL still remains entrapped near the upper end of the gel tube. Of course, the distance between VLDL and LDL is thereby shortened by two pH units (cf. Fig. 1A and Fig. 3) (results not shown). Obviously, the resulting isoelectric patterns of HDL and LDL, as visualized by a non-destructive prestaining procedure, are also especially suitable for electrophoresis in the second dimension, in the absence or presence of denaturants, for further study of molecular size, origin and heterogeneity.

Finally, this technique can be scaled up to preparative level for improved separation. The multiphasic electrofocusing column shown in Fig. 4, originally designed for the isolation of serum growth factors (Antoniades *et al.* 1975), is largely based on the same principle as the gel-rod apparatus of Righetti & Drysdale (1974). It offers several advantages (for experimental details, see Stathakos *et al.* 1979) of which some are relevant to the problem discussed here:

(1) The column (I.D. 20 mm) is composed of several gel-units separated by thin aqueous interlayers. The pH gradient is formed throughout the column between top (cathode) and bottom (anode) electrodes.
(2) After electrofocusing, any gel-unit, i.e. actually a chosen ‘segment’ of the pH gradient with the respective focused bands entrapped in it, can be removed intact from the column and be incorporated into a new column containing carrier

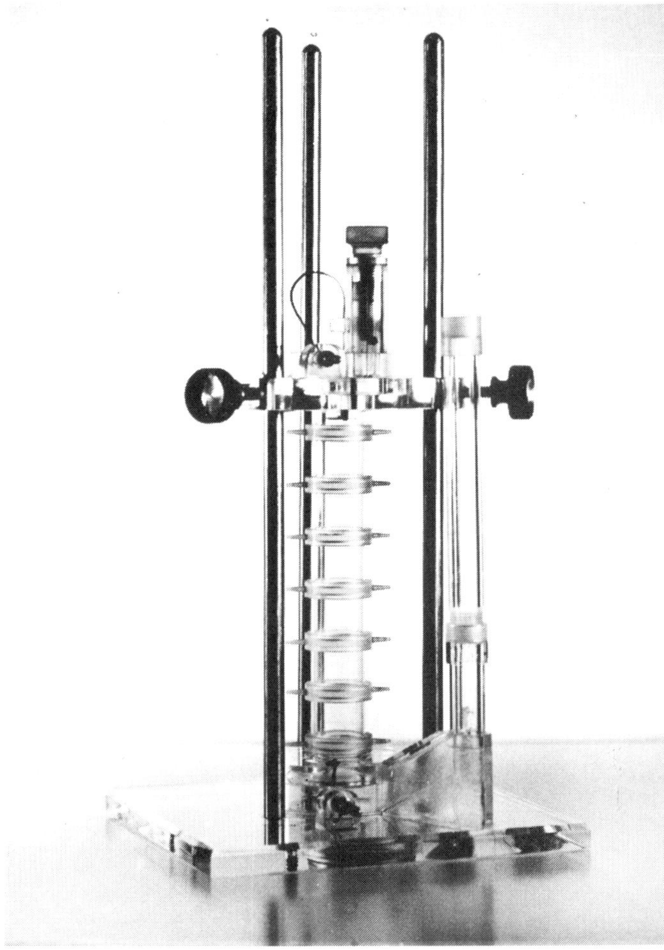

Fig. 4.—Multiphasic column for isoelectric focusing. View of an assembled column with six gel-units; I.D. 20 mm (Stathakos *et al.* 1979).

ampholytes of a narrow pH range. By refocusing in this column a further resolution is achieved. Sequential refocusing is theoretically unlimited and practical dependent on the carrier ampholytes available and their resolving capacity.

Considering the above, a plausible separation strategy for plasma lipoproteins would include initial focusing of the prestained plasma in a multiphasic column (Fig. 4) in a 3.8% polyacrylamide gel, and subsequent separation of the column segments containing the Lp fractions followed by:

(a) subsequent refocusing of the LDL and HDL 'segments' separately, until isolation of each subtraction is attained.
(b) Incorporation of the uppermost gel-unit which contains the practically immobilized VLDL into a new column as lowest unit, anodally, while all other units above it contain a non-restrictive polyacrylamide (e.g. 2.5%) or agarose or a granular

gel which allows the passage of VLDL during refocusing. Assuming that the VLDL molecules are not disrupted or damaged, they are thus forced to reverse their migration in the gel-matrix and move upwards into the 'Lp-free' pH gradient until they focus at their true isoelectric points.

These fractionation experiments will be the subject of a separate report.

ACKNOWLEDGEMENTS

The skilful technical assistance of Mr J. Lagouros and Mrs H. Sevaslidou is gratefully acknowledged.

REFERENCES

Antoniades, H. N., Stathakos, D., & Scher, C. D. (1975). Isolation of a cationic polypeptide from human serum that stimulates proliferation in 3T3 cells. *Proc. Natl. Acad. Sci. USA* **72,** 2635–2639.

Busbee, D. L., Payne, D. M., Jasheway, D. W., Carlisle, S., & Lacko, A. G. (1981). Separation and detection of lipoproteins in human serum by use of size-exclusion liquid chromatography: a preliminary report. *Clin. Chem.* **27**(12), 2052–2058.

Carlson, L. A., Holmquist, L., & Nilsson-Ehle, P. (1986). Deficiency of hepatic lipase activity in post-heparin plasma in familial hyper-α-triglyceridemia. *Acta Med. Scand.* **219,** 435–447.

Coulhon, M. P., Tallet, F., Yonger, J., Agneray, J., & Raichvarg, D. (1985). Changes in human high density lipoproteins in patients with extrahepatic biliary obstruction. *Clin. Chim. Acta* **145,** 163–172.

Gotto, A. M. Jr., Pownall, H. J., & Havel, R. J. (1986). Introduction to the plasma lipoproteins. *Methods Enzymol.* **128A,** 3–41.

Luley, C. H., Puchois, P., & Kloer, H. U. (1985). The effect of different isolation procedures on high density lipoprotein subfractions obtained by isoelectric focusing. *Clin. Chim. Acta* **146,** 185–193.

McVicar, J. P., Kunitake, S. T., Hamilton, R. L., & Kane, J. P. (1984). Characteristics of human lipoproteins isolated by selected-affinity immunosorption of apolipoprotein A-I. *Proc. Natl. Acad. Sci. USA* **81,** 1356–1360.

Marcel, Y. L. & Weech, P. K. (1986). Isoelectric focusing of plasma lipoproteins. *Methods Enzymol.* **128A,** 432–441.

Masket, B. H., Levy, R. I., & Fredrickson, D. S. (1973). The use of polyacrylamide gel electrophoresis in differentiating Type III hyperlipoproteinemia. *J. Lab. Clin. Med.* **81,** 794–802.

Righetti, P. G. & Drysdale, J. W. (1974). Isoelectric focusing in gels. *J. Chromatogr.* **98,** 271–321.

Stathakos, D., Vellios, A., & Koussoulakos, S. (1979). Multiphasic column electrofocusing: an approach to composite fractionation problems. In: *Electrophoresis 79* (ed Radola, B. J.), Walter de Gruyter & Co., Berlin–New York, 517–528.

Stathakos, D., Rekoumis, G., Avgerinos, A., Kalantzis, N., & Kanaghinis, T. (1983). Isoelectric focusing of plasma lipoproteins prestained with tetrazolium blue: a promising diagnostic tool. In: *Electrophoresis 82* (ed Stathakos, D.), Walter de Gruyter & Co, Berlin–New York, 665–674.

Stathakos, D., Rekoumis, G., Avgerinos, A., & Kanaghinis, T. (1984). Isoelectric focusing of plasma lipoproteins in the diagnosis and prognosis of liver disease. In: *Electrophoresis 83* (ed Hirai, H.), Walter de Gruyter & Co, Berlin–New York, 579–583.

Stinson, R. A. (1975). Protein staining and pH gradient determination on the same gel in isoelectric focusing. *Anal. Biochem.* **69,** 278–282.

Taketa, K. & Watanabe, M. (1981). EElectrophoretic abnormalities of high density lipoproteins in liver diseases. In: *Electrophoresis 81* (eds by Allen, R. C. & Arnaud, P.), Walter de Gruyter & Co, Berlin–New York, 1981, 447–452.

10.9 Mitochondrial DNA expression in liver and brain of ageing rat

M. N. Gadaleta†, V. Petruzzella†, M. Renis‡, F. Fracasso†, A. Giovine§, & P. Cantatore†

(1) Highly labelled, single-stranded probes for specific mitochondrial transcripts have been prepared and used in hybridization experiments with total mtRNA in order to quantitate the expression of mtDNA in the liver and in the cerebral hemispheres of adult and ageing rats.
(2) The mtRNA species analysed are the 16S ribosomal RNA (16S rRNA) and the messenger RNA for the subunit I of cytochrome oxidase (CoI mRNA).
(3) The relative content of 16S rRNA does not change either in the liver or in the synaptic mitochondria extracted from cerebral hemispheres, whereas the content of CoI mRNA decreases in ageing rats.

10.9.1 INTRODUCTION

Animal cells are endowed with two genetic systems, one localized in the nucleus and the other in the mitochondrion. Mammalian mitochondrial (mt) DNA is a small, double-stranded, circular molecule of about 16 000 base pairs (bp), carrying the information for part of the cell energy machinery. It codes in fact for 11 mRNAs specifying 13 out of 60 polypeptides of the inner mitochondrial membrane respiratory complexes, other than for two rRNA and 22 tRNAs (Fig. 1) (Cantatore & Saccone 1987). MtDNA is inherited in a maternal non-mendelian way, and on this basis several hereditary mitochondrial diseases have now been recognized (Wallace 1987). Alterations of mtDNA seem also to play a role in senescence. Of the several molecular theories on ageing (Dubitsky *et al.* 1985) the free-radical theory directly involves mitochondria and mitochondrial DNA. In fact, according to Miquel & Fleming's 'oxygen-radical mitochondrial injury' hypothesis of ageing in post-mitotic cells (1986), the fundamental cause of senescence is the accumulation of damaged mitochondria, due to the release in the organelles of the toxic by-products of respiration.

These by-products, apart from altering mitochondrial membrane permeability, mutagenize mitochondrial DNA which is in close spatial relationship to the

† Dipartimento di Biochimica e Biologia Molecolare e 'Centro di Studio sui Mitocondri e Metabolismo Energetico', Universitá di Bari, ‡ Dipartimento di Biologia Cellulare, Universitá della Calabria, § Ospedale Riuniti 'Don Uva', Casa delle Divina Provvidenza, Bisceglie, Italy

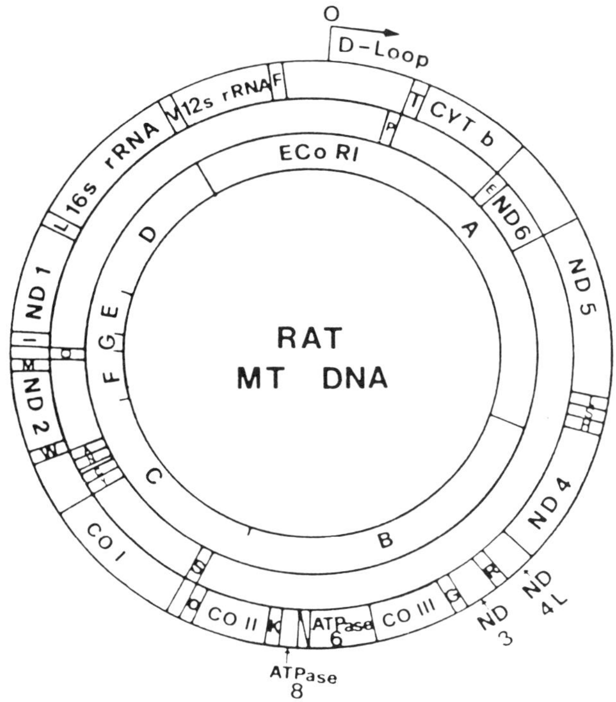

Fig. 1.—Gene organization and restriction map of rat mtDNA. The circles show the position of the genes and of the EcoRI fragments. H strand genes are in the outer circle, L strand genes in the middle circle. Ribosomal RNA genes are indicated as 16S rRNA and 12S rRNA. tRNA genes are indicated with one letter amino acid notations. Protein genes are as follows: ND1, ND2, ND3, ND4, ND4L, ND5, ND6 indicate subunits of NADH dehydrogenase; COI, COII and COIII indicates subunits I, II and III of cytochrome oxidase; ATPase 6 and ATPase 8 indicates subunits 6 and 8 of the Fo ATPase. O indicates the origin of H-strand replication. D-loop indicates the D-loop region, that is the only non-coding region of mammalian mtDNA, and contains the signals for the regulation of H strand replication and of H and L strand transcription. The fragments obtained by cutting rat mtDNA with EcoRI restriction enzyme are indicated as A, B, C, D, E, F, G in the inner circle.

mitochondrial inner membrane and is unprotected by histone-like proteins. The lack of mtDNA repair mechanisms leads to an accumulation of mutated mtDNA with consequent impaired replacement of mtDNA coded polypeptides and of mitochondria, decline in ATP synthesis, energy production, protein synthesis, and physiological performance. Experimental support for this theory comes at the moment mainly from studies on insects, particularly *Drosophila* (Dubiksky *et al.*, 1985), whereas data in the literature on age-related changes in mamalian mitochondria are controversial (Miquel & Fleming 1986, Hansford 1983). Ultrastructural alterations of mitochondria, decrease of cytochrome oxidase activity, decrease of cytochromes, of protein synthesis, and loss of mitochondria and of mitochondrial DNA have been reported.

In the present paper mtDNA expression in ageing rats has been studied. Highly labelled single-strand probes for specific mt transcripts have been prepared, and the relative quantity of these has been measured in liver and cerebral hemispheres of adult and ageing rats.

10.9.2 MATERIALS AND METHODS

Materials

Nitrocellulose filters were obtained from Schleicher and Schull (F.R.G.); RNAse A and T1 were from Boehringer and BRL respectively [α^{32}P] dCTP (3000 Ci/mmol) was from Amersham; the restriction enzymes were from New England Biolabs or Amersham.

Animals

Male albino rats of the Wistar strain 4 and 28 months old were used.

Mitochondrial isolation and nucleic acid extraction

Animals were killed by decapitation. All further operations were carried out at 4°C with sterile solutions and glassware. Liver mitochondria were isolated as previously reported (Cantatore *et al.* 1986). Cerebral hemispheres' synaptic mitochondria were isolated as reported by Lai *et al.* (1977). Nucleic acids were extracted as described by Cantatore *et al.* (1986).

Probes labelling

To prepare the single-stranded hybridization probes, DNA fragments coding for 16S tRNA and CoI mRNA were cloned in the plasmid vector Bluescribe (Stratagene), which has the promoters for T-3 and T-7 RNA polymerase in a position adjacent to the cloning sites. The probes used were a fragment of 855 bp, containing part of the CoI gene and coming from the digestion of the ECoRI, C, mtDNA fragment with Taq I and a piece of 1304 bp, containing part of the 16S gene, resulting from the cleavage of ECoRI D with HhaI (see Figs 1, 2). The CoI probe was inserted in the AccI site of the vector. The 16S probe, contained in the plasmid pUC8, was digested with Eco RI and Bam HI and inserted in the same sites of Bluescribe. To deduce the mode of the insertion, the recombinant clones were transcribed with T-3 and T-7 RNA polymerase in the presence of a radioactive precursor and the transcripts hybridized with a filter transferred cold mtRNA. The results of such experiments (not shown) indicated that the CoI and 16S probes are given by T-7 and T-3 RNA polymerase transcription, respectively. For the transcription 1 μg of the recombinant clone, containing the CoI probe, was first linearized with Hind III (this site is placed downstream from the 3′ end of the insert) and then labelled in the presence of 0.4 mM ATP, 0.4 mM CTP, 0.4 mM GTP, 40 μCi of [α^{32}P] UTP (800 Ci/mmole), 40 mM TRIS-HCl pH 7.5, 6 mM $MgCl_2$, 2 mM spermidine, 10 mM DTT, 30 units of RNAsin (Boehringer), 10 units of T-7 RNA polymerase (Stratagene) for 1 h at 37°C. At the end of the reaction 30 units of RNAsin and 20 μg/ml of DNAse (RNAse-free) were added. After a further incubation for 10 min at 37°C the mixture was phenol extracted and ethanol precipitated in the presence of 2 M ammonium acetate and 20 μg of tRNA. After centrifugation the pellet was dissolved in water, reprecipitated twice with ethanol, and then resuspended in a small volume of sterile water. The activity of the synthesized RNA was of about $1 \cdot 10^8$ dpm/μg. In the case

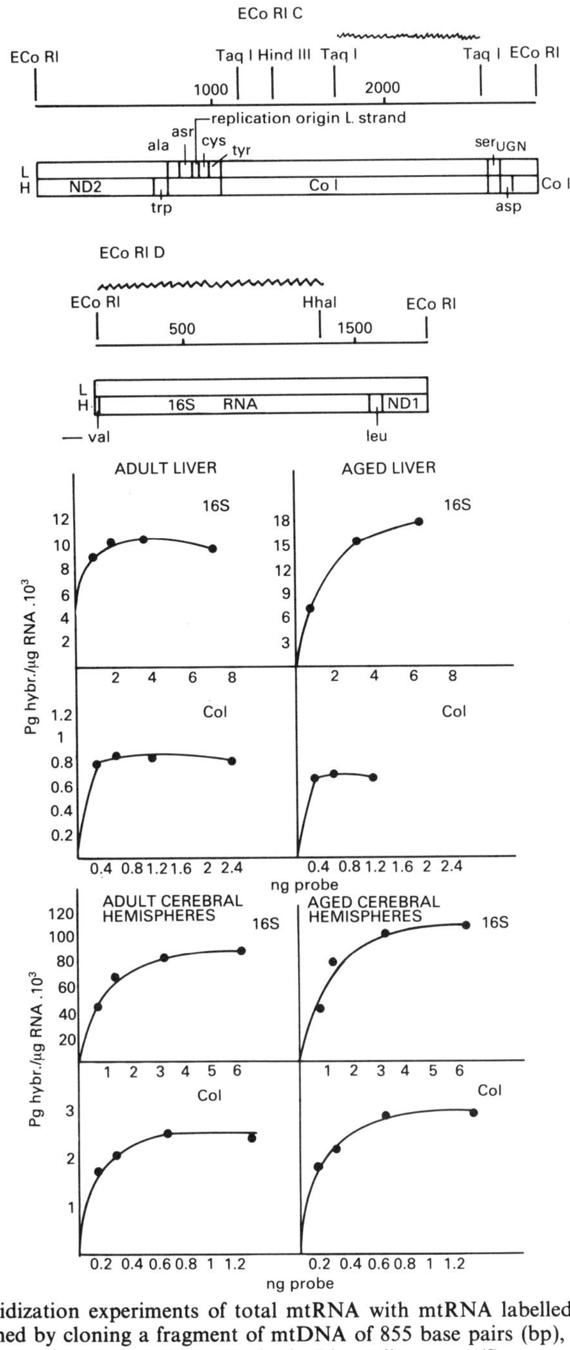

Fig. 2.—Hybridization experiments of total mtRNA with mtRNA labelled probes. The CoI probe is obtained by cloning a fragment of mtDNA of 855 base pairs (bp), resulting from the digestion of ECoRI C fragment with Taq I, in the Bluescribe vector (Stratagene) and transcribed in the presence of T-7 RNA polymerase and $\alpha^{32}P[UTP]$. The 16S probe is obtained by cloning and transcribing in the same vector a fragment of mtDNA of 1304 pb coming from the digestion of ECoRI D fragment with Hha I. The squiggle indicates the labelled RNA obtained. Total mtRNA extracted from mitochondria isolated from liver or cerebral hemispheres of adult and ageing rats was hybridized with increasing quantities of labelled mtRNA probes. Probes had a specific activity high enough to give hybridization signal between 10^3 and 10^4 dpm. Data obtained by a single RNA preparation are reported.

of the 16S probe, the labelling was done essentially with the same procedure except that the [α^{32}P] UTP had final specific activity at 20 Ci/mmol, and T-3 RNA polymerase (instead of T-7) was used. Moreover, owing to lack of useful restriction sites downstream from the insertion site, the reaction was carried out with circular DNA.

Hybridization conditions

Hybridization was performed by combining a fixed amount of mtRNA extracted from cerebral hemispheres and liver of 4- and 28-month old Wistar rats with increasing quantities of labelled RNA probes. After incubation for 20 h at 50°C in a medium containing 80% formamide, 40 mM Pipes pH 6.7, 1 mM EDTA, 0.4 M NaCl, and 10 μg of *E. coli* tRNA, the sample was digested with 7.5 U/ml of RNAse A and 0.198 U/ml of RNAse T1 for 30 min at 30°C in 200 μl of 0.3 M NaCl, 10 mM Tris pH 7.8, 5 mM EDTA. The amount of the hybrid was determined from the difference between the trichloroacetic acid insoluble radioactivity of the mtRNA containing samples and that of the controls. In the experiments reported in this paper the radioactivity contained in the blanks was about 1% that of the hybridized RNA.

10.9.3 RESULTS AND DISCUSSION

The EcoRI restriction map of mtDNA is shown in Fig. 1. Restriction fragments containing the information for one ribosomal RNA, 16S rRNA, and one messenger RNA, the mRNA for subunit 1 of cytochrome oxidase (CoI mRNA), have been selected to obtain highly labelled single-stranded probes as reported in *Materials and methods*. Probes and a representative hybridization experiment are shown in Fig. 2. The amount of 16S rRNA and CoI mRNA present in each preparation of liver or cerebral hemispheres' synaptic mitochondria was calculated by the quantity of total mtRNA hybridized at saturation in the presence of increasing quantity of labelled probes. Hybridization data were normalized with respect to the quantity of mtDNA co-extracted with RNA from isolated mitochondria (Cantatore *et al.* 1986). The relative content of 16S rRNA and CoI mRNA in liver and cerebral hemispheres' synaptic mitochondria of adult and ageing rats are shown in Table 1. The 16S rRNA level does not change either in the liver or in the cerebral hemispheres, whereas the content of CoI mRNA decreases by 33% and 42% in the two tissues, respectively. The decrease of CoI mRNA is in agreement with the decrease of cytochrome oxidase

Table 1—Relative content of 16S rRNA and CoI mRNA in liver and cerebral hemispheres mitochondria of adult and ageing rat

Mt transcript	Liver		Cerebral hemispheres	
	Adult	Ageing	Adult	Ageing
16S rRNA	1.00 ±0.12	0.87 ± 0.15	1.00 ± 0.12	0.82 ±0.09
CoI mRNA	0.075 ± 0.003	0.05 ± 0.004	0.06 ± 0.005	0.035 ± 0.003

The amount of 16S rRNA and CoI mRNA has been measured by solution hybridizaton between total mtRNA and single-strand labelled probes. The pg of hybridized RNA per μg total mtRNA (see Fig. 2) have been normalized to mtDNA content of each preparation. The values reported in the table are referred to the amount of 16S rRNA and CoI mRNA already calculated in adult rat liver (Cantatore *et al.* 1986). Data reported are the mean of three experiments run in duplicate ±SD.

activity in rat liver (Hansford, 1983) and in rat forebrains synaptic mitochondria (Harmon *et al.* 1987). The results are also in agreement with our previous results concerning the differential expression of mtDNA in rat liver and under different physiological conditions. The concentration of CoI mRNA in fact does change both during perinatal development and in the hypothyroid state, whereas the 16S rRNA level remains constant, thus indicating a differential regulation of the two mtDNA transcription units (Cantatore *et al.* 1986, 1987).

In conclusion, damage at the level of mtDNA expression seems to take place in ageing rat. Whether this damage is a primary cause or an effect of senescence, however, remains to be demonstrated.

ACKNOWLEDGEMENTS

This work has been accomplished with funds from Ministero Pubblica Istruzione (40% and 60%), Italy. The authors would like to thank Mr D. Munno for excellent technical assistance and Ms E. Lampugnani for typing and word-processing.

REFERENCES

Cantatore, P., Loguercio Polosa, P., Fracasso, F., Flagella, Z., & Gadaleta, M. N. (1986). Quantitation of mitochondrial RNA species during rat liver development: the concentration of cytochrome oxidase subunit I (CoI) mRNA increases at birth, *Cell Differentiation* **19,** 125–132.

Cantatore, P., Flagella, Z., Fracasso, F., Lezza, A., Gadaleta, M. N., & de Montalvo, A. (1987). Synthesis and turnover rates of four rat liver mitochondria RNA species, *FEBS Lett.* **213,** 144–148.

Cantatore, P. & Saccone, C. (1987). Organization, structure and evolution of mammalian mitochondrial genes, *Int. Rev. Cytol.* **108,** 149–208.

Dubitsky, R., Bensch, K. G., & Fleming, J. E. (1985). Age-related changes in turnover and concentration of a subset of thorax polypeptides from *Drosophila melanogaster*, *Mech. Ageing Development* **32,** 311–317.

Gadaleta, M. N., Loguercio Polosa, P., Lezza, A., Fracasso, F., & Cantatore, P. (1985). Mitochondrial transcription in rat liver under different physiological conditions. In: *Achievements and perspectives of mitochondrial research*, **2,** Biogenesis (eds Quagliariello, E., Slater, E. C., Palmieri, F., Saccone, C., & Kroon, A. M.), Elsevier Science Publishers, Amsterdam, 417–425.

Hansford, R. G. (1983). Bioenergetics in aging. *Biochim. Biophys. Acta* **726,** 41–80.

Harmon, H. J., Nank, S., & Floyd, R. A. (1987). Age-dependent changes in rat brain in mitochondria of synaptic and non-synaptic origins, *Mech. Ageing Development* **38,** 167–177.

Lai, J. C. K., Walsh, M. J., Dennis, S. C., & Clark, J. B. (1977). Synaptic and non-synaptic mitochondria from rat brain: isolation and characterization, *J. Neurochemistry* **28,** 625–631.

Miquel, J. & Fleming, J. (1986). Theoretical and experimental support for an 'oxygen radical-mitochondrial injury' hypothesis of cell aging. In: *Free radicals, aging and degenerative diseases*, *Modern Ageing Research* **8** (eds Johnson, J. E. Jr., Walford, R., Harman, D., & Miquel, J.), Alan R. Liss, New York, 51–74.

Wallace, D. C. (1987). Maternal genes: mitochondrial diseases. In: *Medical and experimental mammalian genetics: a perspective* (ed McKusick, V.), Alan R. Liss, New York, 137–140.

10.10 B cell and phagocytic functions with advancing age

Salvatore Antonaci,† Emilio Jirillo,‡ & Lorenzo Bonomo§

B cell function and phagocytic activities have been analysed in the elderly. Either T cell-independent or T cell-dependent polyclonal B cell responses are significantly impaired, probably owing to an exogenous inhibitory effect of soluble suppressive factors. The same mechanism seems to account for the reduced phagocyte-mediated chemotactic and phagocytic responsiveness. Altogether, these data point out an age-related decline of immunoresponsiveness.

Increased life-span has prompted many studies on factors which can improve the quality of life. In this regard, the immune system seems to play an important role in either the biology of senescence or in the pathogenesis of age-related diseases.

Since 1974 evidence has been provided for a reduction of T-mediated delayed hypersensitivity in the elderly (Roberts-Thompson *et al.* 1974). Additionally, other studies indicate a decrease of aged T cell proliferation likely related to either a diminished capacity of cells to divide in culture or to an impaired synthesis of lymphokines (LKs) which amplify T cell response (Staiano-Coico *et al.* 1984; Rabinowich *et al.* 1985).

In spite of the well-characterized deficiency of T cell activities in aged people, conflicting results are reported on B cell and phagocyte functions with advancing age. Therefore, we will provide an update on recent studies performed by our group on the above topics.

As far as aged B lymphocyte function is concerned, the elderly are characterized by a reduced capacity of spontaneous immunoglobulin (Ig) synthesis following polyclonal B cell activation (Antonaci *et al.* 1983). Adherent cells are selectively involved in the depressed B cell response since monocyte depletion or indomethacin treatment leads to a full recovery of Ig production. The monocyte-mediated inhibitory effect is probably due to an exaggerated release of prostaglandins (PGs) of the E series which may depress B cell activation (Antonaci *et al.* 1983), as observed in other test systems (Goodwin and Ceuppens, 1983). Soluble suppressive factors may also be responsible for the decreased B cell activity in several T lymphocyte

† Medicina Clinica and ‡ Immunologia, University of Bari Medical School, Policlinico, 70124 Bari, Italy. §Clinica Medica III, University of Rome Medical School, Policlinico Umberto I, 00161 Rome, Italy.

driven systems. In this context, elderly individuals exhibit a deficit of their T immunoregulatory capacity which may affect either T helper (Th) or T suppressor (Ts) functions or both (Antonaci *et al.* 1985a). These defects do not represent an age-related cell intrinsic dysfunction, since overnight cell preincubation before culture gives rise to a recovery of T immunoregulatory effects. The soluble suppressive factors may also act by recruiting cell subsets, which *per se* do not exhibit suppressive effect, to act as suppressor cells. This is the case of $CD8^+CD11^-$ lymphocytes which significantly suppress B cell response in the pokeweed mitogen (PWM) differentiation system (Antonaci *et al.* 1987). The abrogation of this paradoxical effect by overnight incubation or indomethacin treatment of aged cells clearly support the role of soluble suppressive factors in the imbalance of B lymphocyte activity in the elderly.

Several observations point out an impairment of phagocyte activity during senescence. Interestingly, monocyte chemotactic activity displays a dual pattern according to the stimulus employed. C5a gives rise to a normal response, while lymphocyte-derived chemotactic factor (LDCF) induces a lower chemotactic responsiveness in comparison with young donors (Antonaci *et al.* 1984). A PG-dependent inhibitory mechanism is also involved in this deficit since indomethacin pretreatment of mononuclear cell suspensions, before activation to induce LDCF release, gives rise to LK production which is able to trigger monocyte chemotaxis to a level similar to that observed in young individuals.

Other factors may be also responsible for the decreased LDCF release. In some individuals, the reduced synthesis is due to a lower frequency of $CD8^+$ cells which is the subset responsible for LDCF production (Antonaci *et al.* 1985b).

Finally, phagocytosis mediated by monocytes and chemotaxis and phagocytosis due to polymorphs are reduced in aged individuals (Antonaci *et al.* 1984), thus supporting the impairment of non-specific immunity in the elderly. PGs may play a role in the imbalance of these latter activities, even if the involvement of metabolic pathway (Antonaci *et al.* 1984) suggests a multifactorial pathogenetic mechanism.

In conclusion, these findings emphasize the decline of immunoresponsiveness in the elderly, thus offering a suitable model for a therapeutical approach in order to correct these deficits in ageing.

ACKNOWLEDGEMENTS

Paper supported by Consiglio Nazionale delle Ricerche (Progetto Finalizzato 'Medicina Preventiva e Riabilitativa'—Sottoprogetto 'Meccanismi di Invecchiamento'), Rome, Italy.

REFERENCES

Antonaci, S., Jirillo, E., Lucivero, G., Gallitelli, M., Garofalo, A. R., & Bonomo, L. (1983) Humoral immune response in aged humans: suppressor effect of monocytes on spontaneous plaque-forming cell generation, *Clin. Exp. Immunol.*, **52,** 387–392.

Antonaci, S., Jirillo, E., Ventura, M. T., Garofalo, A. R., & Bonomo, L. (1984) Non-specific immunity in aging: deficiency of monocyte and polymorphonuclear cell-mediated functions, *Mech. Ageing Dev.*, **24,** 367–375.

Antonaci, S., Jirillo, E., Gallitelli, M., Garolfalo, A. R., & Bonomo, L. (1985a) Impairment of T immunoregulatory activities in the induction of antibody specific response in aged humans, *Mech. Ageing Dev.*, **30,** 251–259.

Antonaci, S., Jirillo, E., Serlenga, E., & Bonomo, L. (1985b) Monocyte chemotactic responsiveness triggered by lymphocyte-derived chemotactic factor in aged donors. Definitive report, *Lymphokine Res.*, **4,** 359–365.

Antonaci, S., Jirillo, E., Gallitelli, M., Garofalo, A. R., & Bonomo, L. (1987) Regulatory effects mediated by $OKT8^+$ subsets on B cell response in the elderly, *Mech. Ageing Dev.*, **41**, 115–124.

Goodwin, J. S. & Ceuppens, J. (1983) Regulation of the immune response by prostaglandins, *J. Clin. Immunol.*, **3,** 295–315.

Rabinowich, H., Goses Y., Reshef, T., & Klajman, A. (1985) Interleukin-2 production and activity in aged humans, *Mech. Ageing Dev.*, **32**, 213–226.

Roberts-Thompson, I. C., Whittingham, S., Young-Chayud, V., & McKay, I. R. (1974) Ageing v. immune response and mortality, *Lancet*, **ii,** 368–370.

Staiano-Coico, L., Darzynkiewicz, Z., Melamed, M. R., & Weksler, M. E. (1984) Immunological studies of aging. IX. Impaired proliferation of T lympocytes detected in elderly humans by flow cytometry, *J. Immunol.*, **132,** 1788–1792.

Index